Infections, Infertility, and Assisted Reproduction

Assisted reproductive technology (ART) treatment is vulnerable to the hazard of potential infection from many different sources: patients, samples, staff, and the environment. Culture of gametes and embryos in vitro provides multiple targets for transmission of potential infection, including the developing embryo, neighbouring gametes and embryos, the couple undergoing treatment, and other couples being treated during the same period. This unique situation, with multifaceted opportunities for microbial growth and transmission, makes infection and contamination control absolutely crucial in the practice of assisted reproduction, and in the laboratory in particular.

This unique and practical book provides a basic overview of microbiology in the context of ART, providing an up-to-date guide to infections in reproductive medicine. The relevant facets of the complex and vast field of microbiology are condensed and focused, highlighting information that is crucial for safe practice in both clinical and laboratory aspects of ART. This is an essential publication for all ART clinics and laboratories.

Kay Elder is Director of Continuing Education at Bourn Hall Clinic, Bourn, Cambridge, UK.

Doris J. Baker is Chair and Professor, Department of Clinical Sciences at the University of Kentucky.

Julie A. Ribes is Associate Professor of Pathology and Laboratory Medicine at the University of Kentucky.

T0185907

Infections, Infertility, and Assisted Reproduction

Kay Elder, M.B., Ch.B., Ph.D.

Director of Continuing Education, Bourn Hall Clinic,
Cambridge, UK

Doris J. Baker, Ph.D.

Professor and Chair, Department of Clinical Sciences and
Director of Graduate Programs in Reproductive Laboratory
Science, University of Kentucky, Lexington, KY, USA

Julie A. Ribes, M.D., Ph.D.

Associate Professor of Pathology and Laboratory Medicine, and
Director of Clinical Microbiology, University of Kentucky,
Lexington, KY, USA

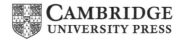
CAMBRIDGE
UNIVERSITY PRESS

CAMBRIDGE UNIVERSITY PRESS
Cambridge, New York, Melbourne, Madrid, Cape Town,
Singapore, São Paulo, Delhi, Tokyo, Mexico City

Cambridge University Press
The Edinburgh Building, Cambridge CB2 8RU, UK

Published in the United States of America by Cambridge University Press, New York

www.cambridge.org
Information on this title: www.cambridge.org/9780521178518

First published 2004
First paperback edition 2011

A catalogue record for this publication is available from the British Library

Library of Congress Cataloguing in Publication data
Elder, Kay, 1946–
Infections, infertility, and assisted reproduction/Kay Elder, Julie Ribes, Doris Baker.
     p.   cm.
Includes bibliographical references and index.
ISBN 0 521 81910 5
1. Human reproductive technology.   2. Infertility – Complications – Treatment.   3. Communicable
diseases.   4. Microbiology.   I. Ribes, Julie, 1960–   II. Baker, Doris, 1950–   III. Title.
RC889.E375   2004
616.6′9206 – dc22   2003060536

ISBN 978-0-521-81910-7 Hardback
ISBN 978-0-521-17851-8 Paperback

To: our families,

Robbie and Bethany
John and Justin
Paul and Maxwell James

With love and thanks for their patience, tolerance, and support.

Contents

Foreword

Roger G. Gosden
*The Jones Institute for Reproductive Medicine
Norfolk, VA.*

Lucinda L. Veeck
*Weill Medical College of Cornell University
New York, NY*

Wolbachia are gram-negative, intracellular bacteria that shelter in the gonads of invertebrates, and have profound effects on the fertility of their hosts. In some species, infected hosts can only reproduce parthenogenetically, in others cytoplasmic incompatibility prevents infected males from breeding with uninfected females, and in some cases genetically determined male embryos are transformed into females. *Wolbachia* engineers effects, as do all parasites, for selfish ends. Although this bizarre pathology is unknown in medical science, the relationships between microbes and human fertility are nonetheless complex, fascinating and important for the practice of reproductive medicine.

Unfortunately, and usually without advance warning, microbes occasionally enter the clinical laboratory through infected semen or vaginal tissue. When this occurs, a patient's treatment outcome may be seriously compromised because microbes can quickly deplete nutrients in culture media and alter the pH, and it would be irresponsible to knowingly transfer an infected embryo or semen to a patient. Bacterial and fungal growth are often obvious and easily tested, but how often do infectious agents go unrecognized and contribute to the problems of infertility, treatment failure and even possibly affect the child-to-be?

This is the first book on medical microbiology that has been written by experts in reproduction for clinical scientists and physicians in their own field. They are to be congratulated on filling a gap in the literature between microbiology and assisted reproduction, which they achieve in three sections. The first serves as a primer of medical microbiology for readers who are unfamiliar or rusty on the subject. The second focuses on microbes that have implications for human reproduction, whether by causing infertility (a familiar example being *Chlamydia*) or by jeopardizing reproductive safety (such as HIV).

In the final section, the practical implications of this knowledge are addressed in the context of infertility, and especially the setting of the clinical embryology laboratory. Every embryologist is trained in sterile techniques, filtration of media and prudent use of antibiotics to keep out the bugs, but a deeper knowledge of the foundations of safe and effective practice is an undervalued safeguard for patient care.

Preface

The world of microbes is intrinsically fascinating. Microbes are abundant in every place on earth where larger living creatures exist, and they can also thrive in habitat extremes where no other kind of organism can survive for long: from deep under the sea to the stratosphere – up to 32 km in the atmosphere, in oil formations and in hot telluric water. It is estimated that the total biomass of microbes probably exceeds that of all the plants and animals in the biosphere. This biomass is predominantly composed of bacteria, and these microorganisms play a crucial role in recycling much of the organic material in the biosphere. Despite their minute size, microorganisms carry out all the fundamental processes of biochemistry and molecular biology that are essential to the survival of all living species. Although their size may give them the illusion of being 'primitive', their range of biochemical and biophysical capabilities is far wider than that of higher organisms. One of their most important properties is adaptability and versatility, a key feature in their long history of evolution. Fossil records suggest that at least some members of the microbial world, oxygen-producing cyanobacter-like organisms, had evolved 3.46 billion years ago (Schopf, 1993); a viable fungus, *Absidia corymbifera*, was recovered from the right boot that accompanied the frozen, well-preserved prehistoric corpse, 'Ice Man', aged approximately 5300 years (Haselwandter & Ebner, 1994).

Records of microbial disease that probably influenced the course of history can be found in archaeological sites of early civilizations, as well as in later periods of history. A hieroglyph from the capital of ancient Egypt dated approximately 3700 BC illustrates a priest (Ruma) with typical clinical signs of a viral infection, paralytic poliomyelitis. The mummified body of the Pharaoh Siptah, who died in 1193 BC, also shows signs of classic paralytic poliomyelitis, and the preserved mummy of Rameses V has facial pustular lesions suggesting that his death in 1143 BC was probably due to smallpox. This virulent disease was endemic in China by 1000 BC, and had reached Europe by 710 AD. Hernando Cortez transferred the disease to the Americas in 1520, and it appears that around 3 500 000 Aztecs died of smallpox within the next two years – arguably precipitating the end of the Aztec empire.

In the early 1330s an outbreak of deadly Bubonic plague occurred in China, one of the busiest of the world's trading nations, and rapidly spread to Western Asia and Europe. Between 1347 and 1352 this plague, 'The Black Death', killed 25 million people – one-third of the population of Europe – with far-reaching social, cultural and economic repercussions.

The world of assisted reproduction is equally fascinating, and is one that also has a long history of evolution. The concept of assisted procreation by human artificial insemination was a topic of discussion between Jewish philosophers as early as the third century AD, and tales exist of fourteenth-century Arab horse breeders obtaining sperm from mated mares belonging to rival groups, using the sperm to inseminate their own mares. Assisted reproduction explores the fundamental principles behind the creation of a new life, the intricate biological mechanisms that are involved when mature gametes come into contact, combine genetically and set in motion a cascade of events leading to the correct expression of genes that form a new individual.

Microbiology and assisted reproduction both deal with a miniature world, magnified for observation with the help of microscopy. Culture of microorganisms and of preimplantation embryos in vitro requires special media and growth conditions to promote cell division, and both are visualized and assessed at various stages following cell division. A knowledge of microbiology is fundamental to the safety and success of assisted reproductive techniques – but the field of microbiology is vast, and continues to increase in complexity with the discovery of new organisms and implementation of new medical treatments. The field of assisted reproductive technology also continues to expand and develop, particularly in areas of science and biotechnology. Members of an assisted reproduction team are not usually also experts in infectious diseases, and may find it difficult to identify and follow significant areas of microbiology that can impact upon their practice.

The purpose of this book is to select areas and topics in microbiology that are specifically relevant to assisted reproductive technology (ART), in order to provide a very basic background of facts and fundamental principles. A background of understanding can help prevent contamination and transmission of disease in ART, and also limit the opportunities for microbial survival in embryo culture and cryopreservation systems. The book is divided into three Parts:

Part I provides an outline of microorganism classification and identification, as a foundation for understanding the relationships and the differences between the types of organisms that may be encountered in routine ART practice. The microorganisms that are human pathogens or resident flora, and those that are routinely found in the environment are introduced. Each chapter includes an Appendix of antimicrobial drugs and their modes of action.

Part II details organisms that cause disease of the reproductive tract and those that are blood-borne pathogens, describing their etiology, pathogenesis, diagnosis, pathology and treatment.

Part III describes the practical application of microbiology principles within an assisted reproduction laboratory.

REFERENCES

Haselwandter, K. & Ebner, M. R. (1994). Microorganisms surviving for 5300 years. *FEMS Microbiology Letters*, **116**(2), 189–93.

Schopf, J. W. (1993). Microfossils of the early Archean apex chart: new evidence of the antiquity of life. *Science*, **260**, 640–6.

Acknowledgements

Digital images for illustrations were produced with the expert help of Stephen Welch and Robbie Hughes. We would like to thank all of our colleagues and friends for their valuable encouragement, input and comments throughout the preparation of this book, with particular acknowledgement of the contributions made by Marc van den Berg, Charles Cornwell, Rajvi Mehta, Rita Basuray, George Kalantzopoulos, Dimitra Kaftani and Kim Campbell. Special thanks to Professor Bob Edwards for his personal reflections on the 'History of IVF' and to Alan Smith for his perspectives on the development of biotechnology.

Barbara and Janet – thank you for your endless patience and moral support.

We are also grateful for the support of Bourn Hall Clinic, Cambridge, and the Departments of Clinical Sciences and Pathology and Laboratory Medicine, University of Kentucky, and the University of Kentucky Clinical Microbiology Laboratory.

Overview of microbiology

Introduction

History of microbiology

The history of microbiology, the scientific study of microorganisms, had its origins in the second half of the seventeenth century, when Anton van Leeuwenhoek (1632–1723), a tradesman in Delft, Holland, learned to grind lenses in order to make microscopes that would allow him to magnify and observe a wide range of materials and objects. Although he had no formal education and no knowledge of the scientific dogma of the day, his skill, diligence and open mind led him to make some of the most important discoveries in the history of biology. He made simple powerful magnifying glasses, and with careful attention to lighting and detail, built microscopes that magnified over 200 times. These instruments allowed him to view clear and bright images that he studied and described in meticulous detail. In 1673 he began writing letters to the newly formed Royal Society of London, describing what he had seen with his microscopes. He corresponded with the Royal Society for the next 50 years; his letters, written in Dutch, were translated into English or Latin and printed in the *Philosophical Transactions of the Royal Society*. These letters include the first descriptions of living bacteria ever recorded, taken from the plaque between his teeth, and from two ladies and two old men who had never cleaned their teeth:

> I then most always saw, with great wonder, that in the said matter there were many very little living animalcules, very prettily a-moving. The biggest sort . . . had a very strong and swift motion, and shot through the water (or spittle) like a pike does through the water. The second sort . . . oft-times spun round like a top . . . and these were far more in number . . . there were an unbelievably great company of living animalcules, a-swimming more nimbly than any I had ever seen up to this time. The biggest sort . . . bent their body into curves in going forwards . . . Moreover, the other animalcules were in such enormous numbers, that all the water . . . seemed to be alive.

His *Letters to the Royal Society* also included descriptions of free-living and parasitic protozoa, sperm cells, blood cells, microscopic nematodes, and a great deal more. In a Letter of June 12, 1716, he wrote:

> . . . my work, which I've done for a long time, was not pursued in order to gain the praise I now enjoy, but chiefly from a craving after knowledge, which I notice resides in me more than in most other men. And therewithal, whenever I found out anything remarkable, I have thought it my duty to put down my discovery on paper, so that all ingenious people might be informed thereof.

At this time, around the turn of the eighteenth century, diseases were thought to arise by 'spontaneous generation', although it was recognised that certain clinically definable illnesses apparently did not have second or further recurrences. The ancient Chinese practice of preventing severe natural smallpox by 'variolation', inoculating pus from smallpox patients into a scratch on the forearm, was introduced into Europe in the early 1800s. The English farmer, Benjamin Justy, observed that milkmaids who were exposed to cowpox did not develop smallpox, and he inoculated his family with cowpox pus to prevent smallpox. Long before viruses had been recognized as an entity, and with no knowledge of their properties, the physician Edward Jenner (1749–1823) was intrigued by this observation, and started the first scientific investigations of smallpox prevention by human experimentation in 1796. Jenner used fluid from cowpox pustules on the hand of a milkmaid to inoculate the 8-year-old son of his gardener, and later challenged the boy by deliberately inoculating him with material from a real case of smallpox. The boy did not become infected, having apparently developed an immunity to smallpox from the cowpox vaccination. Jenner's early experiments led to the development of vaccination as protection against infectious disease and laid the foundations for the science of immunology, which was further developed during the nineteenth century by Pasteur, Koch, von Behring and Erlich.

The nineteenth century was a 'Golden Age' in the history of microbiology. The Hungarian doctor, Ignaz Semmelweiss (1818–1865), observed that puerperal fever often occurred when doctors went directly from the post-mortem room to the delivery room, and seldom occurred when midwives carried out deliveries. He thus introduced the notion that infectious agents might be transmitted, and suggested hand washing with chlorinated lime water. Significant discoveries about bacteria and the nature of disease were then made by Louis Pasteur, Joseph Lister, Paul Ehrlich, Christian Gram, R. J. Petri, Robert Koch (1843–1910) and others. Louis Pasteur and Robert Koch together developed the 'germ theory of disease', disproving the 'spontaneous generation' theory held at the time. Louis Pasteur (1822–1895) developed the scientific basis for Jenner's experimental approach to vaccination, and produced useful animal and human vaccines against rabies, anthrax and cholera. In 1876 Robert Koch provided the first proof for the 'germ theory' with his discovery of *Bacillus anthracis* as the cause of anthrax. Using blood from infected animals, he obtained pure cultures of the bacilli by growing them on the aqueous humour of an ox's eye. He observed that under unfavourable conditions the bacilli could form rounded spores that resisted adverse conditions, and these began to grow again as bacilli when suitable conditions were restored. Koch went on to invent new methods of cultivating bacteria on solid media such as sterile slices of potato and on agar kept in the recently invented Petri dish. In 1892 he described the conditions, known as Koch's Postulates, which must be satisfied in order to define particular bacteria as a cause of a specific disease:

(i) The agent must be present in every case of the disease.

(ii) The agent must be isolated from the host and grown in vitro.

(iii) The disease must be reproduced when a pure culture of the agent is inoculated into a healthy susceptible host.

(iv) The same agent must be recovered once again from the experimentally infected host.

Koch's further significant contributions to microbiology included work on the tubercle bacillus and identifying *Vibrio* as a cause of cholera, as well as work in India and Africa on malaria, plague, typhus, trypanosomiasis and tickborne spirochaete infections. He was awarded the Nobel Prize for Physiology or Medicine in 1905, and continued his work on bacteriology and serology until his death in 1910.

During the 1800s, agents that caused diseases were being classified as filterable – small enough to pass through a ceramic filter (named 'virus' by Pasteur, from the Latin for 'poison') – or nonfilterable, retained on the surface of the filter (bacteria). Towards the end of the century, a Russian botanist, Dmitri Iwanowski, recognized an agent (tobacco mosaic virus) that could transmit disease to other plants after passage through ceramic filters fine enough to retain the smallest known bacteria. In 1898 Martinus Beijerinick confirmed and developed Iwanowski's observations, and was the first to describe a virus as *contagium vivum fluidum* (soluble living germ). In 1908 Karl Landsteiner and Erwin Popper proved that poliomyelitis was caused by a virus, and shortly thereafter (1915–1917), Frederick Twort and Felix d'Herrelle independently described viruses that infect bacteria, naming them 'bacteriophages'. These early discoveries laid the foundation for further studies about the properties of bacteria and viruses, and, more significantly, about cell genetics and the transfer of genetic information between cells. In the 1930s, poliovirus was grown in cultured cells, opening up the field of diagnostic virology. By the 1950s, plasmids were recognized as extranuclear genetic elements that replicate autonomously, and Joshua Lederberg and Norton Zinder reported on transfer of genetic information by viruses (Zinder & Lederberg, 1952).

Following the announcement of the DNA double helix structure by Watson and Crick in 1953, the properties of bacteria, bacteriophages and animal viruses were fully exploited and formed the basis of a new scientific discipline: molecular biology, the study of cell metabolic regulation and its genetic machinery. Over the next 20 years, *Escherichia coli* and other bacterial cell-free systems were used to elucidate the molecular steps and mechanisms involved in DNA replication, transcription and translation, and protein synthesis, assembly and transport. The development of vaccines and antimicrobial drugs began during the 1950s, and antibiotic resistance that could be transferred between strains of bacteria was identified by 1959 (Ochiai *et al.*, 1959). In 1967, Thomas Brock identified a thermophilic bacterium *Thermus acquaticus*; 20 years later, a heat-stable DNA polymerase was isolated from this bacterium and used in the polymerase chain reaction (PCR) as a means of amplifying nucleic acids (Brock, 1967; Saiki *et al.*, 1988). Another significant advance in molecular biology came with the recognition that bacteria produce restriction endonuclease enzymes that cut DNA at specific sites, and in 1972 Paul Berg constructed a recombinant DNA molecule from viral and bacterial DNA using such enzymes (Jackson *et al.*, 1972). The concept of gene splicing was reported by 1977, and in that same year Frederick Sanger and his colleagues elucidated the complete nucleotide sequence of the bacteriophage ϕX174, the first microorganism to have its genome sequenced (Sanger *et al.*, 1977). Berg, Gilbert and Sanger were awarded the Nobel Prize for Chemistry in 1980.

These discoveries involving microorganisms established the foundation for genetic engineering. Gene cloning and modification, recombinant DNA technology and DNA sequencing established biotechnology as a new commercial enterprise: by 2002 the biotechnology industry had worldwide drug sales in excess of 10 billion US dollars. The first genetically engineered human protein, insulin, was available by 1982, and the first complete genome sequence of a bacterium, *Haemophilus influenzae,* was published in 1995. Hormones and other proteins manufactured by recombinant DNA technology are now used routinely to treat a variety of diseases, and recombinant follicle stimulating hormone (FSH), luteinizing hormone (LH) and human chorionic gonadotrophin (hCG) are available for routine use in assisted reproductive technology.

A parallel line of investigation that was also a key feature in molecular biology and medicine during the latter part of the twentieth century came from the study of retroviruses, novel viruses that require reverse transcription of RNA into DNA for their replication. During the 1960s, Howard Temin and David Baltimore independently discovered viral reverse transcription, and in 1969 Huebner and Todaro proposed the viral oncogene hypothesis, subsequently expanded and confirmed by Bishop and Varmus in 1976. They identified oncogenes from Rous sarcoma virus that are also present in cells of normal animals, including humans. Proto-oncogenes are apparently essential for normal development, but can become cancer-causing oncogenes when cellular regulators are damaged or modified. Bishop and Varmus were awarded the Nobel Prize for Medicine or Physiology in 1989. In 1983, Luc Montagnier discovered a retrovirus believed to cause the acquired immune deficiency syndrome (AIDS) – the human immunodeficiency virus (HIV). By the end of the twentieth century, the total number of people affected by this novel virus exceeded 36 million.

Around this same time, another novel pathogen of a type not previously described also came to light: in 1982 Stanley Prusiner discovered that scrapie, a transmissible spongiform encephalopathy (TSE) in sheep, could be transmitted by a particle that was apparently composed of protein alone, with no associated nucleic acid – the prion protein (Prusiner, 1982). This was the first time that an agent with neither DNA or RNA had been recognized as pathogenic, challenging previous dogmas about disease pathogenesis and transmission.

The field of microbiology continues to grow and elicit public concern, both in terms of disease pathology and in harnessing the properties of microbes for the study of science, especially molecular genetics. During the past 25–30 years, approximately 30 new pathogens have been identified, including HIV, hemorrhagic viruses such as Ebola, transfusion-related hepatitis C-like viruses, and, most recently, the coronavirus causing sudden acute respiratory syndrome (SARS). The first SARS outbreak occurred in the Guangdong province of China in November 2002 and had spread as a major life-threatening penumonia in several countries by March 2003. The infectious agent was identified during that month, and a massive international collaborative effort resulted in elucidating its complete genome sequence only 3 weeks later, in mid-April 2003. The genome sequence reveals that the SARS virus is a novel class of coronavirus, rather than a recent mutant of the known varieties that cause mild upper respiratory illness in humans and a variety of diseases in other animals. Information deduced from the genome sequence can form the basis for developing targeted antiviral drugs and vaccines, and can help develop diagnostic tests to speed efforts in preventing the global epidemic of SARS. At the beginning of June 2003, 6 months after the first recorded case, the World Health Organization reported 8464 cases from more than two dozen countries, resulting in 799 deaths.

These new diseases are now being defined within a context of 'emergent viruses', and it is clear that new infectious diseases may arise from a combination of different factors that prevail in modern society:

(i) New infectious diseases can emerge from genetic changes in existing organisms (e.g. SARS 'jumped' from animal hosts to humans, with a change in its genetic make-up), and this 'jump' is facilitated by intensive farming and close and crowded living conditions.

(ii) Known diseases may spread to new geographic areas and populations (e.g. malaria in Texas, USA).

(iii) Previously unknown infections may appear in humans living or working in changing ecologic conditions that increase their exposure to insect vectors, animal reservoirs, or environmental sources of novel pathogens, e.g. prions.

(iv) Modern air transportation allows large numbers of people, and hence infectious disease, to travel worldwide with hitherto unprecedented speed.

Other areas that can contribute to pathogen emergence include events in society such as war, civil conflict, population growth and migration, as well as globalization of food supplies, with changes in food processing and packaging. Environmental changes with deforestation/reforestation, changes in water ecosystems, flood, drought, famine, and global warming can significantly alter habitats and exert evolutionary pressures for microbial adaptation and change. Human behaviour, including sexual behaviour, drug use, travel, diet, and even use of child-care facilities have contributed to the transmission of infectious diseases. The use of new medical devices and invasive procedures, organ or tissue transplantation, widespread use of antibiotics and drugs causing immunosuppression have also been instrumental in the emergence of illness due to opportunistic pathogens: normal microbial flora such as *Staphylococcus epidermidis* cause infections on artificial heart valves, and saprophytic fungi cause serious infection in immunocompromised patients.

Microorganisms can restructure their genomes in response to environmental pressures, and during replication there is an opportunity for recombination or re-assortment of genes, as well as recombination with host cell genetic elements. Some viruses (e.g. HIV) evolve continuously, with a high frequency of mutation during replication. Retroviruses are changing extraordinarily rapidly, evolving sporadically with unpredictable patterns, at different rates in different situations. Their genetic and metabolic entanglement with cells gives retroviruses a unique opportunity to mediate subtle, cumulative evolutionary changes in host cells. Viruses that are transmitted over a long time period (HIV) have a selective advantage even when their effective transmission rates are relatively low.

Assisted reproduction techniques are now being used to help people who carry infectious diseases (including those that are potentially fatal and may have deleterious effects on offspring) to have children. This potential breach of evolutionary barriers raises new ethical, policy and even legal issues that must be dealt with cautiously and judiciously (Minkoff & Santoro, 2000).

History of assisted reproduction

Assisted reproduction may also be said to have its origin in the seventeenth century, when Anton van Leeuwenhoek first observed sperm under the microscope and described them as 'animalcules'. In 1779, Lazzaro Spallanzani (1729–1799), an Italian priest and scientist was the first to propose that contact between an egg and sperm was necessary for an embryo to develop and grow. He carried out artificial insemination experiments in dogs, succeeding with live births, and went on to inseminate frogs and fish. Spallanzani is also credited with some of the early experiments in cryobiology, keeping frog, stallion and human sperm viable after cooling in snow and re-warming. The Scottish surgeon, John Hunter (1728–1793), was the first to report artificial insemination in humans, when he collected sperm from a patient who sufferered from hypospadias and injected it into his wife's vagina with a warm syringe. This procedure resulted in the birth of a child in 1785. The next documented case of artificial insemination in humans took place in 1884 at Jefferson Medical College in Philadelphia, USA:

A wealthy merchant complained to a noted physician of his inability to procreate and the doctor took this as a golden opportunity to try out a new procedure. Some time later, his patient's wife was anaesthetised. Before an audience of medical students, the doctor inseminated the woman, using semen obtained from 'the best-looking member of the class'. Nine months later, a child was born. The mother is reputed to have gone to her grave none the wiser as to the manner of her son's provenance. The husband was informed and was delighted. The son discovered his unusual history at the age of 25, when enlightened by a former medical student who had been present at the conception. (Hard, AD, Artificial Impregnation, *Medical World*, 27, p. 163, 1909)

By the turn of the nineteenth century, the use of artificial insemination in rabbits, dogs and horses had been reported in several countries. In 1866 an Italian physician, Paolo Mantegazza, suggested that sperm could be frozen for posthumous use in humans and for breeding of domestic animals, and in 1899 the Russian biologist Ivanoff reported artificial insemination (AI) in domestic farm animals, dogs, foxes, rabbits and poultry. He developed semen extenders, began to freeze sperm and to select superior stallions for breeding. His work laid the foundation for the establishment of artificial insemination as a veterinary breeding technique.

Around this same time in Cambridge UK, the reproductive biologist, Walter Heape, studied the relationship between seasonality and reproduction. In 1891 he reported the recovery of a preimplantation embryo after flushing a rabbit oviduct and transferring this to a foster mother with continued normal development (Heape, 1891). His work encouraged others to experiment with embryo culture; in 1912 Alain Brachet, founder of the Belgian School of Embryology, succeeded in keeping a rabbit blastocyst alive in blood plasma for 48 hours. Pregnancies were then successfully obtained after flushing embryos from a number of species, from mice and rabbits to sheep and cows. Embryo flushing and transfer to recipients became a routine in domestic animal breeding during the 1970s.

Artificial insemination

By 1949, Chris Polge in Cambridge had developed the use of glycerol as a semen cryoprotectant, and the process of semen cryopreservation was refined for use in cattle breeding and veterinary practice. The advantages of artificial insemination were recognized: genetic improvement of livestock, decrease in the expense of breeding, the potential to increase fertility, and a possible disease control mechanism. Almquist and his colleagues proposed that bacterial contaminants in semen could be controlled by adding antibiotics to bovine semen (Almquist *et al.*, 1949). The practice of artificial insemination was soon established as a reproductive treatment in humans. Methods for cryopreserving human semen and performing artificial insemination were refined in the early 1950s (Sherman & Bunge, 1953), and a comprehensive account of Donor Insemination was published in 1954 (Bunge *et al.*, 1954). By the mid-1980s, however, it became apparent that donor insemination had disadvantages as well as advantages, including the potential to transmit infectious diseases. Before rigorous screening was introduced, HIV, *Chlamydia*, Hepatitis B and genital herpes were spread via donor semen (Nagel *et al.*, 1986; Berry *et al.*, 1987; Moore *et al.*, 1989; McLaughlin, 2002).

In vitro fertilization

Advances in reproductive endocrinology, including identification of steroid hormones and their role in reproduction, contributed significantly to research in reproductive biology during the first half of the twentieth century. During the 1930s–40s, the pituitary hormones responsible for follicle growth and luteinization were identified, and a combination of FSH and LH treatments were shown to promote maturation of ovarian follicles and to trigger ovulation. Urine from postmenopausal women was found to contain high concentrations of gonadotrophins, and these urinary preparations were used to induce ovulation in anovulatory patients during the early 1950s.

Parallel relevant studies in gamete physiology and mammalian embryology were underway by this time, with important observations reported by Austin, Chang and Yanagimachi. In 1951, Robert Edwards began working towards his Ph.D. project in Edinburgh University's Department of Animal Genetics headed by Professor Conrad Waddington and under the directon of Alan Beatty. Here he began to pursue his interest in reproductive biology, studying sperm and eggs, and the process of ovulation in the mouse. After 1 year spent in Pasadena at the California Institute of Technology working on problems in immunology and embryology, in 1958 he joined the MRC in Mill Hill, where he worked with

Alan Parkes and Bunny Austin, continuing to explore his interest in genetics, mammalian oocytes and the process of fertilization. During this period he started expanding his interests into human oocyte maturation and fertilization, and with the help of the gynaecologist Molly Rose began to observe human oocytes retrieved from surgical biopsy specimens. In 1962 he observed spontaneous resumption of meiosis in a human oocyte in vitro for the first time. After a brief period in Glasgow with John Paul, he was appointed as a Ford Foundation Fellow in the Physiological Laboratory in Cambridge in 1963. By this time Chang (1959) had successfully carried out in vitro fertilization with rabbit oocytes and sperm, and Yanagamichi (1964) subsequently reported successful IVF in the golden hamster. Whittingham was working towards fertilization of mouse eggs in vitro, and reported success in 1968. In Cambridge, Bob Edwards began on the slow and arduous road that eventually led to successful human in vitro fertilization. He continued his studies using the limited and scarce material available from human ovarian biopsy and pathology specimens, and published his observations about maturation in vitro of mouse, sheep, cow, pig, rhesus monkey and human ovarian oocytes (Edwards, 1965). Working with several Ph.D. students, Edwards fertilized mouse and cow eggs in vitro, and obtained mouse offspring. With his students, he studied the growth of chimaeric embryos constructed by injecting a single or several inner cell mass cells from donor blastocysts into recipient genetically marked blastocysts. The birth of live chimaeras confirmed the capacity of single stem cells to colonize virtually all organs in the recipient, including germline, but not trophectoderm. They also removed small pieces of trophectoderm from live rabbit blastocysts and determined their sex by identifying whether they expressed the sex chromatin body. Embryos with this body were classified as females and the others as males. The sex of fetuses and offspring at birth had been correctly diagnosed, signifying the onset of preimplantation genetic diagnosis for inherited characteristics. At this time, anomalies observed in some rabbit offspring caused them some concern, but a large study by Chang on in vitro fertilization in mice proved that the anomalies were due to the segregation of a recessive gene, and not due to IVF.

In 1968 Edwards began his historic collaboration with Patrick Steptoe, the gynaecologist who pioneered and introduced the technique of pelvic laparoscopy in the UK. Using this new technique in his clinical practice in Oldham General Hospital near Manchester, Steptoe was able to rescue fresh pre-ovulatory oocytes from the pelvis of patients who suffered from infertility due to tubal damage. Bob Edwards and his colleague, Jean Purdy, traveled from Cambridge to Oldham in order to culture, observe and fertilize these oocytes in vitro. The team began to experiment with culture conditions to optimize the in vitro fertilization system, and tried ovarian stimulation with drugs in order to increase the number of oocytes available for fertilization. After observing apparently normal human embryo development to the blastocyst stage in 1970, they began to consider re-implanting embryos created in vitro into the uteri of patients in order to achieve pregnancies: the first human embryo transfers were carried out in 1972. Despite the fact that their trials and experiments were conducted in the face of fierce opposition and criticism from their peers at the time, they continued to persevere in their efforts, with repeated failure and disappointment for the next 6 years. Finally, their 10 years of collaboration, persistence and perseverance were rewarded with the successful birth of the first IVF baby in 1978.

The modern field of assisted reproductive technology (ART) arrived with the birth of Louise Brown on July 25, 1978. After a 2-year lag, when no funds or facilities were available to continue their pioneering work, Steptoe and Edwards opened a private clinic near Cambridge: Bourn Hall Clinic, dedicated solely to treating infertility patients using in vitro fertilization and embryo transfer. The first babies were conceived within days, and many more within 3 months. Their rapid clinical success in achieving pregnancies and live births led to the introduction of IVF treatment worldwide throughout the 1980s and 1990s. The first babies born after transfer of embryos that had been frozen and thawed were born in 1984–85, and cryopreservation of embryos as well as semen became routine. Experiments with cell cultures and

co-culture allowed the development of stage-specific media optimized for embryo culture to the blastocyst stage. Advances in technique and micromanipulation technology led to the establishment of assisted fertilization (intracytoplasmic sperm injection, ICSI) by a Belgian team led by André Van Steirteghem and including Gianpiero Palermo (Palermo et al., 1992) by the mid 1990s. Other microsurgical interventions were then introduced, such as assisted hatching and embryo biopsy for genetic diagnosis. Gonadal tissue cryopreservation, in vitro oocyte maturation and embryonic stem cell culture are now under development as therapeutic instruments and remedies for the future.

The first live calves resulting from bovine IVF were born in the USA in 1981. This further milestone in reproductive biotechnology inspired the development of IVF as the next potential commercial application of assisted reproduction in domestic species, following on from AI and conventional transfer of embryos produced in vivo from superovulated donors. The assisted reproductive techniques continued to be refined so that by the 1990s IVF was integrated into routine domestic species breeding programmes. Equine IVF has also been introduced into the world of horse breeding (although reproductive technology procedures cannot be used for thoroughbreds). China used artificial insemination to produce the first giant panda cub in captivity in 1963, and assisted reproduction is now used in the rescue and propagation of endangered species, from pandas and large cats to dolphins. Artificial insemination, and, in some cases, in vitro fertilization are used routinely in specialist zoos throughout the world.

In the field of scientific research, application of assisted reproductive techniques in animal systems has helped to unravel the fundamental steps involved in fertilization, gene programming and expression, regulation of the cell cycle and patterns of differentiation. Somatic cell nuclear transfer into enucleated oocytes has created 'cloned' animals in several species, the most famous being Dolly the sheep, who was born in Edinburgh in 1997; Dolly was euthanized at an early age in February 2003, after developing arthritis and progressive lung disease.

Advances in molecular biology and biotechnology continue to be applied in ART. Preimplantation genetic diagnosis (PGD), introduced in 1988, is used to screen embryos for sex-linked diseases or autosomal mutations in order to exclude chromosomally abnormal embryos from transfer. Molecular biology techniques can identify chromosomes with the use of fluorescently labelled probes for hybridization, or to amplify DNA from a single blastomere using PCR. This technique is also used for gender selection, now used routinely in animal breeding programmes.

Assisted reproductive technology (ART) and microbiology

Assisted reproduction is a multidisciplinary field that relies on close teamwork and collaboration between different medical and scientific disciplines that must cover a wide range of expertise, including microbiology. Culture media and systems used to process and culture gametes and embryos are designed to encourage cell growth, but this system can also encourage the growth of a wide variety of microbes. Whereas cell division in preimplantation embryos is relatively slow, with each cell cycle lasting approximately 24 hours, microbes can multiply very rapidly under the right conditions. Under constant conditions the generation time for a specific bacterium is reproducible, but varies greatly among species. The generation time for some bacteria is only 15–20 minutes; others have generation times of hours or even days. Spore-forming organisms have the ability to go into 'suspended animation', allowing them to withstand extreme conditions (freezing, high temperatures, lack of nutrients). This important property allows the organisms to survive in central heating and air conditioning systems or cooling towers

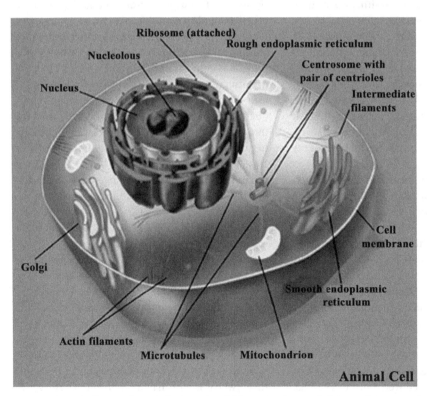

Fig. 1.1. Schematic diagram of a typical eukaryotic cell, illustrating characteristic intracellular organelles.

for indefinite periods: the 'Ice Man' fungus survived at least 5300 years, and live bacterial spores were found in ancient pressed plants at Kew Gardens dating back to the seventeenth century. Viruses do not form spores, but some can survive dry on handkerchiefs, or cleaning or drying cloths if protein is present, e.g. in droplets from a sneeze or cough. These properties presents special problems in the ART laboratory since many agents used to inhibit or destroy microorganisms are toxic to sperm, oocytes and embryos. An ART laboratory must incorporate strict guidelines for maintaining necessary sterile conditions without compromising the gametes and embryos.

Patients presenting for infertility treatment often have a background of infectious disease as a factor in their infertility, and it is now acknowledged that some chronic infectious diseases may be 'silent' or inapparent, but transmissible in some patients (e.g. Herpes, *Ureaplasma*, *Chlamydia*). Some patients may be taking antimicrobial drugs that will have a negative effect on gamete function: for example, bacterial protein synthesis inhibitors affect sperm mitochondrial function, adversely affecting sperm motility. The trend for worldwide travel also introduces new contacts and potentially infectious agents across previous geographic barriers.

There are many factors to be taken into account when assessing the risk from microorganisms, and some that are unique to ART are complex and multifaceted. Formal assessment for quantifying risk requires experimental study data, epidemiological information, population biology and mathematical modelling – this is not possible in assisted reproductive practice. Instead, ART laboratory practitioners need to collate, review and evaluate relevant information, bearing in mind that ART practises breach biological barriers, increasing the risk:

> Wisdom lies in knowing what one is doing and why one is doing it – to take liberties in ignorance is to court disaster – each fragment of knowledge teaches us how much more we have yet to learn. (John Postgate *Microbes and Man*, 2000)

> Chance favours the prepared mind (Louis Pasteur, 1822–1895)

Overview of microbiology

Naturam primum cognoscere rerum
First . . . to learn the nature of things (*Aristotle, 384–322 BC*)

Living things have been traditionally classified into five biological Kingdoms: Animals (Animalia), Plants (Plantae), Fungi (Fungi), Protozoa (Protista) and Bacteria (Monera). Animals, plants, fungi and protozoa are eukaryotic, with nuclei, cytoskeletons, and internal membranes (see Fig. 1.1). Their chromosomes undergo typical reorganization during cell division. Bacteria are prokaryotes, i.e. they have no well-defined nucleus or nuclear membrane and divide by amitotic division (binary fission) (Fig. 1.2). The world of microbes covers a wide variety of different organisms within the Kingdoms of Fungi, Protista and Monera, with a diverse range

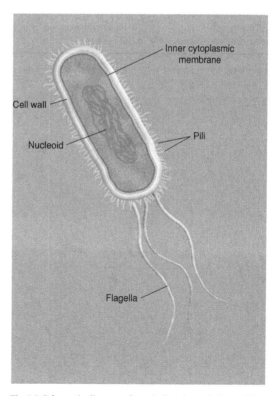

Fig. 1.2. Schematic diagram of a typical prokaryotic (bacterial) cell, illustrating the nucleoid, inner cytoplasmic membrane, cell wall, pili and flagella.

Table 1.1. Relative sizes of microbes and cells

Microbe	Size	Cell	Size
Microbe		**Cells**	
Prion protein	27–55 kD molecular weight,	Red blood cell (yardstick)	7 μm
	243 amino acids, <15 nm	White blood cell ranges	6–25 μm
Small virus	20 nm	Epithelial cells (squamous)	40–60 μm
(Papillomavirus, Poliovirus)			
HIV virus	110 nm	**Human gametes/embryos**	
Large virus (Poxvirus,	250–400 nm	Mature spermatozoon	4.0–5.0 μm in length;
Herpesvirus)		head size	2.5–3.5 μm in width
Bacteria size range	0.25 μm to 1 μm in width and	Mature spermatozoon tail	45 μm
	1 to 3 μm in length	length	
Mycoplasma species	0.3 × 0.8 μm	Round spermatid	7–8 μm
Staphylococcus spp.	1–3 μm	Primary spermatocyte	14–16 μm
Fungi	up to 25 μm	Human oocyte	100 μm–115 μm (including ZP)
Single-celled yeast	8 μm	Zygote pronuclei	~30 μm
Protozoa	10–60 μm	Cleaving embryo	approx. 175 μm, including ZP
Amoeboid cyst	10–20 μm diameter		
Trichomonas vaginalis	13 μm long		
Parasite eggs	50–150 μm diameter		
Parasitic adult worms	2 cm–1 m long		

$1 \, \mu m = 1 \times 10^{-6}$ metre $= 1 \times 10^{-3}$ mm; $\quad 1 \, \eta m = 1 \times 10^{-9}$ metre $= 1 \times 10^{-6}$ mm; $\quad$ ZP: zona pellucida.

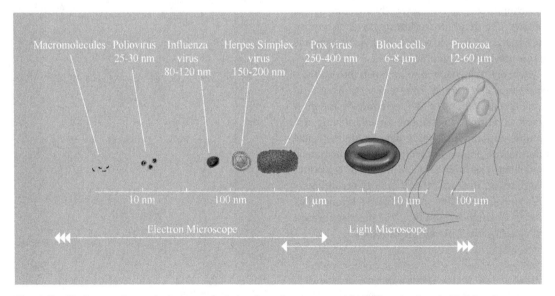

Fig. 1.3. Size of microorganisms and microscope resolution. Bacteria, protozoa and fungi all can be viewed with light microscopy. The average diameter for protozoa is 12–60 μm; the largest parasitic protozoan, *Balantidium coli* is 60 μm × 40 μm. Bacteria range in size from 0.25 to 1 μm in width and 1 to 3 μm in length. Viruses are larger than macromolecules, but smaller than the smallest bacteria. Viruses can be visualized by electron microscopy.

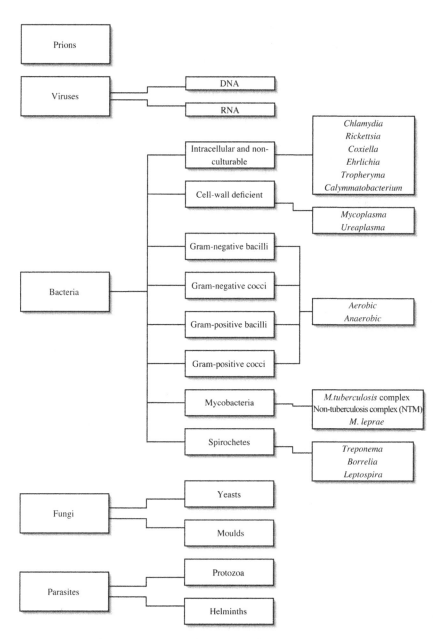

Fig. 1.4. Overview of microorganisms, in order of size and complexity.

of properties. This microcosm is further classified into basic 'families' of phylogenetic classification based upon evolutionary sequence and characteristic properties.

(i) Prokaryotes: Bacteria, Cyanobacteria, Rickettsiae
(ii) Fungi: (eukaryotes) moulds, mushrooms, yeasts
(iii) Viruses
(iv) Eukaryotic protists (protozoa): unicellular or multicellular

A virus is a submicroscopic infectious particle composed of a protein coat and a nucleic acid core. Viruses, like cells, carry genetic information encoded in their nucleic acid, and can undergo mutations and reproduce; however, they cannot carry out metabolism, and thus are not considered 'alive' by the classical definition. Viruses are classified by the type of nucleic acid they contain, and the shape of their protein capsule.

Prions are a recent addition to the list of 'microorganisms'. They do not fit into any of the 'classical' families, and present a further challenge to accepted definitions of 'life': although they apparently show multiplication, heredity and variation, they do not have the ability to react and adjust to environments.

In the late 1970s, a new group of organisms was added to this classification: the Archaea, a group of bacteria that live at high temperatures or produce methane. Because these organisms are biochemically and genetically different from usual bacteria, it was proposed that life be divided into three *domains*: Eukaryota, Eubacteria and Archaea – rather than the classical five kingdoms. Archaeans have been found in the most extreme environments on the planet, and also in plankton of the open sea and as methane-producing organisms inside the digestive tracts of cows, termites, and marine life. They live in the anoxic muds of marshes and at the bottom of the ocean, and even thrive in petroleum deposits deep underground. In May 2002, the discovery of another new member of the Archaea was reported, the Nanoarchaeota. This microbe has one of the smallest genomes known, with 500 000 nucleotide bases. The sequence of these nucleotide bases may point to the minimum number of genes needed for

an organism to sustain itself. The authors speculate that these nanoorganisms may represent an earlier intermediate form of life (Huber *et al.*, 2002). Their finding suggests that there may be other similarly unusual groups of microbes yet to be discovered.

Pathogenic microbiology primarily deals with genera and species within families. Microorganisms that are important in clinical ART practice can be found in all the categories, and they cover a wide range of sizes. Table 1.1 describes the size range of microbes relative to blood cells, gametes and embryos; Fig. 1.3 illustrates the relative sizes of protozoa, bacteria, viruses and macromolecules. An overview of the microorganisms discussed in Part I, in order of size and complexity, is presented in Fig. 1.4.

REFERENCES

Almquist, J. O., Glantz, P. J. & Shaffer, H. E. (1949). The effect of a combination of penicillin and streptomycin upon the viability and bacterial content of bovine semen. *Journal of Dairy Science*, **32**: 183–90.

Berry, W. R., Gottesfeld, R. L., Alter, H. J. & Vierling, J. M. (1987). Transmission of hepatitis B virus by artificial insemination. *Journal of the American Medical Association*, **257**: 1079–81.

Brock, T. D. (1967). Micro-organisms adapted to high temperatures. *Nature* (*London*), **214**: 882–5.

Bunge, R. G., Keeteel W. C. & Sherman J. K. (1954). Clinical use of frozen semen. *Fertility and Sterility*, **5**: 520–9.

Chang, M. C. (1959). Fertilization of rabbit ova in vitro. *Nature (London)*, **184**: 406.

Edwards, R. G. (1965). Maturation in vitro of mouse, sheep, cow, pig, rhesus monkey and human ovarian oocytes. *Nature (London)*, **208**: 349–51.

(1989). *Life Before Birth: Reflections on the Embryo Debate*. London: Hutchinson.

Heape, W. (1891). Preliminary note on the transplantation and growth of mammalian ova within a uterine foster-mother. *Proceedings of the Royal Society*, **48**: 457.

Huber, H., Hohn, M. J., Rachel, R., Fuchs, T., Wimmer, V. C. & Stetter, K. O. (2002). A new phylum of Archaea represented by a nanosized hyperthermophilic symbiont. *Nature*, **417**: 63–7.

Jackson, D. A., Symons, R. H. & Berg, P. (1972). Biochemical method for inserting new genetic information into DNA of simian virus 40: circular SV 40 DNA molecules containing lamda phage genes and the galactose operon of *Escherichia coli. Proceedings of the National Academy of Science, USA,* **69**: 2904–9.

McLaughlin, E. A. (2002). Cryopreservation, screening and storage of sperm – the challenges for the twenty-first century. *Human Fertility,* **5** (Suppl.): S61–5.

Minkoff, H. & Santoro, N. (2000). Ethical considerations in the treatment of infertility in women with human immunodeficiency virus infection. *New England Journal of Medicine,* **343**: 1748–50.

Moore, D. E., Ashley, R. L., Zarutskie, P. W. *et al.* (1989). Transmission of genital herpes by donor insemination. *Journal of the American Medical Association,* **261**: 3441–3.

Nagel, T. C., Tagatz, G. E. & Campbell, B. F. (1986). Transmission of *Chlamydia trachomatis* by artificial insemination. *Fertility and Sterility,* **46**: 959–62.

Ochiai, K., Yamanda, K., Kimura, K. & Sawada, O. (1959). Studies on the inheritance of drug resistance between *Shigella* strains and *Escherichia coli* strains. *Nippon Iji Shimpo,* **1861**: 34–46.

Palermo, G., Joris, H., Devroey, P. & Van Steirteghem, A. C. (1992). Pregnancies after intracytoplasmic injection of single spermatozoon into an oocyte. *Lancet,* **340**: 17–18.

Prusiner, S. B. (1982). Novel proteinaceous particles cause scrapie. *Science,* **216**: 136–44.

Saiki, R. K., Gelfand, D. H., Stoffel, S. *et al.* (1988). Primer-directed enzymatic amplification of DNA with a thermostable DNA polymerase. *Science,* **239**: 487–91.

Sanger, F., Air, G. M., Barrell, B. G. *et al.* (1977). Nucleotide sequence of bacteriophage phi X174 DNA. *Nature,* **165**: 687–95.

Sherman, J. K. & Bunge, R. G. (1953). Observations on preservation of human spermatozoa at low temperatures. *Proceedings of the Society for Experimental Biology and Medicine,* **82**(4), 686–8.

Yanagamachi, R. & Chang, M. C. (1964). IVF of golden hamster ova. *Journal of Experimental Zoology,* **156**: 361–76.

Zinder, N. & Lederberg, J. (1952). Genetic exchange in Salmonella. *Journal of Bacteriology,* **64**: 679–99.

FURTHER READING

http://www.ucmp.berkeley.edu/archaea/archaea.html
http://www-micro.msb.le.ac.uk/Tutorials/Time/Machine.html
http://www.tulane.edu/~dmsander/WWW/224/
    Classification224.html

Advisory Committee on Dangerous Pathogens (2002). Microbiological risk assessment – an interim report, HMSO Publications.

Austin, C. R. (1951). Observations on the penetration of the sperm into the mammalian egg. *Australian Journal of Scientific Research,* **4**: 581–96.

Balen, A. H. & Jacobs, H. S. (1997). *Infertility in Practice.* Edinburgh: Churchill Livingstone.

Bloom, B. R. (2003). Lessons from SARS. *Science,* **300**: 701.

Brackett, R. G., Bousquet, D., Boice, M. L. *et al.* (1982). Normal development following in vitro fertilization in the cow. *Biology of Reproduction,* **27**: 147–58.

Cole, H. & Cupps, P. (1977). *Reproduction in Domestic Animals.* New York: Academic Press.

Dobell, C. (ed.) (1960). *Antony van Leeuwenhoek and his 'Little Animals'.* New York: Dover Publications.

Edwards, R. G. (1972). Control of human development. In *Artificial Control of Reproduction; Reproduction in Mammals,* Book 5, ed. Austin C. R. & Short R. V., pp. 87–113. Cambridge, UK: Cambridge University Press.

Edwards, R. G., Bavister, B. D. & Steptoe, P. C. (1969). Early stages of fertilization in vitro of human oocytes matured in vitro. *Nature (London),* **221**: 632–5.

Epidemiologic Notes and Reports: HIV-1 infection and artificial insemination with processed semen (1990). *Morbidity and Mortality Weekly Report,* **39**(15): 249,255–6.

Ford, B. J. (1991). *The Leeuwenhoek Legacy.* Bristol: Biopress and London: Farrand Press.

Gosden, R. G. (1999). *Cheating Time: Sex, Science and Aging.* New York: W. H. Freeman & Co.

Haselwandter, K. & Ebner, M. R. (1994). Microorganisms surviving for 5300 years. *FEMS Microbiology* (Lett). **116**: 189–94.

Medvei, V. V. (1993). *The History of Clinical Endocrinology.* Carnforth, Lancs. Parthenon.

Morice, P., Josset, P., Charon, C. & Dubuisson, J. B. (1995). History of infertility. *Human Reproduction Update,* **1**(5): 497–504.

Parkes, A. S. (1966). The rise of reproductive endocrinology, 1926–40. *Journal of Endocrinology,* **34**: 19–32.

Polge, C. (1972). Increasing reproductive potential in farm animals. In *Artificial Control of Reproduction, Reproduction in Mammals,* Book 5, ed. Austin C. R. & Short R. V., pp. 1–32. Cambridge, UK: Cambridge University Press.

Postgate, J. (2000) *Microbes and Man,* 4th edition. Cambridge, UK: Cambridge University Press.

Robert G. Edwards at 75 (2002). *Reproductive BioMedicine Online* **4**, suppl. 1.

Schopf, J. W. (1993). Microfossils of the early Archean apex chart: new evidence of the antiquity of life. *Science,* **260**: 640–6.

Steptoe, P. C. & Edwards, R. G. (1970). Laparoscopic recovery of pre-ovulatory human oocytes after priming of ovaries with gonadotrophins. *Lancet*, **i**: 683–9.

(1976). Reimplantation of a human embryo with subsequent tubal pregnancy. *Lancet*, **i**: 880–2.

(1978). Birth after the re-implantation of a human embryo (letter). *Lancet*, **ii**: 366.

Yanagamachi, R. & Chang, M. C. (1964). IVF of golden hamster ova. *Journal of Experimental Zoology*, **156**: 361–76.

Whittingham, D. G. (1968). Fertilization of mouse eggs in vitro. *Nature*, **200**: 281–2.

Appendix: glossary of terms

abscess local collection of pus.

aerobe a bacterium that grows in ambient air, which contains 21% oxygen (O_2) and a small amount (0.03%) of carbon dioxide (CO_2).

aerosol suspension of small solid or liquid particles in air; fine spray of droplets.

anaerobe a bacterium that usually cannot grow in the presence of oxygen, but which grows in atmosphere composed of 5–10% hydrogen (H_2), 5–10% CO_2, 80–90% nitrogen (N_2) and 0% oxygen (O_2).

antibiotic substance produced by a microorganism that suppresses the growth of, or kills, other microorganisms.

antigenaemia the presence of an antigen in the blood.

antimicrobial chemical drug produced by a microorganism that is growth suppressive or microbiocidal in activity.

antiseptic compound that inhibits bacterial growth without necessarily killing the bacteria.

bacteriostatic agent that inhibits the replication of target bacteria, but does not kill the organism.

bacteriocidal agent that kills the target organism.

bacteriophage virus that infects a bacterium.

bacteriuria bacteria in the urine.

BBV Blood-borne viruses.

biotype biologic or biochemical type of an organism. Organisms of a given biotype have identical biologic or biochemical characteristics. Key markers are used to recognise biotypes in tracing spread of organism during epidemics.

candle jar a jar with a lid providing a gas-tight seal in which a small white candle is placed and lit after culture plates are added. The candle will only burn until the oxygen is reduced to a point that burning is no longer supported; at that point the atmosphere in the jar will have a lower oxygen content than room air and ~3% carbon dioxide.

capnophile an organism that requires increased CO_2 (5–10%) and approximately 15% O_2. *Neisseria gonorrhoeae* and *Haemophilus influenzae* are capnophilic bacteria. These organisms will grow in a candle jar with 3% CO_2 or a CO_2 incubator.

carrier a healthy person who is carrying, and usually excreting an infectious agent, but who generally has no symptoms of the infection.

catalase bacterial enzyme that breaks down hydrogen peroxide with release of oxygen.

CD4 an antigen found on the surface of T-helper cells and certain other types of cell such as the monocyte, that acts as a receptor for attachment of HIV.

CFU Colony forming units; numbers of bacterial colonies on agar cultures, each of which started as a single bacterium in the original specimen.

chlamydyospore thick-walled fungal spore formed from vegetative cell.

chronic infection persistence of a replicating infectious agent in the host for longer than 6 months.

commensalism a symbiotic relationship in which one organism benefits without harming the host organism.

community-acquired pertaining to outside the hospital (community-acquired infection).

conidia asexual fungal spores.

conjugation passing genetic information between bacteria via pili.

contaminant an agent that causes contamination or pollution. In laboratory cultures, contaminants generally arise from skin flora or from environmental sources.

CSF cerebrospinal fluid.

culdocentesis aspiration of cul-de-sac fluid requiring puncture of the vaginal wall to enter into the retroperitoneal space.

cystitis inflammation of the urinary bladder.

cytopathic effect (CPE) changes in cell morphology resulting from viral infection of a cell culture monolayer.

dark-field microscopy technique used to visualize very small or thin microorganisms such as spirochaetes; light is reflected or refracted from the surface of viewed objects.

decontamination process of rendering an object or area safe by removing microbes or rendering them harmless using biologic or chemical agents.

definitive host the host in which sexual reproduction of a parasite takes place.

dematiaceous pigmented (dark coloured) moulds, as in those that produce melanin. When examining these moulds, the reverse side of the culture plate appears dark, indicating a pigmented mycelium.

dermatophyte parasitic fungus on skin, hair or nails.

DFA direct fluorescent antibody test.

dimorphic fungi fungi with both mould and yeast phases.

disinfectant agent that destroys or inhibits microorganisms.

dysgonic bacteria that grows poorly in culture.

dysuria painful urination.

edema excessive accumulation of tissue fluid.

Eh oxidation–reduction potential.

endemic occuring in a particular region or population.

elementary body infectious stage of *Chlamydia*.

ELISA enzyme-linked immunosorbent assay.

EMB eosin-methylene blue.

enterotoxin toxin that affects the intestinal mucosa.

endotoxin substance containing lipopolysaccharide found in the gram-negative cell bacterial wall; plays an important role in complications of sepsis (shock, disseminated intravascular coagulation, thrombocytopenia).

epidemiology the study of occurrence and distribution of disease in populations and factors that control the presence or absence of disease.

etiology causative agent or cause of disease.

fastidious an organism with very stringent growth requirements. Certain anaerobes will not grow in the presence of even traces of oxygen.

eugonic growing luxuriantly (refers to bacterial cultures).

fermentation anaerobic decomposition of carbohydrate.

fimbrae fingerlike proteinaceous projections that act as a bacterial adherence mechanism.

flagella structures composed mostly of protein responsible for microbe motility.

FTA fluorescent treponemal antibody A.

fulminant a condition or symptom that is of very sudden onset, severe, and of short duration, often leading to death.

hyaline non-pigmented, used to refer to fungal organisms that do not produce melanin. When examining the reverse side of the culture plate, these organisms appear tan–white.

iatrogenic caused by medical or surgical intervention, induced by the treatment itself.

IFA indirect fluorescent antibody.

immunocompromised a state of reduced resistance to infection and other foreign substances that results from drugs, radiation illness, congenital defect or certain infections (e.g. HIV).

immunoglobulin antibody; there are five classes: IgG, IgM, IgA, IgE and IgD.

inclusion bodies microscopic bodies within body cells thought to be viral particles in morphogenesis.

incubation period the interval between exposure to an infection and the appearance of the first symptoms.

induration abnormal hardness of tissue resulting from inflammation and hyperaemia.

infection invasion and subsequent multiplication of microorganisms, causing disease.

indolent a disease process that is failing to heal or has persisted.

latent infection persistence of a non-replicating infectious agent in the host.

leukocytosis elevated white blood cell count.

leukopenia low white blood cell count.

media

    differential permits recognition of organism or group based on recognition of natural organism product identified by incorporating the appropriate substrate and indicator in media.

    enrichment medium that favours growth of one or more organisms and suppresses growth of competing flora.

    selective medium that contains inhibitory substances or unusual growth factors that allow one particular organism or group to grow while suppressing most others.

meningitis inflammation of the meninges of the brain.

metastatic spreading from primary site to distance focus via the bloodstream or lymphatic system.

microconidia small, single-celled fungal spores.

mixed culture growth of more than one organism from a single culture.

microaerophile grows under reduced O_2 (5–10%). Examples are *Helicobacter pylori* and *Campylobacter jejuni*. It is unlikely that these organisms would be encountered in an ART laboratory.

mycelium mass of hyphae.

mycoses fungal diseases.

myositis inflammation of muscle.

nares nostrils; external openings to nose.

neonatal first 4 weeks after birth.

NGU non-gonococcal urethritis.

non-productive infection failure of a virus-infected mammalian cell to release progeny virions, usually due to the suppression of late gene expression.

normal flora the body's resident microbes, will not cause disease in the 'normal' site, but may if displaced. Some of the organisms that may be encountered in ART may be normal flora (e.g. *E. coli* and *E. faecalis* found in semen that are normal stool flora) can cause a real problem if they contaminate culture medium.

nosocomial (Noso, disease, komeo, hospital) disease acquired by patients during hospitalization–clinical manifestations present at least 72 hours after admission. Organisms are carried on the hands of healthcare providers from colonized patients to newly admitted patients, who then become colonized themselves.

OPF operation protection factor.

O&P ova and parasites.

O–F oxidation–fermentation media.

oncogene regulatory gene of a mammalian cell that has been integrated into the genome of a retrovirus.

oncogenic having the potential to cause normal cells to become malignant.

opportunistic pathogen does not normally produce disease. When the host is immunocompromised due to antibiotic therapy, cancer therapy, steroids or debilitating conditions, opportunists proliferate and cause infection.

pandemic epidemic that covers a wide geographic region or is worldwide.

parasite organism that lives on, or within, another organism, at that organism's expense.

parenteral route of drug administration other than by mouth (intravenous (IV), intramuscular (IM)).

parotitis inflammation of the parotid gland; mumps is the most common cause.

paroxysm rapid onset of symptoms (or return of symptoms); usually refers to cyclic recurrence of malaria symptoms.

pathogen an organism that can cause disease.

pathogenesis process by which an organism causes disease.

pathogenic capable of causing disease.

pathologic caused by, or involving, a morbid condition such as a pathologic state.

PCR polymerase chain reaction.

peptidoglycan murein layer of bacterial cell wall responsible for shape and strength to withstand changes in osmotic pressure.

perineum portion of the body bound by the pubic bone anteriorly and the coccyx posteriorly.

percutaneous through the skin (e.g. bladder aspiration).

petechiae tiny hemorrhagic spots on the skin or mucous membranes.

phage grouping or phagotype bacterial grouping based on the ability of certain strains to be lysed by specific bacteriophages (useful in epidemiological tracing of hospital outbreaks).

PID pelvic inflammatory disease.

pili similar to fimbrae; for transfer of genetic material during bacterial conjugation.

plasmid autonomously replicating DNA molecule found in bacteria; they may be transferred from cell to cell.

pleomorphic having more than one form.

prion proteinaceous infectious agent associated with Creutzfeldt–Jakob disease and other chronic debilitating CNS diseases.

proctitis inflammation of the rectum.

prodrome early manifestations of disease before specific symptoms appear.

prognosis forecast as to outcome of disease.

prostatitis inflammation of the prostate gland, usually caused by infection.

protists eukaryotic microorganisms.

pure culture growth of a single organism in culture.

pus inflammatory material consisting of many white blood cells, other cellular debris and often bacteria.

pyuria presence of eight or more white blood cells (WBCs) per cubic mm in uncentrifuged urine.

purulent containing pus.

reagin an antibody that reacts in various serologic tests for syphilis.

reservoir source from which infectious agent may disseminate.

reticulate body metabolically active form in *Chlamydia* life cycle.

RPR rapid plasma reagin, non-treponemal tests for antibodies to syphilis.

routes of infection may be
direct transmission
   congenital
   sexual contact
   hand-to-hand transmission oral–fecal
   respiratory droplets/secretions
indirect transmission
   fomites
   water and food
   animals, insect vectors, arthropod vectors
   airborne
   nosocomial infections
   community-acquired infections
   endogenous infection
   exogenous infection – obtained or produced outside the body; not part of the body's resident flora. *Clostridium tetani* and *Clostridium botulinum* are acquired from the environment. *E. coli*, on the other hand is resident bowel flora and can cause infection when it reaches another body site (e.g. from ruptured appendix).

saprophytic living off or deriving nutrition from decaying plant or animal matter.

septate having cross walls, as in septate hyphae.

seroconversion the development of antibodies not previously present resulting from a primary infection.

serogroup, serotype or serovar grouping of bacteria based upon the antigenic diversity of their surface or subsurface antigens.

septicemia or sepsis systemic disease pathogens or their toxins in the blood.

spore reproductive cell of bacteria, fungi or protozoa; may be inactive in bacteria.

sensitivity ability of a test to detect all true cases for condition being tested; absence of false-negatives.

specificity ability of a test to correctly yield a negative result when condition being detected is absent; absence of false-positive results.

STD sexually transmitted disease.

substrate substance on which enzyme acts.

suppuration pus formation.

synergism combined effect of two or more agents that is greater than the sum of each separately.

syndrome set of symptoms occurring together.

teichoic acids part of gram-positive bacteria cell wall consisting of glycerol or ribitol phosphate polymers combined with various amino acids and sugars.

teleomorph sexual stage of fungi.

thrush *Candida* infection producing white lesions, usually in the oral cavity.

tolerance a form of induced resistance to antimicrobials.

transduction moving of genetic material from one prokaryote to another via a bacteriophage.

transformation organism takes up free DNA in environment when another organism dies.

transposon genetic material that can move from one genetic element to another (plasmid to plasmid or plasmid to chromosome); called 'jumping genes'.

Tzanck test stained smear of cells from the base of vesicles, examined for inclusion bodies produced by herpes simplex or varicella-zoster viruses.

true pathogen causes disease when it enters target body site in sufficient numbers, e.g. hemorrhagic viruses or syphilis.

viremia the presence of virus in the blood.

Bacteriology

Bacteria are unicellular organisms that belong to the kingdom of Prokaryotae. Whereas eukaryotes have membrane-bound cytoplasmic organelles designed to carry out specific functions, bacteria have no well-defined nucleus, nuclear membrane or membrane-bound organelles. Their bacterial genome consists of a single, double-stranded, closed circular DNA molecule that lies within the cytoplasm, along with mesosomes, ribosomes, and various cytoplasmic granules, all of which are enclosed within a thin elastic trilaminar membrane. The majority of bacteria also lack the cytoskeleton that gives support and structure to eukaryotes. With the exception of the mycoplasmas, bacteria contain a cell wall of unique chemical composition. They are microscopic in size, with species ranging from 0.25 μm to 1 μm in width and 1 μm to 10 μm in length. Some bacterial species have capsules, flagella, or pili, and some species produce endospores.

Bacteria are divided into Orders, Families, Genera, and species, and named according to genus and species: e.g. *Escherichia* (genus) *coli* (species). Bacteria within the same genus and species also may be designated as subspecies, based upon differences in geographic distribution, transmission, clinical manifestation, and pathogenicity, e.g. *Treponema pallidum* subsp. *pallidum*, and *T. pallidum* subsp. *pertenue*. They may also be classified in serogroups, serotypes, or serovars based upon surface or subsurface antigens or according to the type of capsule surrounding the bacterium. For example, streptococci are grouped on the basis of specific cell wall polysaccharide antigens (Lancefield groups).

Structure and function of bacteria

Bacterial structure

Cell wall

The bacterial cell wall lies close to the cytoplasmic membrane, and gives the organism shape and rigidity. It also acts as a barrier to low molecular weight substances (<10 000 kD), allowing the organism to withstand changes in osmotic pressure that would cause cell lysis, and serves as an attachment site for bacteriophages and appendages such as pili, fimbriae, and flagella. The cell wall is made up of a three-dimensional peptidoglycan lattice, a biopolymer with alternating units of N-acetyl-D-muramic acid and N-acetyl-D-glucosamine linked to short peptides, the murein layer. Differences in cell wall structure between bacteria are reflected in their staining properties, and the gram stain is used to separate bacteria into groups for identification. Gram-positive and gram-negative bacteria differ in the amino acid composition of the peptides, and also have different lipoproteins, phospholipids, and lipopolysaccharides (Fig. 2.1). Bacteria without cell walls (mycoplasmas), or those lacking the peptidoglycan layer (chlamydiae), are referred to as gram-null. Since this cell wall structure is unique to bacteria, antimicrobial agents that are targeted towards its synthesis (e.g. penicillin), or towards triggering of cell wall autolysis will have selective activity against bacteria, with little or no host toxicity. Some bacteria such as *Mycobacterium tuberculosis* and members of the *Nocardiae* have mycolic acid

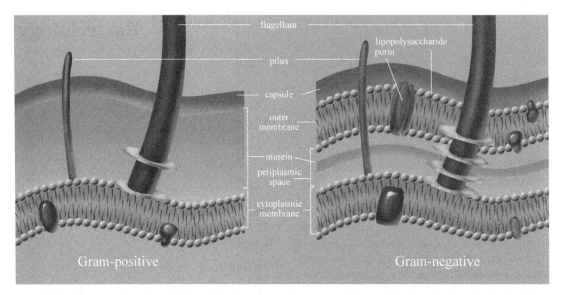

Fig. 2.1. Gram-positive and gram-negative bacterial cell envelopes. The outer membrane and periplasmic space are present only in the gram-negative envelope. The murein layer is thicker in gram-positive envelopes.

in the cell wall, which allows them to retain the crystal violet primary stain after acid decolorizing. These organisms are 'acid-fast' or partially acid-fast, depending on the amount of mycolic acid in the cell wall.

Outer membrane

Gram-negative, but not gram-positive, bacteria have an outer membrane adjacent to the cell wall that serves as a selective permeability barrier to hydrophilic and hydrophobic compounds. This bilayered membrane is composed of lipopolysaccharide (LPS), and is important in the pathogenicity of gram-negative organisms. The lipopolysaccharide layer contains porins, which allow passage of nutrients and solutes, as well as antibiotics. Porins aid in the attachment of the outer membrane to the cell wall, and they vary among bacterial species. Gram-negative bacteria have a periplasmic space between the inner surface of the outer membrane and the outer surface of the cell membrane. This space is filled with the murein layer, a gel-like substance that helps secure nutrients from the outside, containing enzymes that degrade large molecules and detoxify

solutes (including antibiotics) that enter the space from the environment.

Inner cytoplasmic membrane

Both gram-negative and gram-positive bacteria have an inner cytoplasmic membrane. This typical cell membrane is a lipid bilayer of 7 nm thickness studded with proteins, many of which are enzymes that catalyse metabolism within the cell. The membrane serves as an osmotic barrier, allows transport of solutes in and out of the cell, and is the site of many of the functions that are performed within the organelles of eukaryotic cells, including generation of adenosine triphosphate (ATP), cell motility, sensing of environmental changes, housing enzymes for synthesis of cellular building materials, and mediation of chromosome segregation during replication.

Appendages

Capsules

Capsules are well-defined mucoid structures that surround the murein layer of gram-positive bacteria and the outer membrane of gram-negative bacteria.

They are composed of high molecular weight polysaccharides, and their secretion may depend on environmental conditions, especially the nutritional environment. Unlike the cell wall, the capsule does not provide physical strength, and does not function as a permeability barrier. The mucoid capsule, sometimes referred to as the 'slime layer', provides protection from drying, and helps the coated bacteria to evade the host immune system by preventing their engulfment by phagocytic cells. The capsule may also inhibit the immune system, and can facilitate bacterial colonization by attaching to surfaces on teeth and inanimate devices such as prosthetic heart valves. The capsule contributes to the virulence of certain bacteria: the virulence of both *Streptococcus pneumoniae* and *Haemophilus influenzae* are dependent on encapsulation. Capsules also give bacteria a wide antigenic diversity, which contributes to the invasiveness of the organism, and makes effective vaccine preparation more difficult.

Flagella

Some bacteria have **flagella** embedded in the cell envelope that can enhance their invasive properties by making them highly motile. The surface of the flagellum is made up of protein antigens with diverse epitopes that are useful in the identification and classification of some organisms such as *Salmonella*. Spirochetes have periplasmic flagella in the space between the cytoplasmic and outer membranes, and this unusual location is responsible for their helical movement. Bacterial flagella can be arranged in several different ways, including:

(i) polar: one flagellum located at one end of the cell
(ii) monotrichous: several flagella located at one end of the cell
(iii) lophotrichous: flagella located at both ends of the cell
(iv) peritrichous: the entire cell covered with flagella.

Pili or fimbrae

Pili or **fimbrae** are hairlike rigid structures up to 2 μm in length, composed of protein. They originate in the cytoplasmic membrane, and extend to the outside environment. There are two types of pili, known as sex (F) pili, and common pili (fimbriae), and when they are present, cells usually have hundreds of pili. Sex pili may participate in deoxyribonucleic acid (DNA) transfer, mediating the conjugation of donor and recipient cells. Common pili serve as virulence factors by mediating adherence to host cell surfaces, often a first step in establishing infection. Once piliated bacteria are established within the host, the pili can then undergo antigenic variation that allows them to evade the host cell immune system.

Interior of the cell

The inner cytoplasmic membrane surrounds the cytosol, which contains polysomes, inclusions, nucleoid, plasmids, and endospores. The cytosol is abundant in enzymes, and nearly all cell functions are carried out here, including protein synthesis. The granular appearance of the cytosol is due to the many polysomes (messenger ribonucleic acid (mRNA) molecules linked with several ribosomes) that are present during translation and protein synthesis, and inclusions or storage granules, composed primarily of nutrient and energy reserves such as glycogen and polyphosphates. The nucleoid contains highly coiled DNA, intermixed with RNA, polyamines and structural proteins. There is usually only one chromosome per bacterial cell, but during certain stages of cell division, separate extrachromosomal genetic elements known as plasmids may be present independently, in various numbers or not at all.

Endospores

Certain gram-positive bacteria can sporulate to produce endospores when under adverse physical and chemical conditions (including ultraviolet radiation). Endospores are produced by vegetative cells as a survival strategy in situations of nutritional depletion. The metabolically active and growing cell transforms to a dormant state, with a decrease in cytosol and an increase in the thickness of the cell envelope. Endospores are highly resistant to heat and chemical agents, and can survive for years in the environment. Under favourable conditions, the spore will germinate to produce a single vegetative cell that can then multiply. Both environmental contaminants (species of *Bacillus*) and human pathogens (species of *Clostridium* and some species of *Bacillus*, e.g. *B. anthracis*) produce endospores. These highly resistant structures present a problem in sterilization procedures.

Bacterial chromosomes

Bacteria have a single circular chromosome that contains all the genes necessary for the viability of the organism. Unlike chromosomes in the membrane-bound nucleus of eukaryotes, the bacterial chromosome is 'naked' in the cytoplasm. The single chromosome contains double-stranded, supercoiled DNA with a composition and structure identical to that of eukaryotic DNA. The DNA is composed of nucleotides, i.e. purine (adenine and guanine) and pyrimidine (thymine and cytosine) bases linked to deoxyribose sugar and a phosphate group. Via molecular hydrogen bonds, adenine pairs with thymine, cytosine pairs with guanine, and groups of paired bases code for specific genes. The sequence of DNA bases represents the genetic code. All genes collectively comprise the organism's genome, which is usually expressed as the number of base pairs. Genes are widely distributed among bacteria, and similarities or differences in DNA sequence are used to develop molecular tests for detection and identification of pathogenic microorganisms.

Bacteria also contain extrachromosomal genetic material, located on plasmids and transposable elements, both of which can reproduce. Like the bacterial chromosome, plasmids are double-stranded and circular, but there are several differences between them.

(i) A plasmid ranges in size from 1–2 kilobases to 1 megabase or more, whereas the bacterial chromosome is about 1300 μm in length (a single base is 3.4×10^{-4} μm long or 0.34 nanometres in length).

(ii) There is only one chromosome per bacterium, whereas the numbers of plasmids vary.

(iii) The bacterial chromosome is preserved during reproduction, but plasmids may be lost.

(iv) Bacterial chromosomal genes code for proteins essential for viability, while plasmids code for products that mediate transfer between bacterial cells, or for survival determinants such as resistance to antibiotics.

Unlike plasmids, transposable elements do not exist separately in the cell, but are attached either to chromosomes or to plasmids. These entities move from one location to another: from plasmid to chromosome and from chromosome to plasmid. There are two types of transposable elements, insertion sequences and transposons. Insertion sequence genes code for information required for movement along plasmids and chromosomes, and transposons contain genes that code for movement and for drug resistance markers. Genetic exchange among bacteria is due to these extrachromosomal pieces of DNA.

Bacterial reproduction

The process of reproduction in bacteria is similar to that of eukaryotic cells: proteins and enzymes are produced in preparation for DNA replication, DNA is replicated and cytoplasmic division follows. The DNA double helix uncoils, each parent strand then serves as a template for synthesis of a complementary daughter strand, and two new duplicate chromosomes are produced prior to cell division.

Bacterial growth occurs through an asexual vegetative process known as binary fission, with each parent cell producing two daughter cells. The cell enlarges, elongating at designated growing zones, and cellular components are synthesized and assembled into a mature cell structure that resembles the parent. Once it reaches a critical size, the cell begins to divide, and produces two daughter cells; these may or may not separate physically, depending on the species. About half of each new cell consists of newly synthesized material, and the other half is made up of pre-existing material from the parent cell. Each daughter cell has a newly replicated copy of the bacteria's genome. Some species grow in filamentous and cordlike structures (e.g. *Mycobacterium*), or as filamentous or branching mycelia that eventually lead to spore formation and a budding or branching process of cell growth (e.g. *Nocardia*). In eukaryotic cells, new combinations of genes occur via segregation of gametes during sexual reproduction and by recombination of genes on homologous chromosomes during the process of meiosis. Gene exchange in bacteria can occur via recombination, and also by three additional mechanisms: transformation, transduction and conjugation.

Transformation

During transformation bacteria that are competent can take in DNA that is free in the environment from the lysis of dead bacteria, creating new genetic combinations. Transformation is not limited to transfer of genes among bacteria of the same species, and thus genetic traits can be disseminated to a variety of medically important microbes. Among the human pathogens, *Haemophilus*, *Neisseria* and *Streptococcus* have competence characteristics.

Transduction

Transduction is mediated by bacteriophages (viruses that infect bacteria). Viruses integrate their DNA into the bacterial chromosome and direct replication of viral DNA, which is then packaged and released from the bacterial cell during lysis. The virus packages some bacterial DNA along with its own viral DNA, and the bacterial DNA from the previous host is released when the virus infects another bacterium, introducing foreign bacterial DNA into the newly infected cell.

Conjugation

Conjugation is an exchange of genetic material between two strains of living bacteria, with one strain donating DNA to a recipient strain. During this process the pilus of the donor forms a bridge with the recipient bacterium, and this bridge acts as a conduit for DNA to be transferred from the donor bacterium to the recipient. Formation of the bridge triggers DNA replication; the donor cell produces one new DNA strand and passes this to the recipient, where a complementary strand is made. The new DNA is now available to recombine with the recipient cell's genetic material. Bacterial chromosomes, plasmids and transposons may participate in conjugation.

Transcription and translation

When cells are not reproducing or preparing to reproduce, they are carrying out routine cellular activities that are dependent on synthesis of proteins and enzymes. Protein synthesis occurs in two stages: transcription and translation. Transcription is the process by which DNA, carrying the genetic code, is copied onto a complementary strand of mRNA. Usually only one of the two DNA strands serves as a template for RNA transcription. When mRNA is transcribed from DNA, cytosine bases pair with guanine, but uracil is substituted for thymine in pairing with adenine. A sequence of three bases is a triplet, and each triplet encodes for a specific amino acid. This sequence is referred to as a codon. Since there are four bases and the codon consists of three bases, there are 64 (4^3) possible codons, with some amino acids coded for by more than one triplet. In bacteria, the mRNA molecule will code for several genes whose protein products are involved in similar functions. Transfer RNA (tRNA) and ribosomal RNA (rRNA) are also produced during transcription. All three RNA molecules are required for translation when mRNA is decoded by the ribosomes for polypeptide synthesis. Each mRNA codon matches an anticodon located on a specific transfer RNA (tRNA) molecule. The mRNA associates with subunits on the ribosomes, and translation is initiated. As the ribosome moves along the mRNA, it deciphers the mRNA code and matches it with the corresponding anticodon on a tRNA molecule. The tRNA molecule picks up the specific amino acid corresponding to the anticodon and attaches it to a

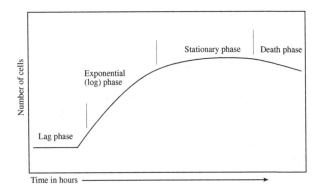

Fig. 2.2. Bacterial growth curve. When a culture of microorganisms is transferred into a new container, there is an initial 'lag phase', while the bacteria adjust to their new environment. Having adapted to the new source of nutrients and new temperature, they then enter an 'exponential', or log phase of rapid multiplication. A 'stationary phase' begins when the bacteria have exhausted the nutrient supply, or have produced toxins that limit their growth; metabolism is adjusted to maintain cells only, without growth. In non-spore forming species, cells enter a 'death phase', where the number of viable cells decreases and the dead cells undergo autolysis.

growing chain of amino acids to form a polypeptide. Translation is terminated when the 'stop' codon (UAA) is reached.

Bacterial growth

Bacterial growth generally occurs very rapidly, with three predictable and recognizable phases over time (Fig. 2.2).

Lag phase: when a bacterium is introduced into a favourable new growth environment, the cell adapts to its new surroundings by synthesizing any new cellular machinery required. Once it has adjusted optimally, there is then a phase of rapid cell growth and division: the exponential or log phase. Bacterial cell numbers increase exponentially, until an essential nutrient is depleted, or toxic metabolites accumulate. Cell growth then slows down and usually stops within a single generation time: the bacteria then enter a stationary phase. The cells are still viable, but metabolism is readjusted in order to maintain the cells only, without growth. Certain bacteria can then

undergo a process of differentiation to form resting stages, spores or cysts that can survive for months or years with no apparent metabolic activity. In non-spore-forming species, if necessary substrates are absent cellular energy supplies are depleted, and the cells enter a death phase. The number of viable cells decreases until no living cells are left, and these dead cells undergo autolysis.

Bacterial metabolism

Bacterial metabolism involves four major processes: acquisition of nutrients, metabolism of acquired nutrients, energy production to support all cellular activity, and synthesis of new materials.

Acquisition of nutrients

Nutrients are transported across the bacterial cell membrane. Oxygen, water and carbon dioxide diffuse into the cell, but energy-requiring active transport is required for the uptake of sugars, amino acids, and organic and inorganic acids. The majority of nutrients are carried across the membrane by carrier molecules.

Metabolism

Once inside the cell, nutrients serve as raw materials for precursor metabolites required for synthesis. The metabolites are produced by three central pathways: the Embden–Meyerhof–Parnas (EMP) pathway, the tricarboxylic acid (TCA) cycle, and the pentose phosphate shunt. Medically important bacteria are often identified by measuring products and byproducts of these metabolic pathways.

Energy production

Energy production is coupled to the breakdown of nutrients, and involves oxidation–reduction reactions. Energy, primarily in the form of ATP is produced in the bacterial cell by the breakdown of nutrients via two general mechanisms: oxidative phosphorylation and fermentative metabolism, which does not require oxygen. The pathways used during fermentative metabolism and the end products produced vary among bacteria, and bacteria can be identified by detecting these end products. For example, the methyl-red test detects use of the mixed acids pathway, and the Voges–Proskauer test detects production of 2,3 butylene glycol. During aerobic respiration, oxidative phosphorylation involves the electron transport chain and requires oxygen as a terminal electron acceptor. During anaerobic respiration, the terminal electron acceptor is not oxygen. The mechanism used to produce ATP is important when cultivating organisms in the clinical microbiology laboratory.

Synthesis

When precursor molecules and energy are available, bacteria assemble the materials into larger molecules or polymers for cellular structures. Bacteria vary widely in their biosynthetic capabilities – this also is important for cultivation in the clinical microbiology laboratory. Some organisms can synthesize the majority of their requirements, while others may be unable to synthesize a particular material, such as an amino acid, and this must be supplied in the laboratory culture medium in order to ensure growth. Synthesis and assembly of macromolecules within the bacterial cell is enzyme driven, and the ability of a bacterium to produce certain enzymes is another means of laboratory identification. For example, members of the genus *Staphylococci* produce the enzyme catalase, and this differentiates the genus from the morphologically similar *Streptococcus* species, which cannot produce catalase. Detection of catalase is an early test for identification of bacteria shown to be gram-positive cocci on the Gram stain.

Bacterial classification and identification

Nomenclature

Bacteria are classified on the basis of shared properties, including genetics, morphology, and physiology. The basic taxonomic group is the species. Occasionally a subspecies is recognized within a species and biotype, and serotype or phagotype may be used to describe groups below the subspecies level. Species with several features in common are grouped into a genus. Similar genera are grouped into families. Bacteria are generally referred to by genus and species: *Escherichia* is the genus and *coli* is the species for the common bacterium *E. coli*.

Family: *Enterobacteriaceae*
Genus: *Escherichia*
  species: *coli*
    Serotype: O157:H7
Genus: *Vibrio*
  species: *cholera*
    Biotype: Classical or El Tor

Both genus and species are used routinely in pathogenic microbiology, with names typed in italics. The genus is always capitalized, and the species is written in lower case, as in *Escherichia coli*. The first letter of the genus name may be used as abbreviation: *E. coli*. When family names are used, they are capitalized, typed in italics or underlined. *E. coli* is in the family *Enterobacteriaceae*. Groups of organisms are often referred to generically. For example, 'streptococci' refer to all members of the genus *Streptococcus*. Generic groupings are never capitalized, italicized or underlined. Organism names change when new information becomes available for better classification of species, and these changes are documented in the *International Journal for Systematic Bacteriology*.

Identification of bacteria

Bacteria are identified by genotypic and phenotypic features, and identification of bacteria by a clinical microbiologist is still based primarily on phenotypic features and physiologic requirements, although molecular technology is now being used more frequently. Bacteria can be grown on a variety of artificial media under various environmental conditions in the microbiology laboratory, and this provides information about the organism's nutritional requirements and ability to grow at various temperatures, pH levels, and atmospheric conditions. The macroscopic appearance observed on artificial media and the microscopic appearance, observed on stained and/or unstained specimens, are critical for the identification of an organism. Antigenic properties are useful for serologic identification of bacteria, and antibiotic susceptibility and resistance profiles also aid in identification. More advanced assays may be necessary for the definitive identification of some bacteria, such as the use of gas liquid chromatography to identify metabolic end products for certain anaerobes, or molecular analysis of cell wall components to place an organism in a particular genus.

The process of identifying a bacterium involves the routine assessment of specific features by the microbiologist:

(i) initial macroscopic examination;
(ii) direct microscopic examination, using the Gram stain and wet preparation;
(iii) cultivation
    (a) nutritional requirements
    (b) environmental requirements
    (c) colony appearance on artificial media (e.g. size);
(iv) post-culture microscopic morphology, including size, shape and arrangement of cells and other physical features noted, such as endospores;
(v) results of the Gram stain or other stain such as acid-fast;
(vi) special stain for endospores, flagella, capsule;
(vii) results of biochemical tests, which may be performed manually or run as a battery using automated instrumentation.

Initial macroscopic examination of clinical specimens

When a specimen arrives in the clinical microbiology laboratory, it is examined macroscopically and evaluated initially by direct microscopic examination. Preliminary data obtained from the initial macroscopic and microscopic examinations provide direction for culture and future testing. The macroscopic appearance of the specimen is noted, along with additional information such as the presence of blood, pus or a foul odor that may assist

with identification. Anaerobic infections are usually characterized by foul odor and the presence of pus.

Microscopic examination

The direct microscopic evaluation is usually a Gram stain, but may include a wet mount preparation. Since the specimen may contain multiple organisms and other materials, the following information is noted:

- presence of inflammatory cells, blood or debris
- Gram reaction
- morphology and arrangement of cells
- relative number of bacterial cells
- additional information for specific identification, e.g. presence of endospores or granules.

The Gram stain (Fig. 2.3) is used to divide bacteria into two main groups, based upon cell wall structure and content. The majority of clinically significant organisms react to the Gram stain; exceptions include those that do not contain a cell wall (*Mycoplasma* spp. and *Ureaplasma urealyticum*), those lacking the peptidoglycan layer (chlamydiae) and those too small to be visualized by light microscopy (spirochetes). For Gram staining, the specimen must be fixed to a glass slide by heat or methanol: methanol fixation preserves the morphology of host cells as well as bacteria. Slides are overlaid with 95% methanol for 1 minute and air dried before staining. Crystal violet is added as the primary stain, followed by a mordant, Gram's iodine, that chemically bonds the alkaline dye to the bacterial cell wall. Treatment with Gram's decolorizer then distinguishes bacteria as either gram-positive or gram-negative. Following decolorization, safranin is added as counterstain. All organisms take up crystal violet, but only gram-negative organisms will decolorize and incorporate the pink-red safranin stain.

Differential staining is based upon differences in the cell wall. Organisms that stain gram-positive have thick cell walls with thick layers of peptidoglycan and many teichoic cross-bridges; organisms that stain gram-negative have a very thin layer of peptidoglycan, and teichoic cross-links resist alcohol

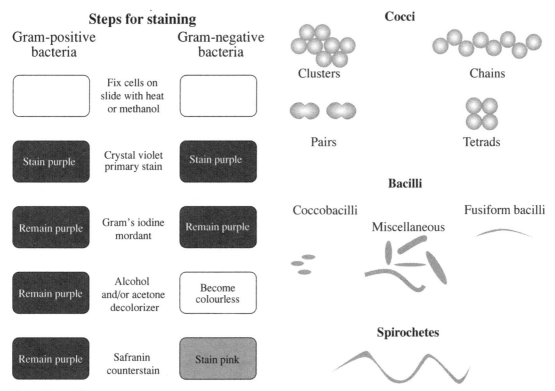

Steps for staining

Gram-positive bacteria | Gram-negative bacteria

Gram-positive		Gram-negative
	Fix cells on slide with heat or methanol	
Stain purple	Crystal violet primary stain	Stain purple
Remain purple	Gram's iodine mordant	Remain purple
Remain purple	Alcohol and/or acetone decolorizer	Become colourless
Remain purple	Safranin counterstain	Stain pink

Fig. 2.3. Gram stain

Cocci

Clusters   Chains

Pairs   Tetrads

Bacilli

Coccobacilli   Miscellaneous   Fusiform bacilli

Spirochetes

Fig. 2.4. Bacterial morphologies. Common shapes and arrangements of bacteria.

1. Heat-fix material on a slide and allow to cool; material also can be fixed using methanol.
2. Flood slide with crystal violet and leave for 10–30 seconds (check staining instructions and run control slides to determine optimum time). Rinse with tap water and shake off excess.
3. Flood slide with Gram's iodine to increase affinity of the primary stain and leave for twice as long as the crystal violet remained on the slide. Rinse with tap water and shake off excess.
4. Flood with alcohol or acetone decolorizer for 10 seconds; rinse with tap water immediately. Repeat this step until blue dye no longer runs off the slide when the decolorizer is added; rinse with tap water and shake off excess.
5. Flood with safranin counterstain and leave for 30 seconds. Rinse with tap water and gently blot the slide dry with absorbent paper or air dry. Air drying is recommended for delicate smears (e.g. certain body fluids).
6. Examine microscopically under oil immersion at a magnification of 1000×. Note bacteria, white blood cells and other cellular material.

decolorization. Crystal violet stain washes out of host cells, including erythrocytes and white blood cells, allowing the cells to absorb the safranin. These cells should stain pink.

Gram staining should be performed on young cultures. Gram-positive bacterial cell walls that are compromised due to age, damage or antibiotic treatment will lose the ability to retain crystal violet and will appear as gram-negative or gram-variable. Gram-negative bacteria, on the other hand, rarely retain crystal violet, if the staining procedure is carried out correctly.

The Gram stain also allows description of morphology, or shape: bacterial shape can take the form of cocci, bacilli or spirochetes, and the various cellular arrangements provide clues to their identification (Fig. 2.4).

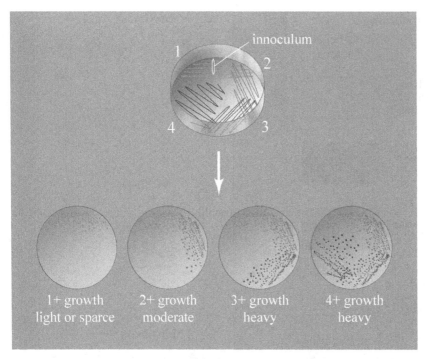

Fig. 2.5. Dilution streak method for isolation and semiquantitation of bacterial colonies. (*a*) = 1+ bacterial growth limited to the first quadrant; (*b*) = 2+ or moderate bacterial growth extends to the second quadrant; (*c*) = 3+ or 4+ heavy bacterial growth extends to the fourth quadrant.

Cocci are arranged in pairs, tetrads, or clusters. These arrangements suggest particular genera (e.g. *Staphylococcus aureus* will form grape-like clusters and streptococci will form chains, particularly when grown in liquid medium). Bacilli vary in length and width: some are so short that they are easily confused as cocci, and are thus referred to as coccobacilli. This cellular morphology is typical for species of *Haemophilus*. Bacilli may also be fusiform, with pointed ends typical of the anaerobic genus *Fusobacterium*. Vibrios are bacilli in the shape of a comma. Two *Campylobacter* bacilli often align to resemble the wings of a seagull. The presence of endospores also provides a key to identification: only two common genera of bacteria form endospores, the aerobic genus, *Bacillus*, and the anaerobic genus *Clostridium*.

Cultivation

Cultivation refers to growing microorganisms in culture: samples are taken from the site of infection in vivo and grown in the laboratory in vitro on artificial media. Bacterial cells in a colony all have the same genotypic and phenotypic characteristics (a clone). Cultures derived from a single bacterium are pure, and those derived from more than one bacterium will be mixed. Biochemical testing and other identification procedures can only be carried out on pure colonies. Figure 2.5 illustrates a technique for obtaining isolated colonies.

Nutritional requirements

The nutritional requirements for most human pathogens are fairly basic, and commercial media have been developed for the cultivation of pathogenic bacteria. Organisms that grow well in a basal medium are considered to be non-fastidious. A typical basal medium consists of a beef extract that provides carbohydrates, nitrogen, vitamins and salts, as well as peptone to control pH. Pathogens that require complex growth factors are considered to be fastidious and require additional substances, usually blood or serum products or vitamins. *Neisseria gonorrhoea* requires hemin and nicotine adenine dinucleotide (NAD), and some nutritionally variant streptococci require vitamin B6 or thiol for growth. Some intracellular bacteria can be cultured only in a cell line (*Chlamydia*) and others cannot be cultured in vitro at all (*Calymmatobacterium granulomatis*).

Types of media

Commercial media are supplied in the form of a liquid broth or a solid agar. Bacterial growth in liquid is determined by turbidity and growth on agar is visualized as a colony derived from a single bacterium. Commercial media not only support bacterial growth, but are also used to grow and isolate the disease-causing pathogens while minimizing the contaminants or colonizers. Colonizers or normal flora/resident flora are defined as organisms that normally inhabit a given body site. *Staphylococcus epidermidis* is resident skin flora; *Lactobacillus* is present in high numbers in the healthy vagina. Contaminants are organisms that 'contaminate' a specimen. They may be from the environment (*Bacillus* spores from the air) or from a body site. For example, semen is easily contaminated with fecal flora (members of the *Enterobacteriaceae* or *Enterococcus* species). Media also have been developed to select for certain pathogenic organisms and to differentiate between organisms as an aid in early identification.

There are four general categories of media: supportive, enrichment, selective and differential (see Appendix 2.1).

Supportive media contain nutrients to support the growth of non-fastidious organisms, providing no advantage to any specific group. For example,

thioglycollate broth supports the growth of a range of organisms, including aerobes, microaerophiles, facultative organisms and anaerobes.

Enrichment media contain nutrient supplements required for the growth of a particular bacterial pathogen, and supports the growth of a particular pathogen from a mixture of organisms based on the pathogen's requirements. Trypticase soy agar (TSA) supports the growth of many fastidious and non-fastidious organisms. Other examples include the following.

Sheep blood agar (SBA) contains blood, and is used for cultivation of most gram-positive and gram-negative organisms. The blood agar plate also supports the growth of most yeasts, but will not support growth for *Haemophilus* spp. and other fastidious organisms that require heme and reduced nicotinamide adenine dinucleotide phosphate (NADPH).

Chocolate agar (CA) contains lysed blood cells; NAD and heme are released. This medium is used for cultivation of *Neisseria* and *Haemophilus*.

IsoVitaleX contains dextrose, cysteine, vitamin B12, thiamine, ferric nitrate, and is also used for cultivation of *Haemophilus*.

Selective media 'select' for particular organisms, inhibiting all organisms except those being sought. Inhibitory agents include dyes, alcohols, acids and antibiotics, e.g.

Modified Thayer–Martin agar (MTM) is composed of chocolate agar supplemented with antibiotics. It is selective for *Neisseria gonorrhoeae* and *Neisseria meningitides* because it supports these *Neisseria* pathogens while inhibiting most other organisms, including gram-positive organisms, gram-negative bacilli, and yeast. The vancomycin in the medium inhibits gram-positive bacteria, the colistin inhibits gram-negative organisms, nystatin inhibits yeasts and trimethoprim inhibits swarming of *Proteus*.

Hektoen enteric media (HE), Salmonella–Shigella agar (SS), and xylose–lysine–deoxycholate agar (XLD) inhibit gram-positive bacteria, and have differential biochemical reactions that permit the distinction between pathogenic and non-pathogenic coliform bacteria.

Differential media incorporate an element or factor that allows colonies of one species to exhibit a metabolic trait that distinguishes or differentiates the species from other organisms growing on the medium. Examples include the following.

MacConkey agar contains a neutral red indicator: lactose fermenters are purple and non-lactose fermenters are clear or light pink. All members of the family *Enterobacteriaceae* grow on MacConkey agar: some ferment lactose and others do not. Crystal violet and bile salts in this medium also inhibit the growth of gram-positive organisms as well as some gram-negative bacilli. Whether or not a gram-negative bacillus grows on MacConkey is a first step in differentiating gram-negative bacilli that are not members of the *Enterobacteriaceae*.

The media selected for inoculation of a specimen will depend on: (i) the body site to be cultured; (ii) information from the direct prep; and (iii) physician order based on his/her observations, patient profile and any current epidemiology information. Appendix 2.1 at the end of this chapter includes media typically used in clinical microbiology and gives examples of enrichment, supportive, selective and differential media. Appendix 2.2 lists biochemical tests used for further identification.

Environmental requirements

Gases: oxygen and carbon dioxide
Genetic make-up determines the oxygen requirements of microbes. Some organisms require oxygen for metabolism, whereas it may be toxic to other species; some grow better in an environment with increased carbon dioxide (CO_2).

An **obligate aerobe** (fungi and mycobacteria) cannot grow unless the atmosphere contains 15–21% oxygen, the concentration found in air (21% oxygen and 0.03% CO_2), or in a CO_2 incubator with 15% oxygen and 5–10% CO_2.

Organisms that require increased carbon dioxide are referred to as **capnophilic**. *Neisseria gonorrhoeae* and *Haemophilus influenzae* are capnophiles.

Organisms that grow best in an oxygen concentration lower than that of ambient air (5–10% oxygen) are **microaerophilic**. *Helicobacter pylori* and *Campylobacter jejuni* require microaerophilic conditions for cultivation.

Anaerobes usually cannot grow in the presence of oxygen, and grow in an atmosphere composed of 5–10% hydrogen (H_2), 5–10% CO_2, 80–90% nitrogen (N_2) and 0% oxygen (O_2).

Obligate anaerobes or strict anaerobes require a strict anaerobic environment where oxygen is totally absent. Most *Bacteroides* spp., *Clostridium*, *Eubacterium*, *Fusobacterium* spp. *Peptostreptococcus* spp., *Porphyromonas* spp., and most strains of *Veillonella parvula*, an organism found in the female genital tract, are obligate anaerobes. Some anaerobes are **aerotolerant**, i.e. they can survive for short periods in the presence of oxygen, but cannot reproduce under these conditions. The *Actinomyces* spp. and *Bifidobacterium* spp. can grow in the presence of reduced or atmospheric oxygen, but thrive under anaerobic conditions.

Facultative anaerobes have enzyme systems that allow them to grow under either aerobic or anaerobic conditions. They preferentially use oxygen as a terminal electron acceptor, but in the absence of oxygen can ferment sugars anaerobically. The *Enterobacteriaceae*, most staphylococci and streptococci are facultative organisms.

Temperature
Microorganisms also have temperature requirements. Human pathogens are **mesophilic**, thriving at a temperature range between 30 °C and 45 °C. Some strict pathogens, such as *N. gonorrhoeae* require a temperature at or near human body temperature for growth. Other bacteria that may be pathogenic to humans (staphylococci and members of the *Enterobacteriaceae*) grow well in vitro at room temperature as well as at 37 °C. Some organisms, including some human pathogens, can grow at temperatures above and below this range. Psychrophilic bacteria grow between 4 °C and 20 °C. *Yersinia enterocolitica*, an organism known to contaminate blood products used for transfusion, can grow in refrigerated units

of red blood cells. In the laboratory, the relatively good growth of this organism in the cold is used to enhance detection of *Yersinia enterocolitica* by 'cold enrichment'. Thermophilic organisms, such as some *Campylobacter* spp. and *Rhizomucor* (fungus) spp. grow best at temperatures >40 °C.

Special requirements
Organisms have an optimal pH range. Since most clinically relevant bacteria grow best at or near a neutral pH (6.5–7.5), commercial media are buffered for neutral pH. Bacterial growth requires moisture, and incubation systems have been designed to prevent loss of water from the medium. Water is necessary for bacterial metabolism, and loss of water increases the relative concentration of solutes leading to osmotic shock and cell lysis. Some bacteria have special environmental requirements, e.g. species of *Vibrio* require varying concentrations of salt for growth.

Post-culture evaluation

Post-culture evaluation documents information gained from the type of media and environmental conditions that have supported growth, and this provides important clues in identifying the organism. Certain species of *Vibrio* will only grow in 8% sodium chloride, whereas most other organisms will not tolerate a high level of salt. Many pathogens require special media (*Legionella pneumophilia*) and therefore will not be detected on basic media such as sheep blood agar. Colony appearance on differential media is especially important, e.g. if a gram-negative bacillus grows on MacConkey agar, it can be placed in a major group, and if it also ferments lactose in the MacConkey medium, it is likely to be a member of the *Enterobacteriaceae*.

In general, the clinical significance of bacterial growth will depend upon the body site from which an organism was cultured and the relative numbers of bacterial colonies on the agar. For example, any organism isolated from a sterile body site (e.g. blood) is significant if not due to contamination, whereas a certain number of organisms must be isolated

from urine to be significant. The isolation of a strict pathogen (e.g. *Yersinia pestis*) is always significant, regardless of the site or number of microorganisms present.

The appearance of organisms growing on media can provide keys to identification, and a report of colony morphology should include the following information.

(i) Colony size: *Bacillus* colonies are large; those of *Haemophilus* are small.

(ii) Pigment: *Pseudomonas aeruginosa* secretes a green pigment and several non-fermenting gram-negative bacilli are pigmented. Pigment may provide important clues for identification of anaerobes: the genus *Porphyromonas* and species of *Prevotella* are pigmented; *Clostridium difficile* fluoresces yellow–green on blood agar.

(iii) Description of the colony shape (form, elevation) and surface (mucoid, dry). Colony shape may be unique: *Actinomyces israelii* colonies have a 'molar tooth' appearance, *Clostridium septicum* has irregular margins resembling a 'Medusa head'; *Actinobacillus actinomycetemcomitans* forms a four- to six-pointed star-like configuration in the centre of a mature colony when grown on clear medium. Colonies of *Eikenella* are sticky and may pit the agar, and colonies of *Proteus* swarm over the entire plate.

(iv) Alterations in medium including pitting of the agar or hemolysis on blood agar. Hemolysis patterns are the key to identifying species of *Streptococcus*, and β-hemolysis around a large, feathered colony suggests *Bacillus cereus*.

(v) Odour is a further clue to organism identification. *Pseudomonas aeruginosa* smells of grapes or tortillas, *S. aureus* smells like dirty athletic socks, and *Clostridium difficile* has the odour of a horse stable.

Clinical specimens often reveal mixed cultures, with organisms that may represent pathogens, contaminants or normal flora. Organisms suspected of being pathogenic, based on the macroscopic appearance and conditions that support

(a) Pus from a boil is Gram-stained and plated to sheep blood agar (SBA), chocolate agar (CA) and MacConkey agar (MAC). The following results were obtained:

Gram stain → gram-positive cocci; clusters suggests staphylococci

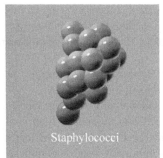

Note: Staphylococci do not always appear in clusters.

Culture results:
SBA = yellow-white, round colonies exhibiting a narrow zone of β-hemolysis.
This appearance on SBA suggests *Staphylococcus aureus*

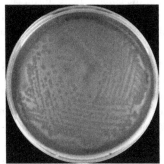

Note: Not all strains of *S. aureus* are beta-hemolytic.

CA = heavy growth; expected for *Staphylococcus aureus*
MAC = no growth; expected for *Staphylococcus aureus*

Since this is a gram-positive coccus and the appearance on SBA suggests *Staphylococcus aureus*, the following tests would be run to confirm:

Catalase = positive
Modified oxidase = negative
Mannitol reduction = positive
Coagulase = positive[a]
[a]most important test since *S. aureus* is the only staphylococcal species pathogenic to humans that produces the enzyme coagulase.

Note: Latex agglutination tests also could be used for identification.

Fig. 2.6. Identification of *Staphylococcus aureus* recovered from an infection site. (*a*) Method and (*b*) flowchart.

(b)

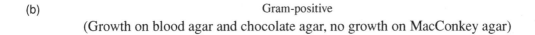

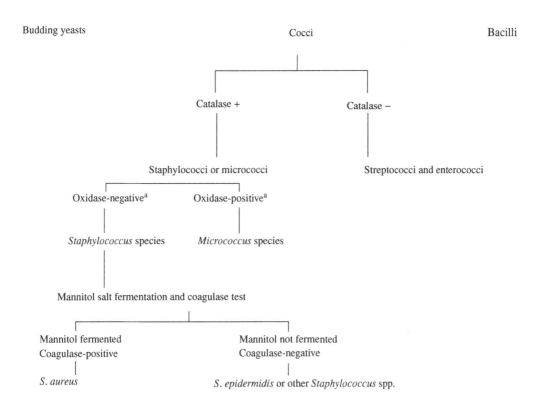

Gram-positive
(Growth on blood agar and chocolate agar, no growth on MacConkey agar)

Budding yeasts   Cocci   Bacilli

Catalase +   Catalase −

Staphylococci or micrococci   Streptococci and enterococci

Oxidase-negative[a]   Oxidase-positive[a]

Staphylococcus species   *Micrococcus* species

Mannitol salt fermentation and coagulase test

Mannitol fermented   Mannitol not fermented
Coagulase-positive   Coagulase-negative

S. aureus   *S. epidermidis* or other *Staphylococcus* spp.

[a]modified oxidase

Note: a gram-positive, β-hemolytic, catalase-positive organism recovered from pus is presumptively
   S. aureus.

Fig. 2.6. (cont.)

organism growth (e.g. chocolate agar, but not blood agar), should be tested. Testing must be performed on organisms obtained from an isolated colony, and the tests should include:

(i) Repeat Gram stain, denoting all morphologic characteristics (e.g. gram-positive cocci in clusters).

(ii) Additional staining if indicated: although not a routine procedure in the clinical laboratory, flagella, capsules, spores and inclusions can be visualized using special stains. When mycobacteria or organisms that are partially acid-fast are suspected (e.g. *Nocardia* and *Rhodococcus*), an acid-fast stain is performed.

(iii) A wet prep to examine motility can provide information in many cases: *Helicobacter pylori* has a corkscrew movement and *Listeria monocytogenes* displays a tumbling motility.

(*a*) A semen specimen with a foul odour was Gram-stained and plated to sheep blood agar (SBA), chocolate agar (CA) and MacConkey agar (MAC). The following results were obtained:

Gram stain → Gram-negative, straight bacilli

Culture media:

SBA = grey, mucoid colonies

CA = growth

MAC = pink, lactose-fermenting colonies

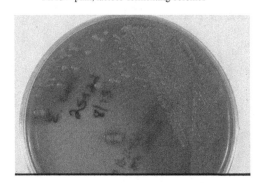

A gram-negative, lactose-fermenting bacillus is likely to be a member of the *Enterobacteriaceae*. All members of the family *Enterobacteriaceae* are oxidase-negative. A series of tests were run to speciate the organism and the following results were obtained:

Oxidase = negative

Indole = positive

Motility medium = positive

Voges–Proskauer = negative

Simmon's citrate = negative

Hydrogen sulfide production = negative

Urease = negative

Note: testing is usually automated or performed using a panel of multiple tests such as the API strip for the *Enterobacteriaceae*.

The organism is identified as *Escherichia coli*, a common fecal contaminant in semen.

Fig. 2.7. Identification of *Escherichia coli* recovered from a semen specimen. (*a*) Method and (*b*) flowchart.

(iv) Preliminary further testing can be carried out based upon culture and microscopy.

    (a) Gram-positive cocci should be tested for catalase. All members of the *Micrococcaceae* (this includes staphylococci) are catalase-positive, streptococci and enterococci are catalase-negative.

    (b) All gram-negative bacilli should be tested for oxidase. Members of the *Enterobacteriaceae*, the most common gram-negative bacilli encountered in the clinical laboratory, are oxidase-negative. The gram-negative bacilli *Pseudomonas* and *Burkholderia* species are oxidase positive.

Definitive organism identification requires additional testing. Biochemical tests to determine metabolic activity (e.g. glucose utilization and enzyme production) may be performed manually or with the use of automated systems. Biochemical reactions are listed in Table 2.2 of the Appendix to this chapter. Additional media-based testing may also be indicated. Vibrios are placed in increasing solutions of sodium chloride to help speciate the genus, and pseudomonads may be subcultured to media containing heavy metals for speciation. Antibiotic resistance profiles are also useful for organism identification. *Staphylococcus saprophyticus* is resistant to novobiocin, whereas

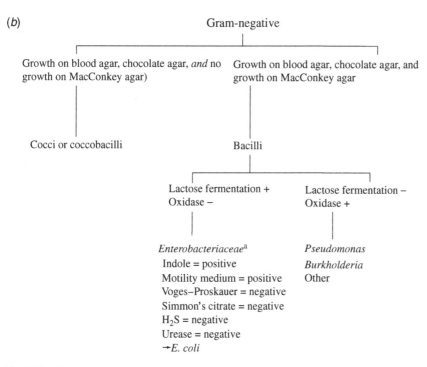

(b)

Gram-negative

Growth on blood agar, chocolate agar, *and* no growth on MacConkey agar)

Growth on blood agar, chocolate agar, and growth on MacConkey agar

Cocci or coccobacilli

Bacilli

Lactose fermentation +
Oxidase −

Lactose fermentation −
Oxidase +

Enterobacteriaceae[a]
Indole = positive
Motility medium = positive
Voges–Proskauer = negative
Simmon's citrate = negative
H_2S = negative
Urease = negative
→*E. coli*

Pseudomonas
Burkholderia
Other

Fig. 2.7. (*cont.*)

other species of coagulase-negative staphylococci are sensitive. Sensitivity to a panel of antibiotics (kanomycin, vancomycin and colistin) helps differentiate anaerobic bacilli. Figures 2.6 and 2.7 illustrate flowcharts and methods for the isolation and identification of organisms in two different specimens.

Physical characteristics observed on stains and in culture and results of metabolic characteristics provide phenotypic information that identifies an organism. Other tools are also used to identify bacteria, including molecular techniques to characterize part of the bacterium's genome, and other analytical methods such as electrophoretic analysis and gas–liquid and high-performance liquid chromatography. Immunochemical methods are important in identifying organisms that cannot be cultured (e.g. *Treponema pallidum*). Immunochemical techniques include detection of antigens using polyclonal and monoclonal antibodies, precipitin and agglutination tests, immunofluorescent assays and

enzyme immunoassays, as well as other immunoassays targeted at antigen detection. Antibodies to antigens associated with infectious disease can be detected by a variety of serodiagnostic methods: agglutination assays, flocculation tests (e.g. rapid plasma reagin (RPR) and Venereal Disease Research Laboratory Slide test (VDRL) tests for syphilis), counterimmunoelectrophoresis, immunodiffusion, hemagglutination inhibition assays, neutralization assays, complement fixation, enzyme-linked immunosorbent assays (e.g. for human immunodeficiency virus (HIV)), indirect fluorescent antibody tests (e.g. fluorescent treponemal antibody absorption test for *T. pallidum*) radioimmunoassays, fluorescent immunoassays, and Western blots (e.g. for *T. pallidum*, HIV and herpes simplex virus types 1 and 2).

The results obtained from the battery of identifying tests place the organisms into their major groups, as illustrated on the overview flowchart (Fig. 1.4).

Table 2.1. Bacteria: Gram-negative bacilli

Grow on MacConkey Oxidase-positive	Grow on MacConkey Oxidase-negative	No growth on MacConkey Oxidase-positive	No growth on MacConkey Oxidase-negative (variable)	Special media for recovery
Pseudomonas[1]	*Acinetobacter*[1]	*Moraxella*[1]	*Haemophilus*[3]	*Campylobacter*[2]
Burkholderia[1]	*Chryseomonas*[1]	Elongated *Neisseria*[1]	*H. ducreyi*[3*]	*Helicobacter*[1]
Achromobacter grp[1]	*Flavomonas*[1]	*Eikenella*[3]		*Arcobacter*[3]
A. xylosoxidans	*Stenotrophomonas*[1]	*Pasteurella*[3]		*Legionella*[1]
A. dentrificans	*Escherichia*[3]	*Actinobacillus*[3]		*Brucella*[1]
	*E. coli*****	*Kingella*[1]		*Bordetella pertussis*[1]
Chryseobacterium[1]	*Shigella*[3]	*Cardiobacterium*[3]		*Bordetella parapertussis*[1]
C. meningosepticum[1]	*Salmonella*[3]	*Capnocytophaga*[1]		*Francisella*[1]
Sphingobacterium[1]	*Citrobacter*[3]	*Sphingomonas paucimobilis*[3]		*Bartonella*[1]
Alcaligene[1]*s*	*Klebsiella*[3]	*Weeksella virosa*[3]		*Afipia*[1]
Bordetella	*Enterobacter*[3]	*Methylobacterium*[3]		*Streptobacillus*[3]
(non-pertussis)[1]	*Serratia*[3]	*Bergeyella zoohelcum*[3]		*Spirillum minus*[1]
Comomona[1]	*Hafnia*[3]			
Vibrio[3]	*Proteus*[3]			
Aeromonas[3]	*Providencia*[3]			
Plesiomonas[3]	*Morganella*[3]			
Chromobacterium[3]	*Yersinia*[3]			
Ralstonia picketti[1]	*Edwardsiella*[3]			
Oligella[3]				
Ochrobacterium[3]				
Shewanella putrefaciens[1]				

Aerobic = [1]; Aerobic, microaerophilic = [2]; Facultative = [3]
urogenital pathogen*.
prenatal/neonatal pathogen**.
urogenital pathogen and prenatal/neonatal pathogen***.

Major groups of organisms

Gram-negative bacilli and coccobacilli

Gram-negative bacilli and coccobacilli are outlined in Table 2.1.

Grow on MacConkey agar, oxidase-positive

Pseudomonas	*Burkholderia*
Ralstonia pickettii	*Achromobacter group*
Chryseobacterium,	*A. xylosoxidans*
Sphingobacterium	*A. dentrificans*
Oligella	*Ochrobacterium*
Non-pertussis *Bordetella*	*Alcaligenes*
Vibrio	*Shewanella putrefaciens*
Plesiomonas shigelloides	*Comomonas*
	Aeromonas
	Chromobacterium violaceum

These organisms are differentiated by specimen source and by further testing.

Pseudomonas, Burkholderia and *Ralstonia*

Species of *Pseudomonas, Burkholderia* and *Ralstonia* are important contaminants found in the environment and in water. *Burkholderia cepacia, Ralstonia pickettii* and *Pseudomonas aeruginosa* are common contaminants of medical devices and solutions. *Pseudomonas aeruginosa* is an opportunistic pathogen that is a leading cause of hospital-acquired infections. These organisms are straight, slender, aerobic bacilli that use a variety of carbohydrates; although they are mesophilic, they can survive at low temperatures (to 4 °C).

Achromobacter and *Ochrobacterium*

Achromobacter and *Ochrobacterium* are all environmental flora, but may occasionally inhabit the human gastrointestinal tract.

Sphingobacterium and *Chryseobacterium*

Sphingobacterium and *Chryseobacterium* are environmental flora that may occasionally be encountered in human specimens, and may contaminate solutions and surfaces in the laboratory setting. *Chryseobacterium meningosepticum* is associated with nursery meningitis. The majority of organisms in this group oxidizes glucose, and display a yellow pigment.

Oligella, Alcaligenes, Shewanella putrefaciens, Comomonas, non-pertussis *Bordetella* and *Achromobacter*

Oligella, Shewanella putrefaciens, Comomonas and non-pertussis *Bordetella* do not utilize glucose, and their morphologies and physiologic requirements vary. These organisms are found in the environment (soil and water), the upper respiratory tract of some mammals, and in humans. The habitat of some species remains unknown. *Achromobacter xylosoxidans, Alcaligenes fecalis* and species of *Comomonas* are found as contaminants in medical devices and solutions, including intravenous and irrigation fluids. *Achromobacter xylosoxidans* has been documented to contaminate soaps and disinfectants. *Oligella* species infect humans as the result of manipulations (e.g. catheterization) of the urinary tract.

The organisms listed in above are commonly seen contaminating fluids, sinks, and incubators in a laboratory setting.

Vibrios, Plesiomonas Aeromonas and *Chromobacterium violaceum*

Vibrios, Plesiomonas and *Aeromonas* inhabit seawater and therefore are associated with diarrhoea or with water wounds. *Vibrio cholera* is a serious toxin-producing pathogen. These genera, along with *Chromobacterium violaceum*, ferment glucose, and all have different morphologies and physiologic features. *Chromobacterium violaceum*, easily identified due to its violet pigment, causes a rare, but very dangerous systemic infection.

Gram-negative bacilli and coccobacilli that grow on MacConkey agar, oxidase-negative

Acinetobacter	*Chryseomonas*
Flavomonas	*Stenotrophomonas*
Enterobacteriaceae:	
Escherichia	*Shigella*
Salmonella	*Citrobacter*
Klebsiella	*Enterobacter*
Serratia	*Hafnia*
Proteus	*Providencia*
Morganella	*Yersinia*
Edwardsiella	

Acinetobacter, Chryseomonas, Flavomonas and *Stenotrophomonas*

These either oxidize or do not utilize glucose. This feature distinguishes them from the largest, and most frequently encountered, organisms, members of *Enterobacteriaceae*, which do ferment glucose. This group of non-fermenters is important because they are associated with nosocomial infections acquired from the colonization of hospitalized patients and contamination of medical devices, equipment and fluids. They are separated by source, enzymes produced and by biochemical testing.

Enterobacteriaceae

Most members of the *Enterobacteriaceae*, including *Escherichia coli*, are normal intestinal flora in humans and other animals. Infections caused by these genera are the result of transmission via the fecal–oral route or from contaminated food and water. The *Enterobacteriaceae* family includes members that are true pathogens: *Yersinia pestis*, the agent of bubonic plague, species of *Salmonella* that cause gastroenteritis, bacteremia and typhoid fever, and *Shigella*, which causes gastroenteritis and dysentery. Members are also associated with water wounds (*Edwardsiella tarda*) and a wide variety of nosocomial infections. Species of *Citrobacter, Enterobacter, Klebsiella, Morganella, Proteus, Providencia* and *Serratia* are spread from person to person and may infect the respiratory tract, urinary tract, blood and other normally sterile sites in hospitalized and debilitated patients. These organisms are of special concern because they are antibiotic resistant. Since members of the *Enterobacteriaceae* are found in feces and in clinical settings, they are encountered in the reproductive laboratory, both as fecal and as environmental contaminants.

Gram-negative bacilli and coccobacilli, do not grow on MacConkey agar, oxidase-positive

Sphingomonas paucimobilis	*Moraxella*
Elongated *Neisseria*	*Eikenella corrodens*
Weeksella virosa	*Bergeyella zoohelcum*
Methylobacterium	*Pasteurella*
Actinobacillus	*Kingella*
Cardiobacterium	*Capnoctyophaga,* and similar organisms

Organisms in this group utilize glucose differently: *Sphingomonas paucimobilis* utilizes glucose oxidatively; *Eikenella corrodens, Weeksella virosa* and *Bergeyella zoohelcum* are asaccharolytic; *Pasteurella, Actinobacillus, Kingella, Cardiobacterium* and *Capnocytophaga* all ferment glucose. These organisms are identified by their morphology and physiologic requirements.

Sphingomonas paucimobilis

An environmental inhabitant that may contaminate medical devices and solutions; infections include catheter-related bacteremia, and wound and urinary tract infections.

Moraxella

Species of *Moraxella* inhabit mucous membranes in humans but rarely cause infections.

Neisseria elongata

Normal upper respiratory tract flora in humans.

Eikenella corrodens

Normal flora in the human mouth; infections with this organism result from trauma from human bites and clenched-fist wounds.

Bergeyella zoohelcum

Oral flora in non-human animals.

Weeksella virosa *and* Methylobacterium

Both *Weeksella virosa* and *Methylobacterium* species are found in the environment and are known to contaminate medical devices and other clinical materials.

Pasteurella

Pasteurella species are normal flora in domestic and wild animals, and infections with these organisms are therefore limited to contact with animals.

Actinobacillus, Kingella, Cardiobacterium, *and* Capnocytophaga

Normal flora in the mouth of humans and animals. Most human infections are due to endogenous flora entering deeper tissues (e.g. dental procedures).

Gram-negative bacilli and coccobacilli that do not grow on MacConkey agar, oxidase variable

This group include the genus *Haemophilus*. There are several species of *Haemophilus*, including *H. influenzae*, which causes life-threatening pneumonia and meningitis, and *H. ducreyi*, associated with chancroid. With the exception of *H. aphrophilus*, species of this genus require either hemin and/or nicotine adenine dinucleotide (NAD) for growth. Species are distinguished based on requirements for these factors, hemolysis on rabbit blood agar and fermentation of sugars. With the exception of *Haemophilus ducreyi*, species of *Haemophilus* are normal upper respiratory flora in humans. All species may cause infection, either from endogenous flora or person-to-person transmission. Only the encapsulated strain of *H. influenzae* is associated with life-threatening infections. *H. ducreyi* is covered in detail in Chapter 7.

Gram-negative bacilli that are optimally recovered on special media

Bartonella	*Afipia*
Campylobacter	*Helicobacter*
Legionella	*Arcobacter*
Bordetella pertussis	*Brucella*
Francisella	*Bordetella parapertussis*
Spirillum minus	*Streptobacillus moniliformis*

Since this group of organisms requires special media for isolation, they are not detected on routine culture in the clinical laboratory and must be specifically sought. The majority cause unusual or atypical infections.

Bartonella

Bartonella species are associated with sand flies, human lice and domestic cats, and may cause zoonotic infections in humans. Trench fever and cat-scratch fever are caused by species of *Bartonella*.

Afipia felis

Once believed to be an agent of cat-scratch fever, but the exact role in causing human disease is not known.

Campylobacter, Arcobacter *and* Helicobacter

Species of *Campylobacter*, *Arcobacter* and *Helicobacter* are small curved, motile bacilli; the majority require microaerophilic conditions for isolation. These organisms may be found in humans and other animals. Both *Campylobacter* and *Arcobacter* cause gastroenteritis and other infections. *Campylobacter jejuni*, subspecies *jejuni* may cause proctitis in homosexual men.

Helicobacter pylori resides in the human gastric mucosa and causes gastritis, peptic ulcer disease and gastric cancer.

Legionella pneumophilia

Causes Legionnaire's disease, a febrile pneumonia. Other *Legionella* species are responsible for pneumonia, endocarditis and wound abscesses.

Brucella

Cattle, sheep, goats, swine and dogs are hosts for *Brucella* species. Although some species will grow on MacConkey agar, many require enriched media and special incubation conditions. *Brucella* is responsible for brucellosis. Although this is a zoonosis, humans can become infected via animal contact (inhalation, direct inoculation or ingestion of unpasteurized and contaminated milk or cheese). In humans the infection may range from asymptomatic to a serious debilitating disease.

Bordetella pertussis *and* Bordetella parapertussis

Special media is required for isolation and for cultivation of *Bordetella pertussis* and *Bordetella parapertussis*, causative agents of whooping cough.

Francisella tularensis

Requires cysteine and a source of iron for growth.

F. tularensis, an extremely virulent organism, causes tularaemia in both animals and humans, a severe systemic infection sometimes referred to as 'rabbit bite fever'.

Francisella phiolmiragia

Present in animals and in ground water and has been associated with infections in near-drowning victims.

Streptobacillus moniliformis *and* Spirillum minus

Agents of rat-bite fever, a serious systemic disease affecting many body sites and associated with complications. *Streptobacillus moniliformis* requires

Table 2.2. Bacteria: gram-negative cocci

Aerobic
Neisseria[1]
*N. gonorrhoeae****[1]
Moraxella catarrhalis[1]

Aerobic = [1]; Aerobic, microaerophilic = [2]; Facultative = [3].
urogenital pathogen*. prenatal/neonatal pathogen**.
urogenital pathogen; and prenatal/neonatal pathogen***.

media with blood or serum and incubation under carbon dioxide for isolation; *Spirillum minus* has never been grown in culture.

Gram-negative cocci

Aerobic gram-negative cocci are shown in Table 2.2.

These species are oxidase positive and do not elongate when exposed to subinhibitory concentrations of penicillin, unlike the elongated *Nesisseria*. *Neisseria gonorrhoeae* and *Neisseria meningitides* are pathogenic; other species of *Neisseria* are normal inhabitants of the upper respiratory tract in humans. *Neisseria gonorrhoeae* is sexually transmitted, and causes gonorrhoea: this organism is described in detail in Chapter 10.

Neisseria meningitides is a leading cause of bacterial meningitis.

Moraxella catarrhalis infections are localized to the respiratory tract, and the organism rarely disseminates: infections include sinus infections, otitis media and pneumonia.

Species of *Neisseria* and *Moraxella catarrhalis* are identified on the basis of appearance (many commensals are pigmented), growth on Thayer–Martin agar, growth on nutrient agar at room temperature and body temperature, utilization of sugars and nitrate reduction.

Gram-positive cocci that are catalase-positive

Gram-positive cocci that are catalase positive are listed in Table 2.3. Those that are catalase-positive include:

Table 2.3. Bacteria: gram-positive cocci

Aerobic	
Catalase-positive	Catalase-negative
Staphylococcus aureus[1]	*Streptococcus*[2] spp.
	S. agalactiae[2]
Coagulase-negative staphylococci	*(Group B***)*
	Enterococcus[2] spp.
Micrococcus[1] spp.	

Aerobic = [1]; Aerobic, microaerophilic = [2]; Facultative = [3].
urogenital pathogen*. prenatal/neonatal pathogen**.
urogenital pathogen; and prenatal/neonatal pathogen***.

- *Staphylococcus aureus* (coagulase positive)
- Coagulase-negative staphylococci
- *Micrococcus* species
- *Stomatococcus mucilaginosus*

Genus identification is based on sheep blood agar colony appearance, reaction to modified oxidase, resistance to bacitracin and susceptibility to lysostaphin.

Staphylococcus aureus

Staphylococcus aureus is normal flora in the respiratory tract and on other mucosal surfaces in some humans (carriers). Many healthcare workers are carriers of *S. aureus*. These organisms are transmitted from person to person via fomites, unwashed hands or when the colonizing organism is introduced to a sterile body site. *S. aureus* is one of the most successful of all bacterial pathogens, because it has a wide range of virulence factors, including toxins and enzymes. These virulence factors are responsible for the numerous *S. aureus* infections, including skin infections (folliculitis, furuncles or boils, carbuncles and impetigo), wound infections, bacteremia, endocarditis, joint infections, scalded skin syndrome in neonates, toxic shock syndrome and food poisoning. Since *S. aureus* colonizes up to 40% of all healthcare workers, and can be spread from unwashed hands, it is a potentially serious problem in the ART laboratory when aseptic technique is not followed. It is resistant to antibiotics, so that infection or contamination with the organism is particularly serious: the penicillin-resistant variant 'MRSA' (methicillin resistant *S. aureus*) has been responsible for serious problems in hospital outbreaks.

Staphylococcus epidermidis

Staphylococcus epidermidis and other coagulase-negative staphylococci are normal skin flora. Infection with these bacteria usually occurs when the patient's endogenous strain reaches a sterile site. *Staphylococcus epidermidis* often appears in large numbers on the human body; it produces slime and can attach to medical devices. Infection often occurs as the result of medical manipulations (e.g. shunt or prosthetic device). *S. epidermidis* is often found in specimens and solutions as a result of contamination from cutaneous sources.

Staphylococcus saprophyticus

Staphylococcus saprophyticus, normal flora on the skin and the genitourinary tract, is a urinary tract pathogen, generally seen in sexually active young women. In comparison to the traditional pathogens such as *E. coli* and others, *S. saprophyticus* may be present in relatively small numbers in pure culture and still be a cause of significant disease. For a clean catch urine, 10 000 cfu/ml would be reported as significant, as opposed to the usual >100 000 cfu/ml.

Staphylococci are speciated based on coagulase production, resistance to novobiocin, growth in salt and mannitol reduction.

Micrococcacae and Stomatococcus mucilaginous

Micrococcus species and *Stomatococcus mucilaginous* are normal flora of human skin and the oropharynx, and rarely cause infection. Both may be isolated as contaminants in clinical specimens. *Micrococcus* species display a variety of pigments.

Gram-positive cocci that are catalase-negative

Examples of gram-positive cocci are listed in Table 2.3. Those that are catalase-negative include *Streptococcus*, *Enterococcus* and related species.

Identification of these genera is based on cellular morphology, hemolysis pattern on sheep blood agar, growth in 6.5% sodium chloride, and hydrolysis of pyrrolidonyl arylamidase (PYR).

Streptococcus pyogenes

Streptococcus pyogenes (Lancefield Group A) produces a large number of virulence factors and causes a wide array of suppurative diseases and toxinoses, as well as some autoimmmune or allergic diseases. At least 55 different strains are known, causing diseases that include acute pharyngitis, impetigo, erysipelas, necrotizing fasciitis and myositis, bacteremia, pneumonia, scarlet fever and streptococcal toxic shock syndrome. The organism cross-reacts with antigens on the heart, leading to rheumatic fever; the deposition of streptococcal antigen-antibody complexes on the glomerulus leads to acute poststreptococcal glomerulonephritis. Although Group A streptococci inhabit skin and the upper respiratory tract in human carriers, this group is not considered part of the normal flora. The bacterium is spread by person-to-person contact via secretions or mucus, or by sneezing and coughing.

Streptococcus agalactiae

Streptococcus agalactiae (Lancefield Group B), normal flora of the female genital tract and lower gastrointestinal tract, has fewer virulence factors than *Streptococcus pyogenes*. Most Group B streptococcal infections are associated with the neonate, often preceded by premature rupture of maternal membranes. Adult infections can occur postpartum, and include endometritis, which can lead to septic shock and additional problems. This species of streptococcus may also cause infections such as endocarditis and arthritis in immunocompromised patients. During pregnancy, mothers are tested to determine if they harbour Group B strep as genital flora, and a positive finding should indicate delivery within 24 h by membrane rupture to prevent neonatal disease. Details of Group B strep infections are covered in Chapter 8.

Other Lancefield groups

Other Lancefield groups of streptococci (C, F and G) are normal flora of human skin, nasopharnyx, genital tract and gastrointestinal tract and cause infections that are similar to *S. pyogenes* and *S. agalactiae*. Group C has been associated with pharyngitis and Group G is associated with underlying malignancies.

Streptococcus pneumoniae

Streptococcus pneumoniae colonizes the naso-pharynx in humans. Exposed individuals (e.g. contact with respiratory secretions) may develop infection. *Streptococcus pneumoniae* has several associated virulence factors, but the polysaccharide capsule is the primary factor. This streptococcus species does not have C-carbohydrate in the cell wall and therefore is not associated with a Lancefield grouping. *Streptococcus pneumoniae* is a leading cause of pneumonia in the elderly, with or without bacteremia, and is also a leading cause of meningitis. Aspiration of the organisms into the lungs leads to pneumonia. *Streptococcus pneumoniae* also causes sinus infections and otitis media.

Viridans streptococci

Viridans streptococci are of low virulence, but they produce an extracellular carbohydrate complex that allows the organism to attach to host cell surfaces and tooth enamel. The organism may cause subacute endocarditis in patients with damaged heart valves, and one member of this group, *S. mutans*, plays a key role in dental caries development. Other streptococci (e.g. *Leuconostoc* spp. and *Aerococcus* spp.) should be first considered as contaminants when encountered in clinical specimens. *Aerococcus urinae* is associated with urinary tract infections.

Enterococcus

Species of *Enterococcus* are found in food, water, soil and as normal flora in humans and other animals. The species associated with human infection, *E. faecalis* and *E. faecium*, are normal flora of the gastrointestinal tract and the female genitourinary tract. Infection tends to occur when the endogenous strains gain access to sterile sites. Transmission may be from person to person or via contaminated medical equipment. There are multidrug resistant strains of *Enterococcus*. Streptococci and enterococci species are differentiated based on cellular arrangement, hemolysis patterns on sheep blood agar (example: Group A is β-hemolytic and *S. pneumoniae* is α-hemolysis), typing for the C-carbohydrate in the cell wall, PYR hydrolysis, growth in 6.5% sodium chloride, hippurate hydrolysis and the CAMP (Christie/Atkins/Munch–Peterson) beta hemolysis enhancement test.

Gram-positive bacilli that are non-branching and catalase positive

Gram-positive bacilli are listed in Table 2.4. *Bacillus*, *Corynebacterium* and *Listeria* (and other related organisms) are non-branching and catalase positive.

Bacillus

Bacillus is an aerobic genus of bacteria that forms environmentally resistant endospores, and this is the primary virulence factor associated with these bacteria. *Bacillus* species are found everywhere in nature. They are commonly found in clinical specimens, and are responsible for contamination in sterile areas. To ensure that bacillus spores are destroyed, sterilization methods must be adequate for their destruction, and endospore destruction must be documented as part of laboratory quality control (e.g. include spore strip indicator in all autoclaving procedures).

The genus includes the well-known *Bacillus anthracis*, which causes anthrax. *Bacillus anthracis* spores are found in the soil. Infection may be caused

Table 2.4. Bacteria: gram-positive bacilli

Aerobic			
Spore-forming	Non-spore-forming		
Non-branching Catalase-positive	Non-branching Catalase-positive	Non-branching Catalase-negative	Branching or Acid-fast
Bacillus[1]	Listeria[1]	Erysipelothrix[1]	Nocardia[1]
	L. monocytogenes**[1]	Lactobacillus[1]	Streptomyces[1]
	Corynebacterium[1]	Arcanobacterium[1]	Rhodococcus[1]
		Gardnerella vaginalis*[1]	

Aerobic = [1]; Aerobic, microaerophilic = [2]; Facultative = [3].
urogenital pathogen*.
prenatal/neonatal pathogen**.
urogenital pathogen; and prenatal/neonatal pathogen***.

by inhalation of spores (pulmonary anthrax), penetration of spores (cutaneous anthrax) or ingestion of spores (gastrointestinal anthrax). This organism is a true human pathogen, and has been used as an agent of bioterrorism.

Bacillus cereus produces toxins that cause food poisoning, the classical 'Chinese rice' gastroenteritis. *B. cereus* may also cause infection when introduced into sterile body sites either by trauma or by exposure to contaminated medical supplies and equipment. These infections often involve immunocompromised patients. Other species of *Bacillus* may be responsible for the same infections caused by *B. cereus*.

Bacillus anthracis can initially be distinguished from the more common *B. cereus* species on the basis of motility: (*B. anthracis* is non-motile, and the more ubiquitous species are motile) and β-hemolysis on sheep blood agar (*B. anthracis* is non-hemolytic and *B. cereus* is β-hemolytic). Definitive identification of *B. anthracis* should take place in an authorized public health laboratory equipped to deal with this serious pathogen. *Bacillus* spp., not otherwise specified, are the most common strains seen in the clinical laboratory. Contaminating strains of *Bacillus* spp. are often identified only to the genus level.

Corynebacterium spp.

The *Corynebacterium* genus does not form endospores, making it easy to distinguish from *Bacillus*. Several species responsible for human disease belong to this genus, including the agent that causes diphtheria, *Corynebacterium diphtheriae*. Corynebacteria are found in the environment and some species are normal human skin flora.

Corynebacterium jeikeium is found on the skin of hospitalized patients, usually in axillary, inguinal and rectal sites. This organism may be introduced via catheters and/or intravenous therapy sites. Multiple antibiotic resistance makes infection with this organism significant, and in compromised patients it can cause septicemia, wound infections and rarely endocarditis. Corynebacteria speciation is based on morphology, colony appearance on selective media, physical characteristics (arrangement of bacteria on Gram stain, pigment) and biochemical reactions.

Listeria monocytogenes

Listeria monocytogenes is a significant reproductive pathogen, distinguishable from species of corynebacteria on the basis of motility (*L. monocytogenes* displays a tumbling motility by direct wet mount and an umbrella-shaped pattern in motility medium), β-hemolysis on sheep blood agar and the ability to survive at 4 °C. *Listeria monocytogenes* colonizes a wide variety of animals and is found in soil and vegetable matter. Infection results from ingestion of contaminated food or dairy products. This organism is intracellular and can cross the placenta of colonized mothers to infect the fetus. Neonatal infection of the CNS at less than one month of age presents as a meningitis syndrome with gram-positive rods (GPR) seen on Gram's stain. Intrauterine infections may also cause spontaneous abortions or stillbirth: granulomatosis infantiseptica is an in utero infection with systemic dissemination that results in stillbirth.

Gram-positive bacilli that are non-branching and catalase-negative

> *Erysipelothrix rhusiopathiae*
> *Arcanobacterium*
> *Gardnerella vaginalis*
> *Lactobacillus* spp.

Identification of these organisms must be considered along with anaerobic gram-positive bacilli, some of which are catalase-negative and will grow on routine media in 5–10% carbon dioxide. They are therefore often described simply as 'gram-positive, catalase-negative, non-spore-forming rods'. Some of these genera can be separated on the basis of biochemical reactions and fermentation of sugars, but gas liquid chromatography is required for the definitive species identification of the majority. Many of these organisms are normal flora in humans and, in general, are rarely encountered in infection.

Erysipelothrix rhusiopathiae

Erysipelothrix rhusiopathiae is carried by, and causes, disease in animals. The organism causes a localized skin infection known as erysipeloid, following a skin puncture wound with animal exposure.

Arcanobacterium pyogenes

Arcanobacterium pyogenes is also carried by, and causes, disease in animals. Infection in humans is usually cutaneous and, like erysipeloid, probably follows an abrasion with exposure to animals. *Arcanobacterium haemolyticum* is normal flora of human skin and pharynx. This organism causes infections similar to those caused by Group A streptococci, including pharyngitis and cellulitis.

Lactobacillus spp. and *Gardnerella vaginalis*

Both *Gardnerella vaginalis* and *Lactobacillus* species are important in discussions involving reproductive microbiology. Lactobacilli are widely distributed in nature, and are found in foods. They are normal flora of the human mouth, gastrointestinal tract and female genital tract. These bacteria are almost always encountered as a contaminant, but may cause bacteremia in immunocompromised individuals. Peroxidase-producing lactobacillus colonization is associated with a healthy vagina. Absence, or a decrease in number of these organisms is associated with an unhealthy state, e.g. lactobacilli numbers in the vagina are decreased in cases of bacterial vaginosis.

Lactobacillus is a highly pleomorphic organism that occurs in long chains as rods, coccobacilli and spirals. It appears as pinpoint, non-hemolytic colonies on sheep blood agar and can be cultured on agar with a low pH (e.g. tomato juice agar).

Gardnerella vaginalis is normal vaginal flora and also may colonize the distal urethra of males. The organism is one of a group contributing to bacterial vaginosis. It is also associated with urinary tract infections, and rarely with bacteremia. *G. vaginalis* organisms are small, pleomorphic and gram-variable. Special media (human blood agar or Columbia colistin-nalidixic acid agar) is required for cultivation of this organism. On human blood agar, the bacteria appear as small, opaque, grey colonies surrounded by a diffuse zone of beta hemolysis. A more complete discussion of *Gardnerella vaginalis* is found in Chapter 8.

Gram-positive bacilli that are branching or partially acid-fast

Table 2.5 outlines gram-positive bacilli. Those that are branching or partially acid-fast include:

- *Nocardia*
- *Rhodococcus*
- *Streptomyces*

This group of organisms, collectively referred to as the actinomycetes, include aerobic, facultative anaerobic and obligate anaerobic bacteria. *Nocardia*, *Streptomyces* and *Rhodococcus* are aerobic. *Nocardia* and *Rhodococcus*, but not *Streptomyces*, contain mycolic acid in the cell wall and are partially acid-fast. *Nocardia* species form branched hyphal filaments that fragment to form rods or coccoid elements.

These genera are separated on the basis of appearance on the Gram stain, colony appearance on routine agar, acid-fastness, lysozome resistance, and urea hydrolysis. Although not frequently encountered in the clinical laboratory, these organisms can cause serious infections in humans.

Nocardia

Nocardia are inhabitants of soil and water. Following traumatic inoculation or inhalation, *Nocardia* may cause infection in both immunocompetent and immunocompromised individuals. Immunocompetent individuals may suffer skin infections, lymphocutaneous infections and mycetoma, a painless chronic, localized, subcutaneous infection. Patients who are immunocompromised may develop an invasive pulmonary infection and various disseminated infections.

Rhodococcus

Rhodococcus is found in soil and water, and as farm animal flora. Infections with *Rhodococcus* are usually opportunistic, with the majority occurring in immunocompromised individuals. Clinical manifestations include pneumonia, bacteremia, skin infections, prostatic abscess, peritonitis and catheter-associated sepsis.

Streptomyces

Streptomyces are found in sand, decaying vegetation and soil. Infection is acquired by traumatic inoculation of organisms, usually in the lower extremities. *Streptomyces* is an agent of actinomycetoma and rarely may cause pericarditis, bacteremia and brain abscess in immunocompromised patients.

Anaerobic bacteria

Anaerobic bacteria include the following genera.

Gram-positive bacilli (Table 2.5)	
Clostridium	*Actinomyces*
Eubacterium	*Bifidobacterium*
Mobiluncus	*Propionibacterium*
Gram-negative bacilli (Table 2.6)	
Bacteroides	*Fusobacterium*
Porphyromonas	*Prevotella*
Gram-positive cocci	
Peptostreptococcus	*Peptococcus*
Gram-negative cocci	
	Veillonella

Anaerobes are normally found in the urethra, vagina, and colon, as well as the oral cavity and upper respiratory tract. Although they may be part of the normal flora, they can be responsible for significant pathology associated with both male and female infertility. Anaerobic infections may be exogenous (usually *Clostridium* spp.) or endogenous (endogenous flora gain access) and endogenous infections are usually polymicrobial. Certain factors predispose the human body to anaerobic infections:

(i) trauma of mucous membranes, especially rectal and vaginal mucosa
(ii) vascular stasis
(iii) tissue necrosis
(iv) decrease in the redox potential of a tissue, when other organisms (facultative anaerobes) scavenge the available oxygen and produce an anaerobic environment.

These infections are often polymicrobial, including streptococci or **Enterobacteriaceae**.

Table 2.5. Bacteria: gram-positive or gram-variable anaerobic bacilli

Anaerobic					
Spore-forming		Non-spore-forming			
Clostridium	*Actinomyces**	*Bifidobacterium*	*Eubacterium*	*Mobiluncus**	*Propionibacterium*
Bacillus; some species curved rods	Bacillus Branching	Curved bacillus Branching	Pleomorphic Some strains have unique morphology	Curved bacillus Gram-variable	Diphtheroid rod Pleomorphic
Some strains aerotolerant	Beaded				
Some strains gram-variable	Variable aerotolerance				

urogenital pathogen*.
prenatal/neonatal pathogen**.
urogenital pathogen; and prenatal/neonatal pathogen***.

Anaerobic infections commonly follow genital tract surgery or traumatic puncture of the genital tract, as well as gastrointestinal surgery or traumatic puncture of the bowel (e.g. during an oocyte retrieval procedure).

The presence of anaerobes in association with an infection is characterized by specific identifying criteria.

(i) Infection is in close proximity to a mucosal surface (anaerobes are the predominant microflora at mucosal surfaces).

(ii) Infection persists despite antimicrobial therapy.

(iii) Presence of a foul odour (*Porphyromonas* and *Fusobacterium* spp. produce foul-smelling metabolic end products).

(iv) Presence of a large quantity of gas (*Clostridium* spp. produce lots of gas).

(v) Presence of black colour or brick-red fluorescence (pigmented species of *Porphyromonas* and *Prevotella* produce a pigment that fluoresces brick-red under long-wave ultraviolet light).

(vi) Presence of sulfur granules (actinomycosis).

(vii) Distinct morphologic characteristics in Gram-stained preps (*Bacteroides* spp. are pleomorphic, *Fusobacterium nucleatum* is fusiform. *Clostridium* spp. are large, gram-positive rods that may or may not contain spores).

Table 2.5 lists examples of gram-positive or gram-variable bacilli.

Gram-positive anaerobic bacilli

Of the gram-positive anaerobic bacilli, *Clostridium* species are easily distinguished by their ability to form endospores. The remaining gram-positive bacilli can be minimally identified based on Gram stain appearance and characteristics on culture media. Definitive identification requires more advanced tests, such as gas liquid chromatography. The genus *Clostridium* includes the serious pathogens *Clostridium tetani*, *C. botulinum*, *C. perfringens* and *C. difficile*.

(i) *Clostridium tetani*, found in soil and manure, releases a potent neurotoxin that is the primary virulence factor leading to tetanus.

(ii) *Clostridium botulinum* causes botulism. The infection is acquired from eating vegetables or meat-based foods containing a preformed neurotoxin.

(iii) *Clostridium perfringens* produces several toxins and may cause gas gangrene and food poisoning. The organism is normal flora in the intestine. In the case of gas gangrene, the infection is usually acquired from a puncture wound, and food poisoning is due to ingestion of

Table 2.6. Bacteria: gram-negative anaerobic bacilli

Anaerobic			
Pleomorphic, non-pigmented Bile-tolerant	Pointed ends, non-pigmented Bile-sensitive	Coccoid or thin rods Pigmented Bile-sensitive	Bacillus, non-pigmented Bile-sensitive or tolerant
Bacterioides fragilis group	*Fusobacterium*	*Porphyromonas* *Prevotella*	*Biophilia*

preformed toxin in food. This organism may be acquired from the use of non-sterile operating instruments and is associated with infections resulting from 'back alley abortions'.

(iv) *Clostridium difficile* produces a toxin that causes a diarrhoea associated with use of antibiotics that may lead to pseudomembranous colitis, a life-threatening disease of the colon. This condition is a nosocomial concern since it is spread from person to person in the hospital setting.

Clostridium is speciated based on Gram stain morphology, arrangement of spores, colony appearance on routine, selective and differential media, aerotolerance, pigmentation, fluorescence, resistance to selected antibiotics and production of lecithinase.

Actinomyces and *Bifidobacterium* are normal flora in the upper respiratory tract and the intestine. *Actinomyces* species are usually involved in mixed infections of the oral, thoracic, pelvic and abdominal regions. Certain species are involved in periodontal disease. *Actinomyces* also are associated with pelvic infections from use of intrauterine devices (discussed in Chapter 11). *Bifidobacterium* may be encountered in mixed infections of the pelvis or abdomen.

Eubacterium spp. are resident flora in the upper respiratory tract, intestine and vagina. *Eubacterium* is associated with mixed infections of the abdomen, genitourinary tract and pelvis.

Propionibacterium is found on skin, in the upper respiratory tract and in the vagina. *Propionibacterium* species are normal skin flora associated with acne.

Mobiluncus species are found in the vagina and contribute to bacterial vaginosis. *Mobiluncus* infections are rarely encountered outside the female genital tract, but the exact role of the organism in gynecologic infections remains unclear.

Gram-negative anaerobic bacilli

Gram-negative anaerobic bacilli (Table 2.6) occur throughout the body and are the organisms most frequently encountered in anaerobic infections. Infections are usually mixed infections with other anaerobes and facultatively anaerobic bacteria, and may be contained, e.g. abscesses. Sites of infection include cranium, periodontium, thorax, peritoneum, liver, and female genital tract. These organisms may also be involved in aspiration pneumonia, decubitus ulcers, sinusitis, septic arthritis and other infections. In general, infections with the gram-negative anaerobes are associated with the body site where they reside as resident flora.

Bacteroides are intestinal flora.

Prevotella are flora in the upper respiratory tract, the intestine, the external genitalia and the vagina.

Fusobacterium is found in the upper respiratory tract and, to a lesser extent, the intestine.

Infections resulting from organisms in the *Bacterioides fragilis* group tend to be below the diaphragm.

Pigmented *Prevotellas*, *Porphyromonas* and *Fusobacterium nucleatum* are involved in infections above the diaphragm.

Anaerobic gram-negative bacilli are identified by aerotolerance, cell shape on the Gram stain, growth on routine, selective and differential media, pigmentation, fluorescence, bile sensitivity, resistance to a selected battery of antibiotics, production of enzymes, and motility.

Table 2.7. Unusual bacteria

Intracellular and non-culturable	Cell wall-deficient	*Mycobacteria*	*Spirochetes*
Chlamydia	*Mycoplasma*	M. tuberculosis complex[1]	*Treponema*[1]
C. trachomatis***	*M. hominis****[3]	NTM (Non-tuberculosis bacteria)[1]	*T. pallidum****[1]
Rickettsia	*M. genitalium****[3]	includes *M. leprae*[1]	*Borrelia*[1]
Coxiella	*Ureaplasma*[3]		*Leptospira*[1]
Ehrlichia	*U. urealyticum*[3]***		
Tropheryma			
Calymmatobacterium			
C. granulomatis*			

Aerobic $=$ [1]; Aerobic, microaerophilic $=$ [2]; Facultative $=$ [3].
urogenital pathogen*.
prenatal/neonatal pathogen**.
urogenital pathogen and prenatal/neonatal pathogen***.

Gram-positive anaerobic cocci

Gram-positive anaerobic cocci are ubiquitous in the human body. *Peptostreptococcus* is found in the upper respiratory tract, intestine and vagina and on skin and external genitalia. *Peptostreptococcus* is often found as part of a mixed anaerobic/facultative infection in cutaneous, respiratory, oral and pelvic sites. The same criteria used to identify gram-positive bacilli are used to identify gram-positive cocci.

Gram-negative anaerobic cocci

Veillonella, genus of anaerobic gram-negative cocci, is resident flora in the upper respiratory tract, the intestine and the vagina. The organism may be involved in mixed infections, but rarely plays a key role. Identification is based on the same criteria used to identify anaerobic gram-negative bacilli. This organism may be confused with *Neisseria gonorrhea* and must be considered when evaluating specimens for the presence of *Neisseria gonorrhoeae*.

N. gonorrhoea should only be presumptively reported if the organisms are kidney-shaped, diplococci and intracellular. *Veillonella* will not be found inside cells and the coccus is larger than *N. gonorrhoeae*.

Mycobacteria and bacteria with unusual growth requirements

Table 2.7 lists examples of bacteria with unusual growth requirements, including:
- Mycobacteria
- Obligate intracellular and non-culturable agents
- Cell wall-deficient bacteria: *Mycoplasma* and *Ureaplasma*
- Spirochetes

Mycobacteria

Mycobacteria are thin, non-motile slow-growing bacilli that have an unusual cell wall; it is rich in lipids and contains N-glycolymuramic acid instead of N-acetylmuramic acid. These properties make it difficult to stain the cells with the aniline dyes used in the Gram stain and also make them 'acid-fast' (resistant to stringent decolorization with 3% hydrochloric acid after application of basic fuchsin dye or after heating following dye application). The stringent acid-fast characteristic makes it easy to distinguish mycobacterium from most other organisms, although other organisms such as the nocardial species may also be acid-fast if a less stringent decolorization step is used (modified acid-fast).

There are more than 70 species of mycobacterium including the pathogens *Mycobacterium tuberculosis* and *Mycobacterium leprae*. These organisms are responsible for a spectrum of infections in humans and animals, ranging from localized lesions to disseminated disease. Mycobacteria are divided into two main groups:

(*i*) *M. tuberculosis* complex, which includes *M. tuberculosis*, *M. bovis* and *M. africanum*. *M. tuberculosis* causes primary tuberculosis lesions in the lung, but can spread to extrapulmonary sites including the genitourinary tract, lymph nodes, brain, bones, joints, peritoneum, pericardium and larynx. Tuberculosis infection of the genital tract is covered in Chapter 11.

(*ii*) Non-tuberculosis mycobacteria (NTMs).

The non-tuberculosis mycobacteria group is subdivided on the basis of growth rate (slow-growing vs. rapid-growing) with the slow-growers further divided based on the organism's ability to produce pigment either in the presence of light (photochromogens) or in the absence of light (scotochromogens). Some mycobacteria do not produce pigments under either light or dark conditions and are referred to as non-photochromogens. *M. leprae* cannot be cultivated in vitro. None of the mycobacteria are associated with reproductive problems, but members of the rapid growing mycobacteria are associated with postoperative infections (*M. abscessus*, *M. chelonae* and *M. mucogenicum*). *M. mucogenicum* also is associated with catheter-related sepsis.

Non-culturable obligate intracellular pathogens

Chlamydia	*Rickettsia*
Ehrlichia	*Coxiella burnetii*
Tropheryma whippelii	
Calymmatobacterium granulomatis	

Chlamydia trachomatis and *Calymmatobacterium* are significant reproductive pathogens. *Chlamydiae* have an unusual life cycle characterized by a small (0.25–0.35 μm) infective elementary body (EB) and a large (0.5–1.0 μm) reticulate body (RB) that multiplies within the host cell. The RBs multiply by binary fission in the host cell and condense to form the elementary bodies, which are released when the host cell lyses and dies. These EBs can then infect additional nearby cells.

Chlamydia

The genus *Chlamydia* contains the species: *C. pneumoniae*, *C. trachomatis* and *C. psittaci*.

C. pneumoniae is a human pathogen transmitted from person to person by aerosol droplets from the respiratory tract. The organism may cause pneumonia, bronchitis, sinusitis, pharyngitis and flu-like illness.

C. psittaci, common in birds and domestic animals, causes infections in humans that are characterized by pneumonia, severe headache, hepatosplenomegaly and changes in mental state. The infection may range from mild to life-threatening.

C. trachomatis has subtypes.

Subtypes A, B, Ba and C cause endemic trachoma by spread of the organism from hand to eye from the environment; it may also be spread by flies.

L1, L2 and L3 subtypes are responsible for the sexually transmitted disease lymphogranuloma venereum, described in Chapter 7.

Subtypes D–K may be spread sexually, from hand to eye by autoinoculation of genital secretions, or from eye to eye. These subtypes can cause urethritis, cervicitis, pelvic inflammatory disease and epididymitis. Neonatal transmission causes pneumonia and conjunctivitis in infants.

Species of *Chlamydia* may be grown on cell cultures in the laboratory or identified by direct methods, including cytologic examination, antigen detection and nucleic acid hydridization. *C. trachomatis* and infections caused by subtypes D–K are covered in detail in Chapter 10.

Rickettsia

Rickettsia are small (0.3 μm × 1.0 × 2.0 μm) fastidious, pleomorphic, obligate intracellular parasites that survive outside the host for only very short periods of time. The rickettsia divide by binary fission in host cell cytoplasm, and mature rickettsiae are released with lysis of the host cell. The organisms infect wild animals and humans; humans are accidental hosts who become infected following the bite of an arthropod vector, e.g. ticks, lice, mites, chiggers. *Rickettsia* are associated with states of crowding and unsanitary conditions including famine, war and poverty. They are responsible for spotted fevers, including Rocky Mountain spotted fever, typhus, and scrub typhus. *Rickettsia* are identified by serology or immunohistology.

Ehrlichia

Ehrlichia, also spread to humans via arthropod vectors, infect leukocytes. Once inside the white blood cells, the organisms undergo a developmental cycle similar to *Chlamydia*: an elementary body infects the cell, then multiplies and clusters to form an initial body, then a morula that ruptures to release the EBs. Species of *Ehrlichia* infect monocytes and granulocytes.

Coxiella burnetti

Coxiella burnetti is harboured in farm animals and is the agent of Q fever, an acute systemic infection that primarily affects the lungs. This organism, which is smaller than the rickettsia, can live outside cells, but can only be cultivated on lung tissue. *C. burnetii* has a spore-like life cycle and can exist in two antigenic states:

Phase I, the highly infectious form, is isolated from animals.

Phase II has been grown in culture and found to be non-infectious.

The organism is found in animal milk, urine, feces and birth products. Human infection follows aerosol inhalation. Once inhaled, *C. burnetti* is phagocytized by host cells and multiplies in vacuoles before being picked up by macrophages and carried through lymph nodes to the bloodstream. The organism is identified by serology.

Tropheryma whippelii

Tropheryma whippelii is the agent of Whipple's disease, found primarily in middle-aged men and characterized by the presence of mucopolysaccharide or glycoprotein in virtually every organ system. A cellular immune defect may be involved in the pathogenesis, characterized by diarrhea and weight loss, lymphadenopathy, hyperpigmentation, arthralgia, joint pain and a distended tender abdomen. This organism is phylogenetically a gram-positive actinomycete, unrelated to any other genus known to cause infection. It is detected by PCR assay.

Calymmatobacterium granulomatis

Calymmatobacterium granulomatis causes the sexually transmitted Donovanosis or granuloma inguinale. Donovanosis is common in many parts of the world, including India, the Caribbean and Australia, but is rare in the United States. Although it is primarily sexually transmitted, *C. granulomatis* may be transmitted via non-sexual modes. The infection is characterized by subcutaneous nodules that form red, granulomatous, painless lesions that bleed easily, and patients often present with inguinal lymphadenopathy. *C. granulomatosis* genital lesions have been mistaken for neoplasms. The organism, a gram-negative, pleomorphic encapsulated bacillus, is observed in vacuoles in large mononuclear cells. Since cultivation of *C. granulomatis* is difficult, identification is based on visualizing the organism in scrapings of lesions stained with Wright's or Giemsa stain. Disease manifestations and diagnosis of this organism are presented in Chapter 7.

Mycoplasma (class Mollicutes)

These include the genera *Mycoplasma* and *Ureaplasma*; they are the smallest (0.3 μm × 0.7 μm) free-living organisms and are widespread in nature. They lack a cell wall, but are related to gram-positive bacteria: they appear to have evolved from gram-positive clostridial-like cells by a drastic reduction of genome size, resulting in the loss of many biosynthetic abilities – they may be considered as the best representatives of the concept of a minimal cell. There are many species of mycoplasma in nature; species of *Mycoplasma* and *Ureaplasma urealyticum* are important reproductive pathogens. They are also a known hazard in cell culture systems, causing 'silent' infections that are not visually obvious, but can alter cell metabolism and induce chromosomal aberrations.

In general, they are aerobic and fastidious, requiring sterols in the medium for membrane function and growth. Due to their size and lack of cell wall, typical methods, e.g. Gram staining cannot be used to identify the organisms. Bacterial colonies must be visualized using a stereo microscope. The bacteria are cultured using indicators for different metabolic activities to detect growth. Serodiagnosis is helpful for certain species.

(i) *Mycoplasma pneumoniae*, spread via respiratory droplets, causes a community-acquired pneumonia, primarily in young adults. Infections with *M. pneumoniae* are associated with closed populations (e.g. families, dormitories, military barracks*). M. pneumoniae* also may cause upper respiratory tract infections in children. This organism may be cultured in the laboratory, or serology can be used for diagnosis.

(ii) *Mycoplasma hominis*, *M. genitalium*, and *Ureaplasma urealyticum* are genital mycoplasmas. *M. hominis* and *U. urealyticum* colonize the newborn, but colonization does not persist beyond the age of two years. Individuals acquire the organisms via sexual contact once they reach the age of puberty. These mycoplasma may cause, or contribute to, urogenital infections, including prostatitis, bacterial vaginosis, pelvic inflammatory disease, non-gonococcal urethritis and amnionitis, and may cause invasive disease in immunocompromised patients. The organisms can cause disease in neonates either by crossing the placenta of a colonized mother or from the birth canal during vaginal delivery. Disease in the neonate is systemic and includes meningitis, abscess and pneumonia.

(iii) *U. urealyticum* also is associated with development of chronic lung disease. *M. hominis* is distinguished from *U. urealyticum* by colony morphology, production of urea and glucose utilization. *M. hominis* is positive for arginine (detected by colour change in liquid medium) and has a 'fried egg' morphology; *U. urealyticum* produces the urease enzyme and the colonies appear as dark clumps. Genital mycoplasma and ureaplasma are discussed in Chapter 10.

Spirochetes

These are long, gram-negative, helically curved bacilli. The helical curves are responsible for organism motility and give the bacteria a corkscrew shape. There are numerous spirochetes in nature, some of which are normal flora in humans, and some of which are serious pathogens.

The genera *Treponema*, *Borrelia* and *Leptospira* include human pathogens. They are distinguished by their metabolic and biochemical characteristics, and by the number and tightness of coils:

Treponema are slender with tight coils.

Borrelia are thicker than *Treponema* and have fewer and looser coils.

Leptospira has thick loose coils and hooked ends.

Borrelia recurrentis is transmitted via the bite of a tick or louse and causes relapsing fever. *Borrelia burgdorferi*, transmitted by the bite of *Ixodes* ticks, is responsible for Lyme disease. The organisms are identified using serology and PCR to detect organism DNA. *Leptospira interrogans* causes leptospirosis that is acquired by contact with infected animals. The organism invades the blood and other sites throughout the body including the kidneys and the central nervous system. *L. interrogans* is identified by direct detection in body fluids, as well as by fluorescent antibody staining and molecular techniques.

The reproductive pathogens in this order are members of the genus *Treponema*.

T. pallidum subspecies *pallidum* causes syphilis, a sexually transmitted (or congenital) disease that is limited to humans (covered in detail in Chapter 7). *T. pallidum* subspecies *pertenue* and *T. pallidum* subspecies *endemicum* also infect only humans, causing non-venereal diseases of the skin. These organisms have not been cultivated in vitro for more than one passage. Detection methods include biopsy and visualization using dark-field or phase-contrast microscopy. Other treponemes inhabit the mouth or genital tract in humans, and these organisms can be cultured in the laboratory under anaerobic conditions. Organisms from this group, along with fusiform anaerobes, cause Vincent's angina, a gum disease referred to as acute necrotizing ulcerative gingivitis.

Normal flora in humans

Internal tissues such as blood, bone marrow, solid organs, muscle, pleural, peritoneal, synovial and cerebrospinal fluid are normally free of microorganisms. Surface tissues, such as respiratory tract, oral cavity, eyes, ears, urinary tract, genital tract, gastrointestinal tract and skin, on the other hand, are in constant contact with the environment, and therefore are readily colonized by microbes. The mixtures of organisms regularly found at any anatomical site are known as 'normal flora'. The microbes present as flora establish a dynamic interaction with their host, which results in a situation of mutualistic symbiosis. Many are specifically adapted to host tissues, with biochemical interactions between the surface components of bacteria and host cell adhesion molecules. From the host, flora derive a supply of nutrients, a stable environment, constant temperature, protection and transport. The host also derives some nutritional benefit from his or her flora. In humans, the microbial flora of the gut, for example, provide the host with Vitamin K and some B vitamins. The flora can also stimulate lymphatic tissue development, producing cross-reactive

antibodies, behaving as antigens to elicit an immune response. Colonization by well-adapted flora also excludes other microorganisms from colonizing the site. They compete for attachment sites, and produce substances that inhibit or kill other bacteria, such as fatty acids, peroxides, or specific bacteriocins. The composition of normal flora varies widely in different animal species, and is invariably related to age, sex, diet and environmental temperature. Some are found regularly at particular sites, and others are present only occasionally. Table 2.8 lists the normal flora that may be found at different body sites in the human.

Fortunately, animals that host this large and varied ecosystem have highly developed and elaborate defense mechanisms, which prevent the organisms from travelling to areas where they can cause disease, and also provide mechanisms for dealing with infection if the normal defence barriers are breached.

(i) *Mechanical barriers* include reflexes, such as coughing, gag reflex, sneezing and swallowing. Intact skin is protected by sebaceous gland secretions, as well as continuous sloughing of epithelial cells. Sweat removes microorganisms, and contains the enzyme lysozyme, which is bacteriostatic for some organisms. The conjuctiva is protected by tears, and by lysozyme. The epithelium of mucous membranes is protected by mucus production (traps organisms), the ciliary transport system, lysozyme production, and nasal hairs (filter).

(ii) In the *gastrointestinal tract*, a number of factors are important in maintaining a normal balance of flora. Saliva, lysozyme, stomach acidity, bile, normal peristalsis and maintaining the integrity of the mucosal layer all serve to protect epithelial cells from the flora inhabiting the gut lumen.

(iii) The *genitourinary tract* maintains its balance with the flushing effect of urine and urine acidity. The vaginal epithelium provides an intact barrier and vaginal secretions that are high in lactose. These secretions promote growth and colonization by the H_2O_2-producing lactobacilli that maintain an appropriate vaginal pH and microbiota in the healthy vagina. Prostatic secretions also contain elements that inhibit some bacteria.

(iv) Physiological *circulating fluids*, such as blood and lymphatic secretions, contain soluble and circulating non-specific factors, including complement (C1–C9) that lyses bacterial membranes, and the complement alternate pathway at C3 stage. Acid and alkaline phosphatase inactivate Herpes viruses, interferon proteins prevent virus re-infection, and fibronectin can act as a non-specific opsonin for some microbes.

(v) Host defence mechanisms also include *cellular non-specific immune* effectors, such as alveolar macrophages in the lung, polymorphonuclear neutrophils, eosinophils, fixed macrophages (histiocytes), lactoferrin that sequesters iron available to invading pathogens, and an elaborate system of cytokines produced by cells of the immune system that can affect the immune response, such as Interleukins 1, 6, 8, and tumour necrosis factor (TNF).

(vi) *Metabolic or natural defences* include body temperature: *T. pallidum* cannot survive in patients with a high fever. Specific host cell receptors are important (such as the CD4 receptor on helper lymphocytes that allows HIV infection to occur), and a compromised nutritional and metabolic state of the host can prevent, or facilitate microbial invasion, e.g. diabetic ketoacidosis results in low pH and high glucose levels, an environment where yeast and fungi thrive. Patients presenting with recurrent yeast/fungal infections should always be tested for diabetes.

(vii) Host defence mechanisms also include the sophisticated machinery of *specific immune response* mechanisms: secretory IgA in mucus secretions can bind some pathogens and prevent attachment, and serum IgG neutralizes viruses, acts as an opsonin for bacteria, fungi, and parasites, initiates the complement cascade when bound to an antigen, and neutralizes some bacterial toxins. Serum IgM similarly has a significant and complex role. IgM antibodies represent the first wave of serum immunoglobulin production during an acute infection; IgM is therefore used as an early marker for infection and its disappearance reflects conversion to a chronic infection or convalescent state.

(viii) The *cellular immune system (CMI)* orchestrates an elaborate system of host defence mechanisms, which include T-lymphocytes (T-helper cells), cytotoxic T-cells that kill infected cells directly, natural killer T-cells (NK) that destroy certain bacteria and attack virus-infected cells, and T-suppressor cells that downregulate antibody production by B-cells.

In contrast to this complex and highly developed system of physiological defence mechanisms, the procedures of assisted reproduction involve removing oocytes from their natural, highly protected environment, placing them in contact with semen samples, and culturing embryos in artificial media in a laboratory environment. The oocytes frequently have their only source of protection, the barrier offered by the zona pellucida, breached with microsurgical techniques. In this scenario, there is no defence against any flora in the environment, and therefore an understanding of the background, the hazards, and the precautions that may be applied to protect the gametes and embryos, is a crucial element of any assisted reproductive practice.

Table 2.8. Normal human flora

Site/Specimen	Colonization if applicable	Organisms which are present or may be present	Comments
Blood		Sterile	Although organisms may appear in the blood transiently (e.g. post-dental manipulation), any organism that multiplies and causes symptoms would be considered pathogenic in this site. Parasites may be found in the blood in transit to another site, but this is not a state of good health.
Cerebral Spinal Fluid (CSF) and CNS		Sterile	
Pleural fluid		Sterile	
Peritoneal fluid		Sterile	
Pericardial fluid		Sterile	
Synovial fluid		Sterile	
Bone		Sterile	
Bone marrow	•	Sterile	
Sinuses		Sterile	
Eyes	sparse flora	*Staphylococcus epidermidis* *Lactobacillus* spp.	Other organisms may colonize: *Propionibacterium acnes* *Staphylococcus aureus* (<30% population) *Haemophilus influenzae* (up to 25% of population) *Moraxella catarrhalis*, some *Enterobacteriaceae*, various streptococci (*S. pyogenes*, *S. pneumoniae*, other α-hemolytic and γ-hemolytic strep) are found in a very small percentage of people
Ears	sparse flora	*Staphylococcus epidermidis* *Lactobacillus* spp.	May also see organisms similar to those found in the conjunctival sac listed in the column above, but the following are seen more often: *Streptococcus pneumoniae* *Propionibacterium acne* *Staphylococcus aureus* *Enterobacteriaceae* *Pseudomonas aeruginosa* is found on occasion *Candida* spp. (non-*Candida albicans*) are also common

Skin

Diphtheroids
Staphylococcus epidermidis
Other coagulase-negative
  staphylococci
Propionibacterium acne

Upper respiratory tract

Actinobacter spp.
Viridans strep.
β-hemolytic strep.
Streptococcus pneumoniae
Staphylococcus aureus
Nesisseria spp.
Mycoplasma spp.
Haemophilus influenzae
Haemophilus parainfluenzae
Moraxella catarrhalis
Candida albicans
Herpes simplex virus
Enterobacteriaceae
Mycobacterium spp.
Pseudomonas spp.
Burkholderia cepacia
Klebsiella ozaenae
Eikenella corrodens
Bacteroides spp.
Peptostreptococcus spp.
Actinomyces spp.
Capnocytophaga spp.
Actinobacillus spp.
Filamentous fungi

These organisms are found in the nasopharynx and oropharynx of healthy people, but are possible pathogens

(*cont.*)

Table 2.8. (*cont.*)

Site/Specimen	Colonization if applicable	Organisms which are present or may be present	Comments
Upper respiratory tract		Non-hemolytic strep. Staphylococci Micrococci *Corynebacterium* spp. Coagulase-negative staph *Neisseria* species other than *N. gonorrheae* *Lactobacillus* spp. *Veillonella* spp. Spirochetes *Rothia dentocariosa* *Leptotrichia buccalis* *Selenomonas* *Wolinella* *Stomatococcus mucilaginosus* *Campylobacter* spp.	These organisms are found in the nasopharynx and oropharynx of healthy people, and may be possible pathogens, but these are rare.
Lower respiratory tract			To cause disease in the lower respiratory tract, organisms (either those potential pathogens in the URT or true pathogens) must possess traits or produce products that promote colonization, multiplication and subsequent infection in the host.

Upper urinary tract – (ureters and kidneys)		sterile	Note: All areas above the urethra are sterile
Lower urinary tract:			
bladder	Bladder	sterile	
urethra	Urethra	Coagulase-negative staphylococci, excluding *S. saprophyticus* Viridans and non-hemolytic strep Lactobacilli Diphtheroids (*Corynebacterium* spp.) Non-pathogenic *Neisseria* saprophytic spp. Anaerobic cocci *Propionibacterium* spp. Anaerobic gram-negative bacilli Commensal *Mycobacterium* spp. Commensal *Mycoplasma* spp.	The short female urethra lies in close proximity to the perirectal region, which has many microbes present. Potential pathogens may be present as transient colonizers. These include gram-negative aerobic bacilli (primarily *Enterobacteriaceae*), and occasional yeasts.
Genitourinary tract **Urethra (covered above)** **Lining of the genital tract**		Commensals Coag-neg staph Corynebacteria Anaerobes	Note: Vulva and penis of the uncircumcised male may harbour *Mycobacterium smegmatis* and other gram-positive bacteria
Pre-pubescent and post-menopausal female	Same flora as seen on surface epithelia	Staphylococci Corynebacteria	The flora of the female genital tract is dependent on pH and estrogen concentration, which are dependent on the age of the female. *Lactobacillus* spp. are the primary organisms in normal, healthy vaginal secretions with hydrogen peroxide-producing lactobacilli associated with a healthy state.

(cont.)

Table 2.8. (*cont.*)

Site/Specimen	Colonization if applicable	Organisms which are present or may be present	Comments
Reproductive age females		Large numbers of facultative bacteria *Enterobacteriaceae* Streptococci Staphylococci Anaerobes *Lactobacilli* Non-spore forming bacilli and cocci	The number of anaerobes remain constant throughout the monthly cycle. Note: Many women carry Group B β-hemolytic strep (*S. agalactiae*) which may be transmitted to the neonate. Note: Although yeasts (from the GI tract) may be found transiently in the female vagina, they are not normal flora.
GI tract		*Clostridia*	
Upper small intestine	Babies are colonized by human epithelial flora (staphylococci, *Corynebacterium* spp., other gram-positive organisms (bifidobacteria,	Sparse flora (10^1 to 10^3/mL)consisting of streptococci, lactobacilli, yeasts 10^6 to 10^7/mL	In the large intestine, anaerobes outnumber aerobes 1000:1
Lower small intestine (distal ileum)	clostridia, lactobacilli, streptococci) a few hours after birth; Over time the content of the intestine changes. The normal flora of the adult large bowel is established relatively early in life.	Predominantly: *Enterobacteriaceae* *Bacterioides*	
Large bowel		Predominantly anaerobic species: *Bacterioides* *Clostridium* *Peptostreptococcus* *Bidifobacterium* *Eubacterium* Facultatives include: *Escherichia coli* Other *Enterobacteriaceae* Enterococci Streptococci	

FURTHER READING

Alberts, B., Johnson, A., Lewis, J. *et al.* (2002). *Molecular Biology of the Cell.* 4th edn. New York: Garland Science.

de la Maza, L. M., Pezzlo, M. T. & Baron, E. J. (1997). *Color Atlas of Diagnostic Microbiology.* St. Louis: Mosby Publishers.

Delost, M. D. (1997). *Introduction to Diagnostic Microbiology.* St. Louis: Mosby Publishers.

Forbes, B. A., Sahm, D. F. & Weissfeld, A. S. (1998). *Diagnostic Microbiology.* 10th edn. St. Louis: Mosby Publishers.

Forbes, B. A., Sahm, D. F. & Weissfeld, A. S. (2002). *Diagnostic Microbiology,* 11th edn. St. Louis: Mosby Publishers.

Leland, D. S. (1996). *Clinical Virology.* W. B. Saunders Co.

Morello, J. A., Mizer, H. E., Wilson, M. E. & Granato, P. A. (1998). *Microbiology in Patient Care,* 6th edn. Boston, MA: McGraw-Hill.

Sarosi, G. A. & Davies, S. F. (1994). Therapy for fungal infections. *Mayo Clinic Proceedings,* **69**: 1111–17.

Schaechter, M., Medoff, G. & Schlessinger, D. (1989). *Mechanisms of Microbial Disease.* Baltimore, MD: Williams & Wilkins.

Appendix 2.1. Media used for isolation of bacteria

Medium	Components	Isolation/primary purpose	Differential appearance of colonies on agar
Bacteroides Bile esculin agar (BBE)	Tryptic soy agar (TSA) with ferric ammonium citrate, hemin, bile salts and gentamicin	Selective and differential for *Bacteroides fragilis* group; presumptive identification based on growth on BBE.	*B. fragilis* = dark colonies
Bile esculin agar (BEA)	Nutrient agar with ferric citrate, esculin, bile and sodium deoxycholate. Sodium deoxycholate inhibits many organisms	Differential isolation and presumptive identification of Group D streptococci and enterococci	Medium turns black if esculin is hydrolysed; if esculin is not hydrolysed there will not be a blackening of the medium. Examples: Group D streptococci and enterococci will grow in the presence of bile salts and hydrolyse esculin, turning the medium black; other groups of streptococci will be inhibited by the bile in the medium.
Bismuth sulfite agar (BS)	Peptone agar with dextrose, ferrous sulfate and brilliant green, Gram-positive organisms and members of the family *Enterobacteriaceae* other than *Salmonella* are inhibited by bismuth sulfite and brilliant green.	Selective for isolation of *Salmonella* spp. from stool	
Blood agar (sheep blood)(BA) (SBA)	TSA with blood (may also have *Brucella* agar or beef heart infusion with 5% sheep blood)	Cultivation of fastidious organisms and demonstration of hemolysis	Non-hemolytic = no zone of hemolysis around colony Alpha-hemolysis = greenish-brown area surrounding colony Beta-hemolysis = clear area around colony Examples: Non-hemolytic = Group D streptococci Alpha-hemolytic = *Streptococcus pneumoniae* Beta-hemolytic = *Streptococcus pyogenes* (Note: Blood agar is required for growth of *Streptococcus pyogenes*)

Medium	Composition	Purpose	Notes
Bordet-Gengou	Potato-glycerol-based medium with defibrinated blood and methicillin	Isolation of *Bordetella pertussis*	
Buffered charcoal yeast extract	Yeast extract, agar, charcoal, salts, L-cysteine HCl, ferric pyrophosphate, ACES-buffer, and alpha-ketoglutarate	Enrichment medium for *Legionella* spp.	
Campy-blood agar	*Brucella* agar base with vancomycin, trimethoprim, polymixin B, amphotericin B, and cephalothin	Selective for *Campylobacter* spp.	
Centers for Disease Control and Prevention anaerobic blood agar	SBA with hemin, L-cysteine and vitamin K	Isolation of anaerobes; enhanced growth of peptostreptococci	
Cefsulodin–igrasan–novobiocin agar (CIN)	Peptone base with yeast extract, mannitol, bile salts, cefsulodin, igrasan, novobiocin; neutral red and crystal violet indicators	Selective for *Yersinia* spp.; isolation of *Aeromonas* spp.	
Chocolate agar (CA)	Peptone base with 2% hemoglobin or IsoVitaleX (BBL)	Cultivation of *Haemophilus* spp. and pathogenic *Neisseria* spp.	
Columbia–Colistin–nalidixic acid (CNA)	Columbia agar base with colistin, nalidixic acid and 5% sheep blood	Selective isolation of gram-positive cocci	
Cycloserine–cefoxitin–fructose agar (CCFA)	Egg yolk base with fructose, cycloserine, and cefoxitin; neutral red indicator	Selective for *Clostridium difficile*	*C. difficile* produces yellowish rhizoid colonies
Cystine–tellurite blood agar	Infusion agar base in 5% SBA with potassium tellurite	Isolation of *C. diphtheriae*	*C. diphtheriae* reduces potassium tellurite, producing black colonies.
Eosin methylene blue (EMB)	Peptone base with lactose and sucrose; eosin and methylene blue indicators	Isolation and differentiation of lactose-fermenting and non-lactose-fermenting enteric bacilli	Fermenters = purple (Note: *E. coli* has green, metallic sheen) non-lactose fermenter (NLF) = clear, pink

(cont.)

Appendix 2.1. (*cont.*)

Medium	Components	Isolation/primary purpose	Differential appearance of colonies on agar
Gram-negative broth (GN)	Peptone base with glucose, mannitol, citrate and sodium deoxycholate inhibits many organisms	Selective (enrichment) liquid medium for enteric pathogens	
Hektoen agar (HE)	Peptone base with bile salts, lactose, and sucrose; bromothymol blue and acid fuchsin indicators	Differential and selective medium for isolation and differentiation of *Salmonella* spp. and *Shigella* spp. from other gram-negative enteric bacilli	*Salmonella* and *Shigella* = blue-green, clear Fermenters = yellow-orange NLF = clear, green
Kanamycin–vancomycin–laked blood agar (KVLB)	Brucella agar base with kanamycin, vancomycin, vitamin K, and 5% laked blood	Selective isolation of *Bacteroides* spp. and *Prevotella* spp.	*Prevotella melaninogenica* produces a pigment on this medium
Lowenstein–Jensen agar (LJ)	Egg-based medium; malachite green inhibitor	Isolation of mycobacteria	
MacConkey agar	Peptone base with lactose, crystal violet and bile salts; neutral red indicator Bile salts and crystal violet inhibit gram-positive organisms	Isolation and differentation of lactose-fermenting and non-lactose-fermenting enteric bacilli	Lactose fermenters = red Non-lactose fermenters = clear, pink (take on colour of the medium) Examples: *Klebsiella* spp. are lactose-fermenters. *Proteus* spp. are non-lactose-fermenters.
Mannitol salt agar (MSA)	Peptone base, mannitol, and 7.5% salt; phenol red indicator	Selective isolation of staphylococci	Medium turns yellow when mannitol is hydrolysed. Examples: *Staphyloccus aureus* hydrolyses mannitol, giving a positive reaction. *Staphylococcus epidermidis* does not hydrolyse mannitol, giving a negative reaction.
Middlebrook 7H10 agar	Complex base with albumin, salts, and digest of casein; malachite green inhibitor	Isolation of mycobacteria; antimicrobial susceptibility testing can be performed on colonies growing on this medium	

Medium	Composition	Purpose	Results
Modified Thayer–Martin agar (MTM)	BA with hemoglobin, supplement B; colistin, nystatin, vancomycin and trimethoprim Colistin inhibits growth of gram-negative organisms other than *Neisseria gonorrhoeae* and *Neisseria meningitidis*; nystatin inhibits yeast, vancomycin inhibits gram-positive organisms and trimethoprim inhibits swarming *Proteus* spp.	Selective for *Neisseria gonorrhoeae* and *Neisseria meningitidis*	
New York City agar (NYC)	Peptone agar with cornstarch, yeast dialysate, 3% hemoglobin, horse plasma, vancomycin, colistin, amphotericin B, and trimethoprim	Selective for *Neisseria gonorrhoeae*; genital mycoplasmas also grow	
Salmonella–Shigella agar (SS)	Peptone base with lactose bile salts, brillant green and sodium citrate; neutral red indicator; brilliant green and bile salts inhibit coliforms	Selective for *Salmonella* spp. and *Shigella* spp.	*Salmonella* = clear with black centres *Shigella* = clear Lactose-fermenters = pink NLF = clear
Selenite broth	Peptone base broth with sodium selenite. Sodium selenite is toxic for most *Enterobacteriaceae*	Enrichment for isolation of *Salmonella* spp.	
Schaedler agar	Peptone and soya base with yeast extract, dextrose, buffers, hemin, L-cysteine and 5% blood	Non-selective for recovery of anaerobes and aerobes	
Skirrow agar	Peptone and soya protein base with lysed horse blood; vancomycin, polymyxin B, and trimethoprim	Selective for *Campylobacter* spp.	
Streptococcal selective agar (SSA)	SBA with colistin, trimethoxazole (SXT) and crystal violet	Selective for *Streptococcus pyogenes* and *Streptococcus agalactiae*	
Tetrathionate broth	Peptone base with bile salts and sodium thiosulfate Bile salts and sodium thiosulfate inhibit gram-positive organisms and *Enterobacteriaceae* spp. other than *Salmonella* and *Shigella*.	Selective for *Salmonella* spp. and *Shigella* spp.	

(cont.)

Appendix 2.1. (*cont.*)

Medium	Components	Isolation/primary purpose	Differential appearance of colonies on agar
Thioglycollate broth	Pancreatic digest of casein, soya broth, and glucose Thioglycollate and agar reduce redox potential (Eh)	Supports growth of anaerobes, aerobes, microaerophilic organisms and fastidious organisms	
Thiosulfate citrate–bile salts (TCBS)	Peptone base with yeast extract, bile salts, citrate, sucrose, ferric citrate, and sodium thiosulfate; bromthymol blue indicator	Selective and differential for vibrios	Sucrose-fermenters = yellow Non-sucrose-fermenters = green
Trypticase soya agar (TSA)	Nutrient agar	For isolation of non-fastidious organisms	Examples: *Bacillus* species and coliforms will grow on this medium
Vaginalis (V) agar	Columbia agar with 5% human blood	Selective and differential for *Gardnerella vaginalis*	*G. vaginalis* produces small, grey, opaque colonies surrounded by a diffuse β-hemolytic zone
Xylose lysine deoxycholate agar (XLD)	Yeast extract agar with lysine, xylose, lactose, sucrose, ferric ammonium citrate; phenol red; sodium deoxycholate inhibits gram-positive organisms	Isolation and differentiation of *Salmonella* and *Shigella* spp. from other gram-negative enteric bacilli	*Salmonella* spp. = pink-red with black centre *Shigella* spp. = clear Lactose-fermenters = yellow NLF = red, yellow or clear with or without black centres

Appendix 2.2. Biochemical tests for identification of bacteria

Test	Principle/major use/examples of key positive and negative organisms when applicable
Acetamide utilization	Determines if an organism can use acetamide as the sole source of carbon. Organisms that grow on this medium are able to deaminate acetamide and release ammonia, causing a change in pH. The change in pH results in a colour change in the medium from green to blue. Interpretation: Positive: Deamination of acetamide results in a blue colour. Negative: No change in colour. Examples: Positive: *Pseudomonas aeruginosa* Negative: *Stenotrophomonas maltophilia*
Acetate utilization	Determines if an organism can use acetate as the sole source of carbon. The organism that is able to utilize acetate as a sole carbon source will break down the sodium acetate in the medium causing an increase in pH that turns the indicator from green to blue. Interpretation: Positive: Growth of the organism results in an alkaline (blue) medium. Negative: No growth or growth without change in indicator (no colour change). Examples: Positive: *Escherichia coli* Negative: *Shigella flexneri*
Bacitracin susceptibility	Determines an organism's ability to tolerate bacitracin (0.04 units). A standard quantity of a bacterial suspension is streaked on agar (either tryptic soya agar or sheep blood agar, depending on the organism's growth requirements) and streaked in three directions to produce a lawn of growth. A bacitracin disc is placed in the centre of the streaked plate. Following incubation and bacterial growth, zones of inhibition are measured around the bacitracin disc to determine susceptibility.

(cont.)

Appendix 2.2. (*cont.*)

Test	Principle/major use/examples of key positive and negative organisms when applicable
	Interpretation: Positive: Zone of inhibition around the disc (must measure size) indicates susceptibility. Negative: No zone of inhibition around the disc indicates resistance. Examples: Positive (any zone of inhibition): Group A streptococci; some strains of Lancefield Groups B, C, and F may be susceptible Positive (with zone > 10 mm): *Micrococcus* species Negative (no zone of inhibition): *Staphylococcus* species
Bile esculin	Determines both an organism's ability to grow in the presence of bile (4% oxgall) and its ability to hydrolyse the glycoside esculin to esculetin and dextrose. Interpretation: Positive for growth in bile: growth, but no change in colour of medium. Positive for growth in bile and esculin hydrolysis: growth plus medium turns black. Negative: No growth in the medium Examples: Positive: Group D streptococci and *Enterococcus* species will grow in the bile and will hydrolyse esculin. Negative: Lancefield Groups other than Group D streptococci
Bile solubility test	Determines if an organism is lysed by bile or a bile salt solution such as sodium desoxycholate. Lysis is dependent on the presence of intracellular autolytic enzymes. Bile salts lower the surface tension between the cell membrane of the bacteria and the medium, activating the organism's natural autolytic process. The amidase enzyme splits the muramic acid–alanine bond in peptidoglycan in the cell wall resulting in cell lysis. This test is used to differentiate *Streptococcus pneumoniae* from other species of α–hemolytic streptococci. Interpretation: Positive: Colonies disintegrate with an imprint of the lysed colony remaining within the zone. Negative: Colonies remain intact. Examples: Positive: *Streptococcus pneumoniae.* Negative: α–hemolytic streptococci other than *S. pneumoniae.*

CAMP test

Determines if an organism produces a diffusible extracellular (CAMP factor) protein that acts synergistically with the beta-lysin strain of *Staphylococcus aureus* to cause enhanced lysis of red blood cells in the sheep blood agar medium when the organisms are streaked perpendicular to each other.

Interpretation:
Positive: Enhanced hemolysis will appear as an arrowhead-shaped zone of β-(clear) hemolysis at the juncture of the two organisms.
Negative: No increased hemolysis.

Examples:
Positive: Group B streptococcus.
Negative: Streptococci other than Group B.

Catalase

Catalase is used to distinguish the families *Streptoccoaceae* from *Micrococcaceae*. The test determines the ability of an organism to produce the enzyme catalase that can be detected by adding a 3% solution of hydrogen peroxide to a suspension of the organism to be tested. A positive is indicated by the formation of bubbles.

Catalase-producing bacteria $+3\%$ H_2O_2 $\longrightarrow$ H_2O and O_2 (bubbles form)

Catalase production may function to inactivate toxic hydrogen peroxide and free radicals formed by the myeloperoxidase system with phagocytic cells after ingestion of the microorganisms.

Interpretation:
Positive: Bubbles are produced when H_2O_2 is added to a bacterial colony.
Negative: No bubbling when H_2O_2 is added to the bacterial colony.

Examples:
Positive: Staphylococci and Micrococci
Negative: Streptococci

Cetrimide

Determines an organism's ability to grow in the presence of cetrimide, a toxic substance that inhibits the growth of most bacteria.

Interpretation:
Positive: Organism growth on the agar.
Negative: No growth on the agar.

Examples:
Positive: *Pseudomonas aeruginosa*
Negative: *Escherichia coli*

(cont.)

Appendix 2.2. (cont.)

Test	Principle/major use/examples of key positive and negative organisms when applicable
Citrate utilization (Simmon's citrate)	Determines an organism's ability to use sodium citrate as the sole source of carbon for metabolism. Bromothymol blue is included in the medium as an indicator to detect the breakdown of citric acid.

Citric acid (citrate) → breakdown products

(green = acid)   (blue = alkaline)

Interpretation:

Positive: Intense blue colour.

Negative: Growth, but no colour change.

Examples:

Positive: *Klebsiella pneumoniae*

Negative: *Escherichia coli*

Coagulase test	Coagulase is an enzyme that acts on fibrinogen to form a clot. This test is used to differentiate *Staphylococcus aureus*, which is positive, from staphylococci that are negative for the enzyme. *S. aureus* produces two forms of coagulase; bound (clumping factor) and free. Bound coagulase is bound to the bacterial cell wall and reacts with fibrinogen, causing it to precipitate the bacterial cell wall. This reaction can be visualized as clumping when bacterial cells are mixed with plasma.

Bound coagulase + fibrinogen → fibrin clot

Interpretation:

Positive: Macroscopic clumping in ≤ 10 seconds in coagulated plasma drop

Negative: No clumping

(*Note*: must confirm negative test for bound coagulase with a tube test for free coagulase)

Free coagulase is an extracellular enzyme that causes clot formation when *S. aureus* colonies are incubated with plasma. Free coagulase first binds with a fibrinogen precursor, prothrombin, to activate a plasma coagulase-reacting factor (CRF), which is a modified thrombin molecule, to form a CRF–coagulase complex. This complex in turn reacts with fibrinogen to produce a fibrin clot.

Prothrombin + free coagulase → CRF

CRF + fibrinogen → clot

Free and bound coagulase may act to coat the bacterial cells with fibrin, rendering them resistant to opsonization and phagocytosis.

Positive: *Staphylococcus aureus.*
Negative: Other species of *Staphylococcus* (e.g. *S. epidermidis*)

CTA sugars

Cysteine trypticase agar (CTA) sugars are used for differentiation of *Neisseria* species by observing the production of acid from metabolism of carbohydrates in the CTA. CTA supports the growth of the fastidious *Neisseria* species. The sugars (glucose, maltose, fructose and lactose) are added to yield a 1% concentration in the CTA medium. Following inoculation of organism to the CTA medium and subsequent incubation in a non-CO_2 incubator, the CTA is examined for the production of acid in the top portion of the tube.

Interpretation:

Positive: Yellow in the top of the tube, indicating that acid has been produced
Negative: No colour change in the medium.

Examples:

Positive for glucose only = *Neisseria gonorrhoeae*
Positive for glucose and maltose = *Neisseria meningitidis*
Positive for glucose, maltose and lactose = *Neisseria lactamica*
Positve (+/−) for glucose, maltose, lactose and sucrose = *Neisseria sicca*
Negative for all four = *Moraxella catarrhalis, Neisseriaflavescens*

Decarboxylase tests

The test measures the enzymatic ability of the organism to decarboxylate or hydrolyse an amino acid to form an amine. Decarboxylase media contains glucose, bromcresol purple, a nitrogen source, cresol red indicator, the enzyme activator pyridoxal and the amino acid to be tested. Decarboxylation results in an alkaline pH change, causing a shift in the pH indicators (bromocresol purple and cresol red) to dark purple (colour of the control is pale purple). The amino acids tested are lysine, ornithine and arginine.

Lysine is decarboxylated to cadaverine; ornithine is decarboxylated to putrescine and arginine undergoes a dihydrolase reaction to form citrulline, which is decarboxylated to ornithine. For each amino acid to be tested, it is necessary to inoculate both a tube with basal medium (control to ensure that the organism does not form alkaline end products in the absence of the amine end product) and one with basal medium plus the amino acid to be tested. An uninoculated control is compared to any positive tubes.

Interpretation:

Positive: Blue-purple colour compared to the uninoculated control (pale purple).
Negative: No colour change or yellow in both the test and inoculated control tubes. Glucose is fermented during the early part of the decarboxylation process, leading to a yellow colour. As the pH rises, an optimal environment for decarboxylation occurs and decarboxylation of the amino acid leads to an increase in pH and a purple colour. If a test result is yellow, it should be reincubated for up to 4 days. At the end of the incubation, the acid from glucose fermentation would not mask the alkaline colour change resulting from a positive decarboxylation reaction.

(*cont.*)

Appendix 2.2. (*cont.*)

Test	Principle/major use/examples of key positive and negative organisms when applicable

Uninoculated control: pale purple

Inoculated control: yellow if the organism is a glucose fermenter.

Examples:

Arginine

Positive: *Enterobacter cloacae*

Negative: *Klebsiella pneumoniae*

Lysine:

Positive: *Klebsiella pneumoniae*

Negative: *Enterobacter cloacae*

Ornithine:

Positive: *Enterobacter cloacae*

Negative: *Klebsiella pneumoniae*

DNA hydrolysis

The test determines if an organism has the DNAse enzyme and is therefore able to hydrolyse DNA. Bacteria are streaked onto a medium containing a DNA–methyl green complex. When DNA is hydrolysed, methyl green is released and combines with the highly polymerized DNA at pH of 7.5, turning the medium colourless around the test organism. If DNA is not degraded, the medium remains green.

Interpretation:

Positive: Medium is colourless around the organism.

Negative: Medium remains green.

Note: If toluidene blue is used instead of methyl green, it complexes with polymerized DNA (control) and a royal blue colour results. Where DNA is hydrolysed by the toluidene blue, the dye complexes with the oligo- and mononucleotides resulting in a change in dye structure and absorption spectrum, yielding a bright pink colour.

Interpretation:

Positive: Medium turns pink.

Negative: Medium remains blue.

Examples:

Positive: *Staphylococcus aureus*; *Serratia marcescens*

Negative: *Staphylococcus epidermidis*

Flagella stain (RYU)

The stain is used to determine the arrangement of flagella for motile bacteria. A wet-mount of organism is stained with RYU flagella stain and the motile bacteria are evaluated for: (1) presence or absence of flagella; (2) number of flagella per cell; (3) location of flagella as either peritrichous, lophotrichous or polar; (4) amplitude of wavelength (short or long) and (5) whether or not tufted.

Interpretation:

Positive: Flagella are present and can be described.

Negative: Organism is non-motile; no flagella present

Examples:

Positive:

Peritrichous: *Escherichia coli*

Polar: *Pseudomonas aeruginosa*

Negative: *Klebisella pneumoniae*

Gelatin hydrolysis

The test determines the ability of an organism to produce proteolytic enzymes (gelatinases) that liquefy gelatin. An inoculated tube along with an uninoculated control is incubated for growth, then removed, placed at 4 °C and subsequently observed for liquefaction.

Interpretation:

Positive: Partial or total liquefaction of the inoculated tube; note: control tube must be completely solidified.

Negative: Complete solidification of the tube at 4 °C.

Examples:

Positive: *Proteus vulgaris*

Negative: *Enterobacter aerogenes*

Growth at 42 °C

Determines an organism's ability to grow at 42 °C. Following inoculation and incubation of two trypticase soy agar tubes, one tube is incubated at 35 °C and the other is incubated at 42 °C. The presence of growth is recorded for each tube after 18–24 hours.

Positive: Good growth at both at 35 °C and 42 °C.

Negative: Good growth at 35 °C but not at 42 °C.

Examples:

Positive: *Pseudomonas aeruginosa*

Negative: *Pseudomonas fluorescens*

(cont.)

Appendix 2.2. (cont.)

Test	Principle/major use/examples of key positive and negative organisms when applicable
Hemolysis patterns	Determines if bacteria produce extracellular enzymes that lyse red blood cells in agar (hemolysis). This can result in complete clearing of the erythrocytes (beta hemolysis) or only a partial clearing (α-hemolysis) around the bacterial colony. Interpretation: Positive for β-hemolysis: Complete lysis of red blood cells seen as clearing around the bacterial colony. Positive for β-hemolysis: Partial lysis of red blood cells seen as green discoloration around the bacterial colony. Negative for hemolysis: No effect on red blood cells and no halo around the colony. This is referred to as non-hemolysis or γ-hemolysis. Examples: Positive for β-hemolysis: Group A streptococcus Positive for α-hemolysis: *Streptococcus pneumoniae* and other alpha streptococci Gamma or non-hemolytic: Group D streptococci and *Enterococcus* species
Hippurate hydrolysis	Tests for the presence of the constitutive enzyme, hippuricase, which hydrolyses the substrate hippurate to produce the amino acid, glycine. Glycine is detected by oxidation with ninhydrin reagent, resulting in a deep purple colour. Ninhydrin is added to hippurate that has been inoculated with colonies of the organism and observed for a colour change. Sodium hippurate → sodium benzoate + glycine Glycine + ninhydrin reagent → purple colour Interpretation: Positive: Deep purple colour. Negative: Light purple or no colour change. Examples: Positive: *Streptococcus agalactiae, Campylobacter jejuni, Listeria monocytogenes* Negative: *Streptococcus pyogenes*; other streptococci

Hydrogen sulfide production

This test detects hydrogen sulfide that is produced from the degradation of sulfur-containing amino acids (in peptone). When H_2S combines with a heavy metal such as iron or lead in the medium, ferrous sulfide, a black precipitate is produced.

Interpretation:

Cysteine or methionine $\rightarrow$ pyruvic acid $+ H_2S +$ ammonia

$H_2S + Fe(NH_4)_2(SO_4)_2 \xrightarrow{\text{Desulfurase enzyme}} FeS(\text{black precipitate})$

Positive: Black

Negative: No colour change in medium.

Examples:
Positive: *Salmonella typhi, Eduardsiella* spp.
Negative: *Shigella* spp.

Indole production

Determines if an organism produces the enzyme tryptophanase and is therefore able to split the amino acid tryptophan to form the compound indole. The test is used to presumptively identify *Escherichia coli*, the gram-negative bacillus most commonly encountered in diagnostic microbiology. A suspension of the organism is added to a tryptophan broth and incubated. Following incubation either Kovak's reagent (for *Enterobacteriaceae*) or Ehrlich's reagent after xylene extraction (for other gram-negative bacilli) is added and the mixture is observed for the presence of a red ring in the upper layer of the aqueous mixture.

Tryptone- $\rightarrow$ tryptophan $\rightarrow$ indole $+$ pyruvic acid $+ NH_3$

Interpretation:
Positive: Red ring at the interface.
Negative: No colour reaction.
Variable: Orange colour (indicates production of skatole, a methylated intermediate that may be a precursor to indole production).

Examples:
Positive: *Escherichia coli*
Negative: *Klebsiella pneumoniae*

Litmus milk

Determines an organism's ability to metabolize litmus milk. Lactose fermentation is noted by the litmus turning pink from acid production. If sufficient acid is produced, casein in the milk will coagulate and solidify the milk. Some organisms will shrink the curd and form whey at the surface; other organisms hydrolyse the casein, producing a straw-coloured turbid product. Some organisms reduce litmus, making the medium colourless at the bottom of the tube. Following incubation of the organism in litmus milk, the product is observed for 7 days and all changes recorded. Multiple changes may occur during the observation period.

(*cont.*)

Appendix 2.2. (cont.)

Test	Principle/major use/examples of key positive and negative organisms when applicable
	Interpretation: Positive reactions for litmus indicator: Alkaline reaction: Litmus turns blue. Acid reaction: Litmus turns pink. Negative reaction for litmus indicator: Purple: Identical to uninoculated control Positive reactions for milk appearance: Coagulation (occurs in acid or alkaline conditions): clot Dissolution of clot: clear, greyish, watery fluid with a shrunken, insoluble pink clot (in acid environment; record as digestion). Dissolution of clot: clear, greyish, watery fluid with a shrunken, insoluble blue clot (in alkaline environment; record as peptonization). Examples: Alkaline: *Alcaligenes faecalis* Acid: *Enterococcus faecium* Peptonization: *Burkholderia cepacia*
Lysostaphin	Determines if an organism is susceptible to lysostaphin. Lysostaphin is an endopeptidase that cleaves the glycine-rich pentapeptide cross-bridges in the staphylococcal cell wall peptidoglycan, rendering the cells susceptible to osmotic lysis. Following the addition of a commercial lysostaphin to a suspension of organisms and subsequent incubation, the tube is observed for clearing of the suspension. Interpretation: Positive: Clearing of the suspension; susceptibility to lysostaphin. Negative: No clearing of the suspension; resistance to lysostaphin. Examples: Positive (Susceptible): *Micrococcus* spp. Negative (Resistant): *Staphylococcus* spp.
Methyl red/Voges–Proskauer (MRVP) tests	Determines ability of an organism to produce and maintain stable acid end products from glucose fermentation and the ability of some organisms to produce neutral end products (acetylmethylcarbinol or acetoin) from glucose fermentation. Following inoculation of MR–VP medium and subsequent incubation, the sample is split and one tube is used to perform the MR test and the other to perform the VP test. Methyl red is added to the MR tube and observed for a colour change to red; Barritt's reagents A (alpha-naphthol) and B (KOH) are added to the VP tube, shaken and observed for a colour change to red. Mixed acids + methyl red → red colour

MR

Intepretation:

Positive: Bright red colour (indicative of mixed acid fermentation).

Weakly positive: Red-orange colour.

Positive: *Escherichia coli*
Negative: *Enterobacter cloacae*

Voges–Proskauer-glucose→ 2, 3 butylene glycol + acetoin → red colour

VP interpretation:

Positive: Red colour indicative of acetoin production.

Negative: Yellow colour.

Delayed reaction: Orange colour at surface; reincubate.

Positive: *Enterobacter cloacae*
Negative: *Escherichia coli*

Motility

Determines motility of bacteria. A bacterial colony is inoculated (using a needle to stab a straight line to the bottom to the agar) to a medium containing a small amount of agar and 1% triphenyltetrazolium chloride, a colourless dye that bacteria incorporate and reduce to a red pigment. Motile bacteria move away from the line of the inoculum, and non-motile bacteria grow only along the line of the inoculation.

Interpretation:

Positive: Motile; diffuse growth extending laterally from the line of inoculation.

Negative: Non-motile; growth only along the line of inoculation.

Examples:
Positive: *Escherichia coli*
Negative: *Klebsiella pneumoniae*

Nitrate reduction

The test is used to determine an organism's ability to reduce nitrate. Reduction of nitrate to nitrite is determined by adding sulfanilic acid and alpha-naphthylamine. Sulfanic acid and nitrite react to form a diazonium salt that couples with the alpha–naphthylamine to produce a red, azo dye. Nitrate broth with a Durham tube (inverted small tube at bottom of large tube to detect gas) is inoculated with organism and incubated. Following incubation, the sample is observed for the presence of bubbles in the Durham tube, indicating gas production, and Reagent solution A (sulfanilic acid) and Reagent Solution B (alpha-naphthylamine) are added and observed for the development of a red colour, indicating the presence of nitrite. If no colour develops, zinc powder is then mixed with the broth to which Solutions A and B have

(cont.)

Appendix 2.2. (*cont.*)

Test	Principle/major use/examples of key positive and negative organisms when applicable
	already been added. If a red colour then develops, this is due to zinc catalysing the conversion of nitrate to nitrite, confirming that nitrate was still present and had not been reduced to nitrite. $$NO_3 + 2e + 2H \rightarrow NO_2 + H_2O \rightarrow N_2$$ nitrate　　　nitrite　　　nitrogen gas Interpretation: Positive: Nitrate to nitrite: Red colour when Reagents A and B are added; no gas. Positive: Nitrate to nitrite and nitrite to gas: Red colour when Reagents A and B are added plus gas. Positive: Nitrate to nitrite and nitrite to nitrogen gas: No red colour when Reagents A and B are added; gas present (nitrate has been reduced to nitrite and nitrite to nitrogen gas). Negative: Nitrate not reduced: No red colour when Reagents A and B are added; no gas. Negative confirmation: Nitrate not reduced: No red colour when Reagents A and B are added, but red colour when zinc is added to catalyse the conversion of nitrate to nitrite. Examples: Positive: NO_3 + (gas): *Pseudomonas aeruginosa* Positive: NO_3 + (no gas): *Escherichia coli* Negative: NO_3 − (no gas): *Acinetobacter* spp.
Novobiocin susceptibility	Determines an organism's susceptibility to novobiocin. This test is used to differentiate *Staphylococcus saprophyticus* from other coagulase-negative species of staphylococci. A standard quantity of a bacterial suspension is streaked on sheep blood agar in three directions to produce a lawn of growth. A 5 μg novobiocin disc is placed in the centre of the streaked plate. Following incubation and bacterial growth, zones of inhibition are measured around the novobiocin disc to determine susceptibility. Interpretation: Positive: Zone of inhibition around the disc that is > 16 mm. Negative: No zone of inhibition or zone of inhibition ≤ 16 mm around the disc. Examples: Positive: *Staphylococcus saprophyticus* Negative: Other coagulase-negative staphylococci

ONPG

The ONPG (*o*-nitrophenyl-β- D-galactopyranoside) test is used to determine the ability of an organism to produce the enzyme, β-galactosidase, which hydrolyses the substrate ONPG to form orthonitrophenol, which is a visible, yellow product. ONPG is a rapid test for the detection of β-galactosidase. The test is used primarily to determine if an organism is a slow lactose-fermenter or a non-lactose fermenter. All lactose fermenters (rapid and slow) produce β-galactosidase, but rapid fermenters also produce the enzyme permease that transports the lactose across the bacterial cell membrane. If permease is not produced, lactose must diffuse into the cell, making fermentation of lactose a much slower process. Beta-galactosidase, if present, acts on the substrate ONPG in the same way the enzyme hydrolyses lactose to form galactose and glucose; the end product of ONPG hydrolysis is a visible (yellow) compound, orthonitrophenol.

Interpretation:

Positive: Yellow.

Negative: Colourless.

Examples:

Positive (rapid lactose-fermenter (with permease): *Escherichia coli*

Negative (non-lactose fermenter (β-galactosidase not produced): *Salmonella typhimurium*

Optochin

This test is used to determine the effect of optochin (ethylhydrocurpreine hydrochloride) on an organism. Optochin lyses pneumococci, but other alpha-streptococci are resistant. Lysis is indicated by a zone of inhibition around an optochin (P) disc. Colonies suspected of being *Streptococcus pneumococci* are streaked on sheep blood agar in three directions to produce a lawn of growth. An optochin (P) disc is placed in the centre of the streaked plate. Following incubation in CO_2 and bacterial growth, zones of inhibition are measured around the optochin disc to determine susceptibility.

Interpretation:

Positive: Inhibition indicated by a zone of hemolysis $\geq$14 mm in diameter for 10 μg P disc and $\geq$ 10 mm in diameter for 6 μg P disc.

Negative: No inhibition zones or zones < those listed as positive.

Examples:

Positive: *Streptococcus pneumoniae.*

Negative: Other alpha-hemolytic streptococci.

Oxidase (Kovac's method)

The test is initially used for differentiating between groups of gram-negative bacteria. The test detects the presence of the enzyme cytochrome oxidase. Cytochrome oxidase reacts with oxygen (terminal electron acceptor) in the process of oxidative phosphorylation in aerobic bacteria. Cytochrome oxidase is detected by using reagents that are normally colourless but become coloured when oxidized. It also is used as a key reaction for the identification of *Neisseria* species. The test detects the presence of the bacterial enzyme cytochrome oxidase using the substrate is 1% *N,N,N'* ,*N'* -tetra-methyl-*p*-phenylenediamine dihydrochloride to indophenol, a dark, purple-coloured end product. A drop of oxidase (1% tetraethyl-*p*-phenylenediamine dihydrochloride in dimethyl sulfoxide) is flooded onto bacterial colonies and observed for a colour change. Alternatively, colonies can be placed onto a filter paper impregnated with the reagent and observed for a colour change.

(*cont.*)

Appendix 2.2. (cont.)

Test	Principle/major use/examples of key positive and negative organisms when applicable
	Interpretation: Positive: Dark purple colour indicating the presence of oxidase. Negative: No colour development, indicating the absence of the enzyme. Examples: Positive: *Pseudomonas* spp, *Aeromonas* spp., *Campylobacter* spp., *Neisseria* spp. Negative: *Enterobacteriaceae*, *Stenotrophomonas maltophilia*, *Acinetobacter* spp.
Modified oxidase	A drop of modified oxidase (6% tetraethyl-*p*-phenylenediamine dihydrochloride in dimethyl sulfoxide) is added to a colony of organism that has been placed on filter paper and observed for a colour change. **Interpretation:** Positive: If oxidase is present the colourless reagent will be oxidized and will turn purple or blue black. Negative: No colour change. Examples: Positive: *Micrococcus* spp. Negative: *Staphylococcus* spp.
Oxidation–fermentation (OF)	Oxidation–fermentation determines the oxidative or fermentative metabolic capabilities of an organism. The test determines whether an organism uses carbohydrate substrates to produce acid byproducts. Typically, non-fermentative bacteria are tested for their ability to produce acid from glucose, lactose, maltose, sucrose, xylose and mannitol. A tube of each type of sugar is inoculated with organism along with a control tube containing OF base, but no carbohydrates. The OF medium contains an indicator, 0.2% peptone and 1% of the carbohydrate to facilitate the oxidative use of carbohydrates by non-fermenting, gram-negative bacilli. The carbohydrate is in the deep portion of the tube and the amines are near the top. OF glucose is used to determine if an organism ferments or oxidizes glucose or if it is a non-glucose utilizer. Two tubes of OF glucose and one OF basal medium are inoculated. One tube is overlaid with mineral oil to create anaerobic conditions. Following incubation all tubes are observed for changes in colour. **Interpretation:** Positive for fermentation: Yellow throughout the medium in both tubes due to acid production from the fermentation of glucose under anaerobic conditions. Positive for oxidation: The tube exposed to oxygen is yellow at the top, indicating oxidative glucose utilization; the tube under anaerobic conditions will remain green in colour.

Negative for glucose utilization. Neither tube shows a colour change in the presence of bacterial growth, indicating that the organism is not breaking down glucose, but instead is utilizing the amines in the top of the tube.

Examples:
Fermentative: *Enterobacteriaceae*
Oxidative: *Pseudomonas aeruginosa*
Non-glucose utilizers: *Alcaligenes faecalis*

Phenylalanine deaminase

Tests for the organism's ability to oxidatively deaminate phenylalanine to phenylpyruvic acid.

Phenylalanine → phenylpyruvic acid + FeCl$_3$ → green end product

Ferric chloride is added to a phenylalanine slant that has been incubated with organism and observed for a green colour.

Interpretation:
Positive: Green colour develops after ferric chloride is added.
Negative: Slant remains original colour after addition of ferric chloride.

Examples:
Positive: *Proteus vulgaris*
Negative: *Escherichia coli*

PYR hydrolysis

Detection of the enzyme pyrrolidonyl arylamidase is useful in differentiating streptococci and enterococci. The enzyme L-pyrroglutamyl-aminopeptidase hydrolyses the substrate L-pyrrolidonyl-β-naphthylamide (PYR) to produce β-naphthylamine. Broth containing substrate L-pyrrolidonyl-β-naphthylamide (PYR) is inoculated with the organism and incubated. During the incubation PYR is hydrolysed to produce free β-naphthylamine which is then detected by addition of a diazo dye coupler, *N,N*-dimethylaminocinnamaldehyde, producing a colour change to red.

Interpretation:
Positive: Red colour.
Negative: Slight orange colour or no colour.

Examples:
Positive: *Streptococcus pyogenes, Enterococcus* spp.
Negative: other streptococci

Pyruvate broth

The test determines if an organism is able to utilize pyruvate. The test aids in the differentiation of *Enterococcus faecalis* and *Enterococcus faecium*. Pyruvate broth with indicator is inoculated with organism and incubated to allow for organism growth. Following incubation, the tube is observed for a change in colour.

(*cont.*)

Appendix 2.2. (cont.)

Test	Principle/major use/examples of key positive and negative organisms when applicable
	Interpretation: Positive: Yellow. Negative: Medium remains green in colour or turns yellow-green (a weak reaction that is interpreted as negative). Examples: Positive: *Enterococcus faecalis* Negative: *Enterococcus faecium*
Salt tolerance (growth in 6.5% NaCl)	Determines the ability of an organism to grow in high concentrations of salt. The test is used to differentiate enterococci from non-enterococci. Organisms are incubated in a tube containing 6.5% NaCl and in a control tube containing broth without salt. Following incubation tubes are examined for growth. Interpretation: Positive: Growth is equivalent in both the control tube and the tube containing 6.5% NaCl. Negative: Growth in the control, but scant or no growth in the tube containing 6.5% NaCl. Examples: Positive: Enterococci Negative: Non-enterococci
SXT (sulphamethoxazole-trimethoprim) resistance	Determines an organism's ability to tolerate SXT (1.25 µg). A standard quantity of a bacterial suspension is placed on sheep blood agar, and streaked in three directions to produce a lawn of growth. A SXT disc is placed in the centre of the streaked plate. Following incubation and bacterial growth, zones of inhibition are measured around the SXT disc to determine susceptibility. Interpretation: Positive: Zone of inhibition of any size indicates susceptibility. Negative: No zone of inhibition around the disc. Examples: Positive with zone of inhibition of any size: Typical for beta-hemolytic non-Group A, non-Group B streptococci. (Groups C, G, and F) Negative: Beta-hemolytic streptococci Group A and Group B

Triple sugar iron (TSI)

TSI is used to differentiate gram-negative bacilli. The test detects the ability of these organisms to utilize glucose, lactose and sucrose fermentatively and also detects the organism's ability to form hydrogen sulfide. TSI contains 1% lactose and sucrose, 0.1% glucose, peptone, phenol red as an indicator of acidification and ferrous sulfate as an indicator of hydrogen sulfide production. The test detects: (1) the inability of the organism to ferment any of the sugars, using peptone for energy instead; (2) fermentation of glucose only; (3) fermentation of lactose and/or sucrose in addition to glucose; (4) production of gas; and (5) production of hydrogen sulfide. The TSI butt and slant are inoculated with organism and incubated. When glucose is fermented, the entire medium becomes yellow (acidic) within 8–12 hours of incubation. The butt of the tube will remain yellow after 24 hours incubation due to the organic acids building up for the anaerobic fermentation of glucose, but the slant will become red or alkaline from oxidation of the fermentation products under aerobic conditions and the oxidation of peptones in the medium. If lactose and/or sucrose are fermented, the large amount of fermentation products (10× amount of lactose/sucrose than glucose in the medium) formed on the slant will more than neutralize the alkaline amines and the slant will become acid or yellow at 18–24 hours. The formation of CO_2 and H_2 (hydrogen gas) is indicated by bubbles or cracks in the agar. The production of H_2S requires an acidic environment and is demonstrated by blackening of the butt of the medium.

Interpretation:

Amines are utilized; the organism is a non-utilizer of carbohydrates. The butt and slant are red at 18–24 hours.

Glucose is fermented: Yellow slant and yellow butt at 8–12 hours; red slant and yellow butt at 18–24 hours.

Glucose, lactose and/or sucrose fermentation: The butt and the slant are yellow at 24 hours.

Black precipitate in butt: Ferrous sulfide and hydrogen sulfide gas are produced.

Bubbles or cracks: CO_2 or H_2 is produced.

Examples:
Acid/Acid with gas = *Escherichia coli*
Alkaline/Acid with hydrogen sulfide production = *Salmonella typhi*
Alkaline/no change in butt = *Pseudomonas aeruginosa*

Urea hydrolysis

The test determines the organism's ability to produce the enzyme urease, which hydrolyses urea to produce CO_2 and ammonia.

$$NH_3 + H_2O \rightleftharpoons NH_3 + CO_2 + H_2O \rightleftharpoons (NH_4)_2 \, CO_3$$

Organisms are inoculated into urea broth containing a phenol red indicator and incubated. Following incubation the medium is observed for a change in colour from yellow to bright pink (magenta) when the alkaline ammonia is produced from the breakdown of urea.

(*cont.*)

Appendix 2.2. (*cont.*)

Test	Principle/major use/examples of key positive and negative organisms when applicable
	Interpretation: Positive: Change in colour from light orange to magenta. Negative: No change in colour. Examples: Positive: *Proteus vulgaris* Negative: *Escherichia coli*
X and V factors	X and V factors are used to speciate *Haemophilus*. X factor (hemin) is derived from the digestion or degradation of blood. V factor (NAD) is obtained from yeast or potato extract and is produced by some bacteria (*Staphylococcus aureus*). These factors are required either singly or in combination by various species of *Haemophilus*. X and V factors are impregnated on filter strips that can be placed on a nutrient-poor medium along with the organism to be speciated. Following incubation, the plates are observed for growth of organism around the factors. **Interpretation:** X factor is required: Growth around the X factor disc and around the XV factor disc; no growth around V factor disc. V factor is required: Growth around V factor disc and around XV factor disc; no growth around X factor disc. X and V are required: Growth around the XV factor disc, but not around the X factor disc nor the V factor disc. Examples: Requires X factor only: *Haemophilus ducreyi* Requires V factor only: *Haemophilus parainfluenzae* Requires both X and V factors: *Haemophilus influenzae*

Appendix 2.3. antibacterial agents

Class	Agents	Mode of action	Spectrum of activity	Limitations/Comments
Cell wall synthesis inhibitors				
Beta-lactams	Penicillins Penicillin Ampicillin Piperacillin Mezlocillin Cephalosporins Cefazollin Cefuroxime Cefotexan Cefotaxime Ceftriaxone Ceftrazidime Cefepime Carbapenems Imipenem Meropenem Monolactams Aztreonam	Peptidoglycan cannot be produced, inhibiting cell wall synthesis	• Gram-positive bacteria • Gram-negative bacteria	Advantages: • Broad spectrum antibiotics; most bacteria have a cell wall and are therefore susceptible • Penicillins are inexpensive Disadvantages: • Many organisms produce penicillinase • Many mutant organisms are resistant to penicillins
Glycopeptides	Vancomycin	Prevents incorporation of precursors into growing cell	• Gram-positive bacteria only	
Bacitracin		Inhibits recycling of metabolites needed for synthesis of cell wall peptidoglycan		• External use only, due to toxicity

(cont.)

Appendix 2.3. (*cont.*)

Class	Agents	Mode of action	Spectrum of activity	Limitations/Comments
Cell membrane function inhibitors				
Polymyxins	Polymyxin B Colistin	Cell membrane disruption	• Gram-negative bacteria	• Ineffective against most gram-positive bacteria • Toxicity is a concern since human cell membranes may be affected
Protein synthesis inhibitors				
Aminoglycosides	Gentamicin Kanamycin Streptomycin Tobramycin Amikacin Netilmicin	Bind to ribosomal 30S subunit and inhibit protein synthesis (bacteriocidal)	• Gram-positive bacteria • Gram-negative bacteria	• Not effective against anaerobes • Used in conjunction with beta-lactams for maximum killing
Tetracyclines	Paromomycin*	Bind (doxycycline) to ribosomal 30S subunit and inhibits protein synthesis (bacteriostatic)	• Gram-positive bacteria • Gram-negative bacteria • Intracellular pathogens (e.g. chlamydia, rickettsia and rickettsia-like organisms)	
Chloramphenicol		Binds to ribosomal 50S subunit and inhibits protein synthesis (bacteriocidal)	• Gram-positive bacteria • Gram-negative bacteria	• Toxicity is a concern
Macrolides-Lincosamides	Macrolides Erythromycin Azithromycin Clarithromycin Lincosamide Clindamycin	Bind to ribosomal 50S subunit and inhibit protein synthesis	• Most gram-positive bacteria • Some gram-negative bacteria	

Nitrofuran	Binds to 30S subunit and block translation	• GI pathogens *Salmonella* *Shigella* *Proteus* *Aerobacter* *aerogenes* *Vibrio cholerae* *Giardia lamblia*	
Streptogramins	Quinupristin/dalfopristin	Binds to ribosomal 50S subunit at two different sites, inhibiting protein synthesis	• Gram-positive bacteria	
Oxazolidinones	Linezolid	Binds to ribosomal 50S subunit and interferes with initiation of protein synthesis	• Gram-positive bacteria	• Effective against organisms resistant to other agents

Inhibitors of DNA and RNA synthesis

Rifampicin		Binds to DNA- dependent RNA polymerase and inhibits synthesis of RNA	• Gram-positive bacteria • Gram-negative bacteria (certain organisms)	• Used only in combination with other drugs because resistance can develop rapidly • Used in treatment of tuberculosis and meningitis due to *Neisseria meningitidis*
Fluoroquinolones	Ciprofloxacin Norfloxacin Ofloxacin	Bind to DNA gyrases to inhibit DNA synthesis	• Gram-positive bacteria • Gram-negative bacteria	• Broad-spectrum but spectrum may vary with individual antibiotics
Metronidazole		Disrupts DNA; exact mechanism not known	• Gram-negative bacteria • Gram-positive bacteria (certain genera only) • Anaerobes (mainly gram-negative)	• Most effective against anaerobes; activation requires low redox potential

(cont.)

Appendix 2.3. (*cont.*)

Class	Agents	Mode of action	Spectrum of activity	Limitations/Comments
Inhibitors of metabolic processes				
Nitrofurantoin		May directly damage DNA; exact mechanism not known	• Gram-positive bacteria • Gram-negative bacteria	• Used only to treat urinary tract infections
Sulfonamides		Interfere with folic acid production	• Gram-positive bacteria • Many gram-negative bacteria	• Not effective against *Pseudomonas aeruginosa*
Trimethoprim		Interferes with folic acid production	• Gram-positive bacteria • Many gram-negative bacteria	• Used in combination with sulfonamide (e.g. sulfamethoxazole) to target two different sites

* Paromomycin is an antiparasitic, not an antibacterial, target two sites

FURTHER READING FOR ANTIBACTERIAL AGENTS APPENDIX 2.3

http://www.doh.gov.ph/ndps/table_of_contents2.htm

http://www.nlm.nih.gov/medlineplus/druginfo/uspdi/202668.html

http://www.usadrug.com/IMCAccess/ConsDrugs/Atovaquonecd.shtml

http://www.vet.purdue.edu/depts/bms/courses/chmrx/parahd.htm

Alvarew-Elcoro, S. & Enzler, M. J. (1999). The macrolides: erythromycin, clarithromycin, and azithromycin. *Mayo Clinic Proceedings*, **74**: 613–34.

Hellinger, W. C. & Brewer, N. S. (1999). Carbapenems and monobactams: imipenem, meropenem, and aztreonam. *Mayo Clinic Proceedings*, **74**: 420–34.

Henry, N. K., Hoecker, J. L. & Hable, R. K. (2000). Antimicrobial therapy for infants and children: guidelines for the inpatient and outpatient practice of pediatric infectious diseases. *Mayo Clinic Proceedings*, **75**: 86–97.

Kasten, M. J. (1999). Clindamycin, metronidazole, and chloramphenicol. *Mayo Clinic Proceedings*, **74**: 825–33.

Marshall, W. F. & Blair, J. E. (1999). The cephalosporins. *Mayo Clinic Proceedings*, **74**: 187–95.

Osmon, D. R. (2000). Antimicrobial prophylaxis in adults. *Mayo Clinic Proceedings*, **75**: 98–109.

Physician Desk Reference, 54th edn. (2000). Des Moines, Iowa: Medical Economics Co.

Smilack, J. D. (1999). The tetracyclines. *Mayo Clinic Proceedings*, **74**: 727–9.

Virk, A. & Steckelberg, J. M. (2000). Clinical aspects of antimicrobial resistance. *Mayo Clinic Proceedings*, **75**: 200–14.

Walker, R. C. (1999). The fluoroquinolones. *Mayo Clinic Proceedings*, **74**: 1030–7.

Wilhelm, M. P., Estes, L. & Pharm, D. (1999). Vancomycin. *Mayo Clinic Proceedings*, **74**: 928–35.

Wright, A. J. (1999). The penicillins. *Mayo Clinic Proceedings*, **74**: 290–370.

Mycology: moulds and yeasts

Introduction

Medical mycology studies fungi that may produce disease in humans and other animals. Fungi are not related to bacteria: bacteria are prokaryotes, without a membrane-bound nucleus or intracellular organelles; fungi are eukaryotes that have both sexual and asexual reproductive phases, and have membrane-bound organelles including nuclei, mitochondria, golgi apparatus, endoplasmic reticulum, lysosomes, etc. Initially, fungi were thought to be part of the Kingdom of Plantae, albeit lower members of this Kingdom. When the Five Kingdom division of life forms came into general use, however, the fungi were separated into their own Kingdom, separate from the plants, due to their lack of chloroplasts or chlorophyll, the composition of their cell wall and their asexual reproduction by means of spores. Whereas eukaryotes such as plants and algae contain chlorophyll that allows them to generate energy by photosynthesis (autotrophic), fungi lack chlorophyll: they are heterotrophic, and must absorb nutrients from their environment or host. They can be **saprophytes**, living on dead organic matter (e.g. mushrooms, toadstools, bread mould) or **parasites** utilizing living tissues (e.g. yeast infections). Fungi are aerobic and non-motile; they have rigid cell walls composed of complex polysaccharides such as chitins or glucans and their plasma membrane contains sterols, principally ergosterol. They grow best at a neutral pH in a moist environment, but can tolerate a range of pH. Fungal conidia (spores) can survive in dry and harsh conditions. Because fungal cell walls and membranes differ from those of bacteria, they are insensitive to antibiotics. Fungal infections require treatment with antifungal agents, many of which are targeted toward sterol production. Changes in the ergosterol composition of the membrane can lead to drug resistance. Since fungi are eukaryotic, side effects are common with many treatments that are targeted towards eukaryotic cells.

Fungi can be unicellular or multicellular / filamentous, bear conidia (spores) and usually reproduce by both asexual and sexual processes. Asexual reproduction involves simple nuclear and cytoplasmic division, and sexual reproduction involves the fusion of nuclei from two cells to form a zygote. The processes are not exclusive, and a fungus may reproduce in either, or both, ways.

Fungi appear in two basic forms: yeasts and moulds.

1. **Yeasts** are unicellular (single vegetative cells) that generally form smooth colonies like bacteria. Like bacteria, identification is based on macroscopic and microscopic morphology and biochemical testing. Yeasts reproduce by simple budding to form blastoconidia. A few species, such as some *Saccharomyces* used in wine-making and baking, reproduce by fission.

2. **Moulds** are multicellular, composed of a vegetative growth of filaments. Fungal filaments are known as **hyphae**, and a mass of hyphae make up the **mycelium**. 'Hyphae' and 'mycelium' are terms that are used interchangeably.

Table 3.1. Mycology overview: moulds and yeasts

Zygomycota	Ascomycota		Basidiomycota	Deuteromycota	
Moulds	Moulds	Yeasts	Moulds	Moulds	Yeasts
Absidia	*Ajellomyces*	*Saccharomyces*	*Amanita*	*Acremonium*	*Candida*
Basidiobolus	(*Blastomyces* and *Histoplasma*		(*Cryptococcus*	*Alternaria*	*Cryptococcus*
Conidiobolus	teleomorph stages)		teleomorph stage)	*Aspergillus*	*Hansenula*
Cunninghamella	*Arthroderma*			*Bipolaris*	*Malassezia*
Mucor	(*Trichophyton* and *Microsporium*			*Chrysosporium*	*Rhodotorula*
Rhizopus	teleomorph stages)		*Filobasidiella*	*Cladosporium*	*Torulopsis*
Saksenaea	*Pseudallescheria*			*Coccidioides	*Trichosporon*
	Emericella			*Curvularia*	
	(*Aspergillus* teleomorph stage)			*Epidermophyton*	
	Eurotium			*Exophilia*	
	(*Aspergillus* teleomorph stage)			*Fonsecaea*	
	Neosartorya			*Fusarium*	
	(*Aspergillus* teleomorph stage)			*Paecilomyces*	
				*Paracoccidioides	
				Philophora	
				Scedosporium	
				Scopulariopsis	
				*Sporothrix	
				Wangiella	

* Thermally dimorphic.

Dimorphic pathogenic fungi express one distinct form in tissue (the parasitic yeast form) and another form (saprobic or mould) when grown in the environment or in the laboratory on artificial medium under appropriate conditions.

Fungal infections may be pathogenic for immunocompetent individuals, with immunocompromised individuals, post-surgery patients, patients undergoing radiation therapy and chemotherapy and those receiving corticosteroids at much greater risk for infection. In medical mycology both laboratory and clinical classification must be considered. Laboratory classification is based on taxonomy and organism characteristics. Four clinical classifications are based on type of infection and body sites involved, and both yeasts and moulds are included in these categories. Medically important organisms may include those that are usually encountered as contaminants, as well as those that are associated with disease. They are a source of contamination in

the ART laboratory and may cause disease in individuals with a compromised immune system.

Classes of fungi

The Kingdom of fungi is divided into five phyla, based on the method of spore production of the perfect or sexual state (known as the **teleomorphic state**). Of these five phyla, only four are known to contain human pathogens outlined in Table 3.1: *Zygomycota, Ascomycota, Basidiomycota* and *'Fungi Imperfecti'*, or *Deuteromycota*. The fifth phylum is the *Mycophycophyta*, or Lichens, which represent a symbiosis of two organisms – a fungus and an algae. Mycologists now suggest eliminating the Lichens as a Phylum, and instead reclassifying each individual lichen according to its fungal component.

The majority of clinically significant fungi are members of *Deuteromycota*, but members of

Zygomycota, *Ascomycota* and *Basidiomycota* also may cause infection.

Zygomycetes

Bread or pin moulds belong to the **Zygomycetes**. They are rapidly growing, normally found in soil and decaying vegetable matter and may be pathogens in immunocompromised patients. Their hyphae are aseptate or sparsely septate, producing profuse grey to white aerial mycelia. They reproduce asexually, but compatible mating strains can reproduce sexually to produce zygospores. Clinically important zygomycetes include those that can produce subcutaneous and systemic infections, such as *Mucor*, *Rhizopus*, *Absidia* and rarely other species.

Ascomycetes

Ascomycetes are mostly terrestial saprophytes or parasites of plants: there are 28 650 known species. They have septate hyphae, can reproduce asexually via conidiospores, fission, or fragmentation or sexually via ascospores produced in sac-like structures known as **asci**. Asci are frequently located in a fruiting body, or **ascocarp**. Examples include the dermatophyte *Trichophyton* spp., *Pseudallescheria boydii*, and the yeast that is such a well-known favourite to cell biologists, molecular biologists and biochemists: *Saccharomyces cerevisiae*.

Basidiomycetes

Mushrooms and toadstools belong to the **Basidiomycetes**. There are 16 000 species, saprophytic or parasitic, especially of plants. Their hyphae are septate and they reproduce sexually via basidiospores. Occasionally they reproduce asexually via budding, conidia or mycelial fragmentation. They are rarely isolated in clinical labs, but the pathogenic species *Filobasidiella neoformans* is the sexual form of the basidiomycete yeast *Cryptococcus neoformans*, a major threat as an opportunistic infection in immunocompromised patients, especially patients with HIV or AIDS.

Deuteromycotia

Deuteromycotia or **Fungi Imperfecti** (also known as **Hyphomycetes** or conidial moulds) contain the largest number of organisms (17 000 species) that are responsible for cutaneous, subcutaneous and systemic mycoses. They have septate hyphae and reproduce asexually via conidia on hyphae (conidiophores) or from spore-bearing (conidiogenous) cells. Sexual spore production has not yet been observed for this group.

Laboratory classification of fungi

Taxonomic classification

Taxonomically the four divisions: *Zygomycetes*, *Ascomycetes*, *Basidiomycetes* and *Fungi Imperfecti* are distinguished on the basis of: (a) type of colony produced; (b) type of mycelia present; (c) reproduction and characteristic spores (conidia) and (d) rate of growth.

Type of colonies

Type of colonies produced can be described in terms of texture, topography, and colour:

Texture describes the height of aerial hyphae, which can be cottony/woolly, velvety, granular/powdery, or glabrous/waxy.

Topography describes hills and valleys seen on fungal cultures; these are often masked by aerial hyphae, but can be seen on the reverse side of the colony. They can be flat, rugose (deep radiating furrows), umbonate (button-like) or verrucose (wrinkled).

Colonies have a wide variety of *colours*, and their front and reverse sides may be of different colours.

Dematiaceous fungi produce melanin pigment in the vegetative mycelium, with dark hyphal elements and a dark colour on the reverse side of the culture plate. Hyaline moulds are non-pigmented, producing white or colourless vegetative mycelia seen on the reverse side of clear agar culture medium. These may, however, have highly pigmented surface fruiting structures (spores).

Type of mycelia

Hyphae may intertwine to form a mycelium. In culture, aerial hyphae extend above the medium and account for the macroscopic appearance of the colony. There are two kinds of hyphae: *septate* hyphae have frequent cross-walls, and *nonseptate* (coenocytic) or *sparsely septate* hyphae have a few irregularly spaced cross-walls. The septae divide hyphae into compartments, but not into cells. Hyphae may be light or dark. *Hyaline* hyphae are clear or non-pigmented whereas *dematiaceous* ones have melanin in their cell walls, and produce highly pigmented dark brown, green-black, or black colonies. This pigmentation refers to the vegetative mycelium, and not the asexual fruiting structures. Both hyaline and dematiaceous moulds may produce pigmented spores, but dematiaceous moulds alone produce melanin pigment in the hyphae. *Vegetative* hyphae extend downwards into the medium and absorb nutrients, and can form specialized structures of different shapes, important for organism identification: antler, racquet, spiral, nodular, or rhizoid (root-like).

Aerial hyphae can be seen macroscopically extending above the surface of the colony, and these may support structures involved in both asexual and sexual reproduction. Asexual reproduction is nuclear, and sexual reproduction and cytoplasmic division occurs when two nuclei of closely related compatible strains fuse to form a zygote.

Reproduction and characteristic spores (conidia)

Asexual reproduction

During **asexual reproduction** conidiogenous parent cells give rise to conidia. Conidia may originate blastically or thalically and all layers of the parent cell may be involved (holo) or only the inner cell layers (entero). In blastic division, the parent cell enlarges and a septum separates the enlarged portion into a daughter cell. This division may occur in differing arrangements:

(i) holoblastic: all layers of the parent cell are involved in developing daughter conidia (e.g. penicillium),

(ii) enteroblastic: only the inner cell wall layers are included (e.g. philoconidia).

During thalic division, the septum forms first, and a growing point ahead of it becomes a daughter cell (e.g. budding yeasts). This may be:

(i) **holothalic**, with the formation of microconidia and macroconidia, or

(ii) **arthric**, where daughter cells fragment within the hyphal stand before dispersing into arthroconidia. Arthric may be holoblastic (e.g. *Geotrichum*) or enteroblastic (e.g. *Coccidioides immitis*).

Specialized fruiting bodies (e.g. **sporangia**) may also be involved.

The different types of conidia formed are described by their shape and the manner in which they are formed.

(i) **Blastoconidia** are produced from budding as in the case of yeasts or moulds such as *Cladosporium.*

(ii) **Poroconidia** are formed when the daughter cells push through a minute pore in the parent cell (e.g. *Dreschlera*). The parent may be a specialized conidiogenous cell or a long stalk, a conidiophore (e.g. *Alternaria*).

(iii) **Philoconidia** are elicited from a tube-like structure called a phialide (e.g. *Penicillium*).

(iv) **Annelloconidia** are grown inside a vase-shaped conidiogenous annelide (e.g. *Scopulariopsis*).

(v) **Macroconidia** arise from conversion of an entire hyphal element into a multi-celled conidium (e.g. *Microsporum canis*). Macroconidia may be thin-walled or thick-walled, spiny or smooth, club-shaped or oval, sessile or supported by conidiophores, and may appear as individuals or in clusters.

(vi) **Microconidia** develop from the conversion of an entire hyphal element, but the new conidium remains aseptate (e.g. *Trichophyton rubrum*). Microconidia are one-celled and may be round or oval, sessile or support, and appear individually or in clusters.

(vii) **Chlamydoconidia** (e.g. *Gliocladium*) are thick-walled survival conidia formed during unfavourable conditions that germinate and produce conidia when conditions are more favourable.

(viii) **Arthroconidia** are produced by fragmenting from hyphae through the septation points (e.g. *Coccidioides immitis*). They may be rectangular or barrel-shaped and maybe separated by disjunctor cells.

(ix) **Sporangiospores** are formed by internal cleavage of a sac, called a sporangium (e.g. *Zygomyces*).

Sexual reproduction

Forms of **sexual reproduction** are important for divisions in taxonomy. Three different types of sexual reproduction (**teleomorphic states**) can be recognized:

(i) A nucleus from a male cell (**antheridium**) passes through a bridge into a female cell (**ascogonium**); male and female cells may be from the same colony, or from two compatible colonies. Following fusion to form the zygote, the female cell becomes an **ascus**. The diploid zygote nucleus divides by meiosis to form 4 haploid nuclei, which then divide by mitosis to form 8 nuclei. Each new nucleus is then walled inside the ascus to form an **ascospore**, e.g. the yeast *Saccharomyces cerevisiae* and the mould *Pseudallescheria boydii*.

(ii) Two compatible **hyphae** or yeast cells can fuse to form a binucleate mycelium; the terminal end of the mycelium enlarges into a club-shaped structure, a **basidium**. The two nuclei within the basidium fuse to form a zygote that then undergoes meiosis to produce 4 haploid nuclei, or **basidiospores** that extend out of the basidium.

e.g. *Filobasidiela neoformans*, the sexual stage of *Cryptococcus neoformans*.

(iii) Two compatible hyphae can each form an extending arm, the **zygophore**. When the zygophores meet, they fuse to form a thick-walled protective zygosporangium, within which **zygospores** develop. This process can happen within the same, or between two different compatible colonies.

e.g. the zygomycetes, including *Mucor*, *Rhizopus*, and *Absidia*.

Growth rate

Fungi may grow rapidly or slowly. Moulds may grow rapidly (3–4 days) or may require 3–4 weeks. Rate of growth is affected by type of media, incubation temperature and inhibitors in the patient's specimen. The majority of yeasts and many of the moulds considered to be clinical contaminants require only 2–3 days for growth.

Clinical classification of fungi

Infections

The majority of fungi are mesophilic, and cannot grow at 37 °C; many are saprophytic, and grow more efficiently on non-living substrates than on living tissue. The human body also has a highly efficient defence mechanism to combat fungal proliferation. Therefore, in general the development of fungal disease is related to the immunological status of the host and environmental exposure, rather than to the infecting organism. The relatively small number of fungi that can cause disease have unique enzyme pathways, exhibit thermal dimorphism, and are able to block cell-mediated immune defences in the host. 'Opportunistic' fungi cause infections in debilitated patients with compromised immune systems. Altogether, around 200 human pathogens have been recognized from among an estimated 1.5 million species of fungi. Human fungal diseases include dermatomycoses (skin, hair and nail diseases), yeast infections, pulmonary mycoses, subcutaneous mycoses (infection is traumatically introduced into tissues) and opportunistic fungal disease.

Superficial

Superficial infections are confined to the outermost layer of skin or hair (e.g. epidermis and hair shaft). Living tissue is not invaded and there is no cellular response from the host. Symptoms are primarily cosmetic: discoloration or depigmentation and scaling of skin. These fungi are usually identified in the practitioner's office on the basis of clinical appearance. Examples of superficial fungi are:

Malassezia furfur, which causes tinea versicolor.

Piedraia hortae, which causes black piedra on scalp hair.

Trichosporon beigelii, a yeast that causes white piedra of facial and genital hair.

Exophilia werneckii, which causes tinea nigra of the soles and palms.

Cutaneous

Cutaneous infections are caused by dermatophytes and affect the keratinized layer of skin, hair, and nails. No living tissue is invaded, but the presence of the fungus and its metabolic products causes itching, scaling, broken hair, and thick and discoloured nails. Three genera are etiologic agents of dermatophytoses:

Trichophyton species affect both endothrix and ectothrix hair, skin and nails. They typically cause 'jock itch' and ringworm, but may be responsible for more serious infections, including pustules covering the entire body as well as permanent alopecia.

Epidermophyton primarily infects adults, causing 'jock itch' and 'athlete's foot'.

Microsporum species primarily infect children, and may be spread from person to person or via cats and dogs.

Subcutaneous

Subcutaneous infections are chronic localized infections affecting deeper skin layers such as muscle and connective tissue, and usually do not disseminate. Infection is frequently the result of traumatic implantation of a foreign object into deeper tissue. Because the etiologic agents are found in decaying vegetation and soil, the extremities are usually involved. Infections are characterized by nodular lesions that can suppurate and ulcerate and by the presence of draining sinus tracts. Subcutaneous infections include:

Sporotrichosis or 'rose gardener's disease' caused by *Sporothrix schenckii*.

Chromoblastomycosis, caused by dematiaceous mould that produces sclerotic bodies such as *Cladosporium carionii* or *Philaphora verrucosa*.

Mycetomas may be caused by bacteria (*Actinomycetes*) or fungi (eumycotic mycetoma). Madura foot is an example of eumycotic mycetoma.

Subcutaneous phaeohyphomycosis, caused by species of *Exophilia* and by *Wangiella dermatiditis*, is a more serious infection than superficial phaeohyphomycosis (tinea nigra and black piedra), and this disease is becoming a major concern for immunocompromised patients.

Systemic

Systemic infections affect internal organs and/or deep tissue. They may be caused by almost any fungus if the patient is immunocompomised, but traditionally the systemic infections refer to infections that initially occur in the lungs and disseminate hematogenously with symptoms of fatigue, fever, chronic cough and chest pain. They are caused by the dimorphic fungi, *Histoplasma capsulatum*, *Coccidioides immitis*, *Blastomyces dermatidis*, and *Paracoccidioides brasiliensis*, all of which have endemic areas.

Atypical fungus

Pneumocystis carinii, an opportunistic fungus that infects immunocompromised individuals, remains unclassified. The organism has several characteristics in common with parasites: it has cyst and trophozoite stages, and responds to antiparasitic agents and not to antifungal agents. It was originally thought to be a trypanosome, but DNA sequencing studies reveal that the organism has greater DNA homology with fungi than with parasites, and is an atypical fungus with cholesterol instead of ergosterol in the cell membrane.

It is now classified somewhere between the ascomycetes and the basidiomycetes. *P. carinii* is found worldwide, and it replicates in the alveoli of the lung to produce pneumonia when it is inhaled by immunocompromised hosts (particularly HIV/AIDS patients). *P. carinii* cysts and trophozoites can be detected on Giemsa-stained BAL or biopsy specimens. Antigen detection systems can also be used for diagnosis, and nucleic acid amplification systems are under development.

Yeasts

Yeasts are classified as 'yeasts', meaning that they reproduce sexually by forming either ascospores or basidiospores or as 'yeast-like fungi', which either cannot reproduce sexually or the sexual stage has yet to be demonstrated. In the laboratory all are referred to simply as yeasts. Yeasts grow on bacteriological media as well as on mycology media, and growth can be seen in 2–3 days at 25–30 °C. They generally form smooth colonies that resemble bacteria, and species have characteristic colours: white to cream or tan, a few pink to salmon or red, and some are dematiaceous (pigmented). Isolates vary in texture, from butter-like to velvety or wrinkled, and some (*Cryptococcus*) are mucoid due to capsule production. Strain variation may be seen; phenotypic switching occurs so that two colony types will be noted on subculture. Evaluation of yeasts in the clinical laboratory generally includes a germ-tube or other assay to rapidly identify *C. albicans*, microscopic exam to determine yeast size, a nitrate and urease test (if *Cryptococcus neoformans* is suspected), a sugar assimilation assay and a Tween Cornmeal (TOC) agar culture to determine tertiary structure formation such as pseudohyphae and chlamydospores.

Candida spp.

The incidence of clinically significant yeast infections has increased dramatically, as a result of immunosuppressive therapies. *C. albicans* is the fourth most common cause of blood-borne infection in the USA, and infections with other *Candida* species is also increasing, e.g. *C. tropicalis, C. parapsilosis*: these are very aggressive and difficult to treat. The clinically significant yeasts include:

Candida albicans	*C. tropicalis*
C. parapsilosis	*C. krusei*
C. guilliermondi	*C. lusitaniae*
Cryptococcus neoformans	*Rhodotorula* spp.
Candida (Torulopsis) glabrata	*Sacccharomyces cerevisiae*
Geotricum sp.	*Trichosporon beigelii*
Malassezia furfur	

and the dematiaceous yeasts, *Wangiella dermatiditis* and *Exophilia*.

Candida albicans occurs naturally as a commensal of mucous membranes and in the digestive tract of humans and animals, but it accounts for up to 70% of *Candida* species isolated from sites of infection. Environmental isolates are usually from sources contaminated by human or animal excreta, such as polluted water, soil, air and plants. It causes all types of candidiasis (also known as moniliasis), with diseases ranging from superficial skin infections, oral infections (thrush) and gastritis, to disseminated disease. Oral thrush may be an indication of immunosuppression, and immunocompromised patients can develop disseminated candidiasis. The majority of HIV patients develop thrush, which leads to retrosternal odynophagia (pain on swallowing) in 80% of cases. Patients undergoing chemotherapy may also acquire thrush that can disseminate. Increased blood glucose levels in diabetic patients predispose to thrush infections, as do riboflavin deficiency, oral contraceptives, and antibiotic therapy. *C. albicans*, and other species of *Candida* are discussed in detail in Chapter 8 as agents of vaginitis.

Microscopic morphology of *C. albicans* shows spherical to subspherical budding yeast-like cells or blastoconidia, 2.0–7.0 × 3.0–8.5 μm in size, with pseudohyphae and true hyphae; it grows at 37 °C, 42 °C, and 45 °C. The majority of cases can be diagnosed by a Germ tube or rapid biochemical *Candida albicans* screen.

Candida tropicalis causes aggressive infections, including oral thrush, vaginitis, endophthalmitis, endocarditis, arthritis, peritonitis and mycotic keratitis. It is a major cause of septicemia and disseminated candidiasis, especially in patients with lymphoma, leukemia and diabetes. It is found as part of the normal human mucocutaneous flora, but is the second most frequently encountered medical pathogen, second to *C. albicans*.

In culture, it resembles *C. albicans*, but has only pseudohyphae, and no true hyphae. Sugar assimilation is required to correlate with the TOC culture for definitive identification of all non-albicans yeasts. Infections are resistant to amphotericin B, and are difficult to treat with traditional antifungal therapy.

Candida glabrata is one of the most common yeast species found on the body surface and is often isolated as an incidental finding from skin and urine. It accounts for about 25% of all non-albicans fungal infections seen in the clinical laboratory. Its microscopic morphology shows numerous ovoid, budding yeast-like cells or blastoconidia, $2.0-4.0 \times 3.0-5.5 \, \mu m$ in size. No pseudohyphae or other tertiary structures are produced on TOC culture. This organism utilizes only glucose and trehalose in sugar assimilation assays.

Candida parapsilosis is a major cause of outbreaks of nosocomial infections in hospitals; it can cause endophthalmitis, endocarditis, vaginitis, external ear infections and septicaemia. Nosocomial infections are frequently associated with prolonged use of central venous catheters and can lead to fungemia in immunocompromised patients. In the laboratory it grows at 37 °C, but not at 42 °C and 45 °C. Sugar assimilation and TOC culture are required for definitive identification.

Other *Candida* spp. are occasionally seen in the clinical microbiology laboratory, either as contaminants or in immunocompromised patients such as those with diabetes, malignancies, patients receiving prolonged corticosteroids or antibiotics and intravenous (IV) drug abusers. Definitive identification requires intravenous (TOC) culture and sugar assimilation.

Cryptococcus neoformans is another important pathogenic yeast that causes pulmonary infection and disseminated infections in immunocompromised patients. This yeast is a soil contaminant from pigeon droppings, and represents a major cause of opportunistic infections in AIDS patients, including meningitis. It is characterized by the presence of a slime capsule with anti-phagocytic properties that serves as a virulence factor. Non-pathogenic strains of the other *Cryptococcus* spp. do not have this capsule. *C. neoformans* is nitrate and urease positive, produces only blastoconidia (budding yeasts) on TOC culture and requires sugar assimilation for definitive identification to separate it from the non-pathogenic cryptococci that are seen as contaminants.

Geotrichum candidum is part of the normal flora in the human mouth and skin and can be found in the stool. It most commonly causes bronchial infections, but can cause oral, intestinal, vaginal, hand and skin and (rarely) systemic infections. It is found as a contaminant in soil, cottage cheese, milk and decaying foods such as tomatoes. Laboratory identification is by direct mount examination, where fragmenting hyphae can be seen – these have non-alternating rectangular arthroconidia with rounded ends. Blastoconidia are not produced.

Wangiella dermatitidis and *Exophilia jensmaleii* are two dematiaceous yeast-like moulds that are pathogenic to humans, and may cause cutaneous and subcutaneous mycoses. They grow very slowly, producing black yeast-like colonies whose reverse is also black after 3–4 weeks. They also colonize the gut and are frequently cultured from stool specimens if mycology cultures are ordered. These two organisms can be differentiated from one another on the basis of their optimal growth temperature (*Exophilia* grows only up to 38 °C, while *Wangiella* grows up to 42 °C), and on the basis of casein, tyrosine and xanthine hydrolysis patterns. They may be found as laboratory contaminants.

Trichosporon beigelii and *Malassezia furfur* are agents of superficial mycoses. *Malassezia furfur* is

Table 3.2. Organisms which are contaminants, but may cause infection

Zygomycetes
Aseptate hyphae, Sexual reproduction via
zygospores
Asexual sporangia (or similar specialized
structures) bear asexual conidia

Mucorales	Endomorphorales	Other hyaline contaminants	Dematiaceous moulds
Rhizopus (#1 cause of infection)	*Basidiobolus* subcutaneous disease	*Penicillium*	*Alternaria*
Mucor	*Conidiobolus* rhinofacial disease	*Paecilomyces*	*Aureobasidium*
Absidia (#2 cause of infection)	• Aseptate (less so than the	*Scopulariopsis*	*Bipolaris*
Rhizomucor	Mucorales)	*Gliocladium*	*Cladosporium*
Apophysomyces	• Splendore–Hoppeli material	*Fusarium*	*Curvularia*
Saksenaea	present	*Acremonium*	*Dreshlera*
Mortiterella	• Infections in	*Chryseosporium* (resembles	*Epicoccum*
Syncephalastrum	immunocompetent	*Blastomyces dermatitidis*)	*Nigrospora*
Cunninghamella	individuals	*Sepedonium* (resembles	*Stemphylium*
Cokeromyces	• Not angioinvasive	*Histoplasma capsulatum*)	*Ulocladium*
• Cause infections in		*Aspergillus fumigatus*	
immunocompromised		*Aspergillus niger*	
individuals		*Aspergillus flavus*	
• Splendore–Hoppeli material		*Aspergillus terreus*	
not present		*Aspergillus nidulans*	
• Angioinvasive			

further implicated in causing line sepsis in neonates receiving lipid supplemented hyperalimentation.

Contaminants

Zygomycetes

Contaminants include members of the *Zygomycetes*, other hyaline contaminants (including *Aspergillus* species and penicillin producers), and dematiaceous or dark moulds (Table 3.2). The *Zygomycetes* are hyaline moulds with aseptate, ribbon-like hyphae with great variation in width. They grow rapidly and produce an abundant mycelium that frequently pushes the lid off the petri dish. The *Zygomycetes* reproduce sexually via zygospores and asexual sporangia (or similar specialized structures) and bear asexual conidia. *Rhizopus, Mucor, Absidia* and *Rhizomucor*

are frequent contaminants. The penicillin producers are hyaline moulds that frequently have pigmented microconidia and surface colony coloration on the reverse side of the plate. They have septate hyphae with rather uniform diameters. Penicillin producers grow rapidly producing flat colonies that are frequently powdery, and all have characteristic microscopic morphology. Members include *Penicillum* spp., *Paecilomyces* spp., *Scopulariopsis* spp. and *Gliocladium* spp.

Aspergillus species are hyaline moulds with septate hyphae. Colonies are low growing and velvety, with highly pigmented surfaces. The *Aspergillus* species reproduce asexually by producing strings of conidia from conidigenous cells arranged in swollen vesicles. *Aspergillus fumigatus, A. niger, A. flavus, A. nidulans,* and *A. terreus* may be seen as contaminants in the laboratory, and are discussed in

Chapter 13. Other hyaline moulds seen as contaminants include species of *Fusarium, Acrimonium, Chrysoporium*, and *Sepedonium*. Each of these moulds produces a septate mycelium and may be differentiated on the basis of their microscopic morphology and sporulation characteristics.

Dematiaceous moulds seen as contaminants include species of *Alternaria, Bipolaris, Cladosporium, Curvularia, Aureobasidium, Dreshlera, Epicoccum, Nigrospora, Stemphylium* and *Ulocladium*. The dematiaceous fungal contaminants are dark on top and dark on the reverse. Both conidia and hyphae are generally pigmented. Organisms are differentiated on the basis of colony characteristics, conidia morphology and distribution of conidia and macroconidia. *Aureobasidium pullans* produces thick-walled dematiaceous fungal hyphae and oval blastoconidia. The organism grows as a yeast-like black colony whose reverse is also black. They have a rapid growth rate, with colonies visible within 7 days. *Aureobasidium pullans* is often seen as a biofilm producer and thus may be cultured from water baths, incubator water pans and other moist environments.

Although the fungi listed in this section are generally considered contaminants in clinical specimens, most can produce disease in humans given the correct conditions (Table 3.2). Many are considered opportunists, producing disease in immunocompromised individuals. AIDS-defining opportunistic pathogens are described in Chapter 12, in Table 12.1.

Laboratory identification of fungi

Specimens must be properly collected for fungal identification and should be transported to the laboratory and processed as quickly as possible. Direct microscopic examination of specimens provides a rapid report to the physician and provides important information leading to identification, including:

(i) documentation of specific morphological characteristics that might provide a clue to genus identification;

(ii) clues as to appropriate media for inoculation;

(iii) possible evidence of a positive culture when the patient is on antifungal medication.

Direct examination

Direct examination for fungal elements generally uses some form of wet preparation, including saline wet preparations, potassium hydroxide (KOH) preps or KOH with calcofluor and India ink preparations. KOH dissolves keratin and other cellular elements in the sample and calcofluor binds to polysaccharides present in the chitin of the fungus cell wall. Since any element with a polysaccharide skeleton will fluoresce, fungal elements must be visualized. India ink stain is used to observe yeast cells and the capsule of *Cryptococcus neoformans* in cerebral spinal fluid, although it should be noted that the capsule may not be present, especially in the strain that tends to infect patients with AIDS.

Several additional stains are commonly used to detect fungal elements in tissue sections.

(i) The Giemsa or Wright's Giemsa stain detects *Histoplasma capsulatum* and other yeast forms in blood or bone marrow.

(ii) The Masson–Fontana stain stains melanin in the cell wall and is used to detect dematiaceous fungi.

(iii) Periodic-acid–Schiff (PAS) attaches to polysaccharides in the fungal wall, staining fungal elements a magenta color.

(iv) The Gormori methenamine–silver (GMS) stain, probably the most commonly used fungal stain, detects fungal elements by staining the fungal wall septations grey-black against a background of green tissue elements.

Culture

Direct examination for fungi should always be linked to appropriate culture techniques, since the direct exam is relatively insensitive and cannot speciate any organisms detected. Because cultures must be held for a long time, specimens from sites that might be colonised with bacteria must be plated onto antibiotic-containing medium. Unlike bacteria, fungi do not have a wide range of nutritional and environmental requirements. Therefore, only a few types of media are needed for primary isolation, such as:

(i) Sabouraud dextrose agar or SDA, a nutritionally poor medium with pH 5.6 used for the initial isolation of pathogens and saprobes.

(ii) Sabouraud brain heart infusion agar (SABHI), more enriched than SDA for initial isolation.

(iii) Brain heart infusion agar with Blood (BHIAB), which is of limited use since contaminants and pathogens will grow (used for the isolation of *Histoplasma* and *Nocardia*).

(iv) BHIAB with antibiotics, used to recover slow-growing dimorphic pathogens while inhibiting the growth of bacteria in clinical specimens.

(v) Inhibitory mould agar contains gentamicin, and is used for initial isolation of fungi, again inhibiting bacteria present in the sample.

(vi) Dermatophyte test medium replaces SDA and is used to recover dermatophytes.

(vii) Cornmeal agar enhances blastoconidia formation of yeasts isolated in culture.

(viii) Birdseed agar is used for the isolation and identification of *Cryptococcus neoformans* from yeast colonies identified on initial culture.

(ix) Chrom-agar is now available for rapid identification of yeasts.

Fungi grow optimally at 25–30 °C, with slower growth at the lower temperature. If a dimorphic fungus is suspected, cultures should also be incubated at 37 °C. Cultures are maintained for 4–6 weeks, and for 12 weeks if *Histoplasma capsulatum* is suspected, with twice weekly examination to record rate of growth and gross morphology of the colony (e.g. colour, topography).

Microscopic examination for fungal structures

Several types of preparations can be made, including tease preparation, cellophane tape preparation and slide culture. Slide culture is ideal for observing fungal structures, but since it requires culture it is more difficult and delays the clinical report. Regardless of the type of preparation, the following characteristics should be observed:

(i) septate vs. non-septate hyphae,

(ii) hyaline or dematiaceous hyphae,

(iii) types, size, shape and arrangement of conidia.

Yeasts are cultured on cornmeal agar medium, and identification includes their biochemistry as well as the appearance of specific structures.

Germ tubes, hyphal-like extensions of yeast cells are formed with no constriction at the point of origin of the cell. They have parallel sides, and are non-septate. These differ from pseudohyphae, formed when blastoconidia elongate. Pseudohyphae constrict at the point of origin and true hyphae do not; they may elongate, and may be septate.

Blastoconidia are formed from true budding. Further identification relies on capsule and ascopore production, as well as assimilation reactions, urease and nitrate production, temperature sensitivity and cycloheximide tolerance.

Special media (Birdseed agar) is used to culture *Cryptococcus neoformans*. Oxidase production by *C. neoformans* is observed as a brown colour on the agar.

Mycology in ART

In the context of ART treatment, there are two areas of mycology that must be considered:

(i) contamination of laboratory equipment or culture systems by moulds or yeasts, from the environment or via clinical/laboratory staff. This topic is covered in Chapter 13;

(ii) clinically significant yeasts, especially those responsible for vaginitis are discussed in Chapter 8. Culture systems can easily be infected with yeasts transferred during oocyte retrieval procedures (see Chapter 13, Fig. 13.2).

FURTHER READING

Anaissie, E. J., McGinnis, M. R. & Pfaller, M. A. (2003). *Clinical Mycology*. New York: Churchill Livingston, Elsevier Science.

Chandler, F. W. & Watts, J. C. (1987). *Pathologic Diagnosis of Fungal Infections*. Chicago: ASCP Press.

Ellis, D. H. (2001). An introduction to medical mycology. Mycology Unit, Women's and Children's Hospital, Adelaide. From: *Mycology Online*, http://www.mycology.adelaide.edu.au

Fisher, F. & Cook, N. (1998). *Fundamentals of Mycology*. Philadelphia, PA: W. B. Saunders Co.

Forbes, B. A., Sahm, D. F. & Weissfeld, A. S. (2002). *Diagnostic Microbiology*, 11th edn. St. Louis: Mosby Publishers.

Kern, M. E. & Blevins, K. S. (1997). *Medical Mycology: A Self-Instruction Text*, 2nd edn. Philadelphia, PA: F. A. Davis Co.

Kwon-Chung, K. J. & Bennett, J. E. (1992). *Medical Mycology*. Philadelphia, PA: Lea & Febiger.

Koneman, E. W., Allen, S. D., Janda, W. M., Schreckenberger, P. C. & Winn, W. C. (1997). Mycology. In *Color Atlas and Textbook of Diagnostic Microbiology*, 5th edn, pp. 983–1070. Philadelphia PA: Lippincott.

Larone, D. H. (1993). *Medically Important Fungi: A Guide to Identification*, 2nd edn. Washington, DC: ASM Press.

Ribes, J. A., Vanover-Sams, C. V. & Baker, D. J. (2000). Zygomycetes in human disease. *Clinical Microbiology Reviews* **13**, 236–301.

St-Germain, G. & Summerbell, R. (1996). *Identifying Filamentous Fungi: A Clinical Laboratory Handbook*. Belmont, CA: Star Publishing Co.

Appendix 3.1. antifungal agents

Class	Agents	Mode of action	Indications	Limitations/comments
Polyenes	Amphotericin B deoxycholate	Binds to ergosterol in cell wall of susceptible fungi resulting in alteration of membrane permeability; leakage of cellular contents leads to cell death.	Most species of fungi causing human infection are susceptible to amphotericin B deoxycholate; main indications are: • Candidiasis • Cryptococcosis • Aspergillosis • Blastomycosis • Histoplasmosis • Coccidioidomycosis	Resistance is a problem with *Pseudallescheria boydii*, *Fusarium* species, *Candida lusitaniae*, *Trichosporon* species and some agents of chromoblastomycosis and phaeohyphomycosis as well as occasional isolates of other *Candida* species, including *C. albicans* and *Aspergillus* species • Toxicity is a problem, especially nephrotoxicity
	Amphotericin B lipid complex		Treatment of invasive fungal infections in patients refractory to, or intolerant of, amphotericin B deoxycholate	Lipid vehicles; less nephrotoxic than amphotericin B deoxycholate
	Amphotericin B cholesteryl sulfate		Invasive aspergillosis in patients with renal impairment, those where amphotericin B deoxycholate has failed, or toxicity precludes use	Lipid vehicles; less nephrotoxic than amphotericin B deoxycholate
	Liposomal amphotericin B		Aspergillosis, candidiasis or cryptococcosis in patients who cannot tolerate or who have not responded to amphotericin B deoxycholate	Lipid vehicles; less nephrotoxic than amphotericin B deoxycholate
	Mycostatin		*Candida* species	Topical use
Flucytosine		Two primary mechanisms: 1. Conversion by cytosine deaminase into 5-fluorouracil with subsequent conversion through intermediates into 5-fluorouridine triphosphate; incorporation into fungal RNA leads to miscoding. 2. Conversion by uridine monophosphate phophosphorylase into 5-fluoro-deoxyuridine monophosphate, inhibits thymidylate synthetase and DNA synthesis.	*Cryptococcus neoformans* and *Candida* species In conjunction with amphotericin B deoxycholate for invasive aspergillosis.	Usually administered with amphotericin B for systemic mycoses, especially cryptococcal meningitis Possible role as sole therapy for the treatment of chromoblastomycosis
Azoles	Ketoconazole	Interfere with synthesis and permeability of fungal cell membranes. Inhibits the cytochrome P-450 enzyme responsible for conversion of lanosterol to ergosterol, the major sterol found in most fungal cell membranes.	Histoplasmosis – second line agent Blastomycosis – second line agent Candidiasis – as alternative to fluconazole Coccidioidomycosis – second line agent Paracoccidioidomycosis – second line agent *Pseudallescheria boydii*	Due to newer triazoles, ketoconazole is now used infrequently for systemic fungal infections; considered an alternative agent. Not recommended for patients with *C. immitis* meningitis or those who are seriously ill with any type of *Coccidioides* infection. Not available in parenteral form.

	Drug	Mechanism	Clinical uses	Comments
	Fluconazole (triazole derivative)		Esophageal, oropharyngeal, vaginal, peritoneal, genitourinary and disseminated candidiasis; Cryptococcal meningitis; Superficial dermatophyte infections (tinea cruris and tinea versicolor); Coccidioidomycosis; Paracoccidioidomycosis	Broad spectrum; Generally safe and well tolerated; No advantage over topical agents for superficial infections; Can be administered intravenously; May be alternative to amphotericin B in patients with coccidioidal meningitis, disseminated histoplasmosis in AIDS patients, blastomycosis, sporotrichosis; Studies suggest this as the drug of choice for paracoccidioidomycosis
	Iatraconazole (triazole derivative)		Superficial mycoses, including dermatophytosis, oral and vaginal candidiasis, mucocutaneous candidiasis and tinea versicolor; Onychomycosis; Sporotrichosis; Histoplasmosis; Blastomycosis; Aspergillosis; Cryptococcosis; Coccidioidomycosis; Candidiasis; Paracoccidioidomycosis; Chromoblastomycosis	Broad spectrum; Highly lipid soluble; Studies suggest use for chromoblastomycosis due to *Fonsecaea*, especially *Cladosporium*; Some success in treatment of HIV-positive patients with disseminated *Penicillium marneffei* infection; Drug of choice for paracoccidioidomycosis
	Clotrimazole		Broad spectrum for topical use	Vaginal cream
	Miconazole		Broad spectrum for topical use	Vaginal cream
Other	Terbinafine	Hypothesized to inhibit squalene epoxidase, blocking biosynthesis of ergosterol, an essential component of the fungal cell wall.	Nail infections – topical form	
Other	Ciclopirox		Nail infections	
Other	Tolfinafine		Treatment of tinea pedis	
Other	Nafidine		Dermatophyte infections, especially ringworm; *Candida* infections	
Other	Griseofulvin	Inhibits synthesis of hyphal cell walls; binds to RNA, inhibiting microtubule function and nucleic acid synthesis.	Dermatophyte infections	

FURTHER READING

ANTIFUNGAL AGENTS

http://www.doh.gov.ph/ndps/table of contents2.htm

http://www.nlm.nih.gov/medlineplus/druginfo/uspdi/202668.html

http://www.usadrug.com/IMCAccess/ConsDrugs/Atovaquonecd.shtml

Henry, N. K., Hoecker, J. L., Rhodes, K. & Hable, M. D. (2000). Antimicrobial therapy for infants and children: guidelines for the inpatient and outpatient practice of pediatric infectious diseases, *Mayo Clinic Proceedings*, **75**, 86–97.

Patel, R. (1998). Antifungal agents part I, Amphotericin B preparations and Flucytosine. *Mayo Clinic Proceedings*, **73**, 1205–25.

Physician Desk Reference. (2000). 54th Edn, Des Moines, IA: Medical Economics Co.

Sarosi, G. A. & Davies, S. F. (1994). Therapy for fungal infections. *Mayo Clinic Proceedings*, **69**, 1111–17.

Terrell, C. L. (1999). Antifungal agents II, the azoles. *Mayo Clinic Proceedings*, **74**, 78–100.

Virk, A. & Steckelberg, J. M. (2000). Clinical aspects of antimicrobial resistance. *Mayo Clinic Proceedings*, **75**, 200–14.

4

Virology

Introduction

Viruses are obligate intracellular parasites, i.e. they require an animal, plant or bacterial cell for growth, survival and replication. The virus genome can consist of either DNA or RNA, and they use the host cell replication and protein synthesis machinery for their own growth and replication. Viruses do not have features that previously were thought to be necessary for any living organism: they do not respire, move or grow, produce waste products, utilize energy or display irritability; they do, however, have the ability to replicate inside eukaryotic or prokaryotic host cells. Viruses that infect bacteria are known as bacteriophages, and there are large numbers of viruses that infect plants, with significant impact on horticulture and crops.

Until the recent discovery of prions, viruses were described as the smallest known entities that can cause disease. Their size ranges from 20 nm (poliovirus) to around 400 nm (poxviruses). The smallest known bacterium is around 200 nm (mycoplasma), and the larger ones such as staphylococci are around 500 nm in size. Viruses therefore pass readily through bacterial filters (normally 220 nm) and they can only be visualized by electron microscopy, using negative staining (see Fig. 1.3).

Virus structure

The viral nuclei acid **genome** may consist of DNA or RNA (but never both), and this can be double-stranded, single-stranded, segmented or non-segmented, with positive or negative strand orientation. Viruses have no ribosomes, enzymes or ATP synthesizing machinery and use those of their host cell to carry out the functions necessary for their replication. The viral genome is enclosed by a protein coat, the capsid, which is made up of morphologic protein subunits, the capsomeres. The combination of the viral genome inside the capsid is known as the nucleocapsid. Some viruses have an additional outer membrane, the viral envelope, and viruses that have a viral envelope require this membrane for infectivity. The combination of nucleocapsid and viral envelope is referred to as the complete virion. For non-enveloped viruses, the nucleocapsid alone represents the infective virion. The viral envelope is derived from either the nuclear or the cytoplasmic membrane of the host cell, and it has embedded virus-specific proteins. It is gathered at the end of the replication process when the virus exits the cell. Some envelopes contain 'spikes' (peplomers), which are used to attach to the host cell. Peplomers determine host specificity, and also induce neutralizing antibody. Stripping off the envelope results in loss of virus infectivity.

Virus morphology can take polygonal, helical or complex forms. The virus capsid is usually symmetrical, either icosahedral (shell-like) or helical (tube-like). The capsid may determine host specificity, and it increases efficiency of infection, protects nucleic acids from degradation, and can also induce the formation of virus-neutralizing antibodies in the host.

Host range and specificity

Viruses infect and multiply in specific host cells only. This specificity is determined by specific interaction in virus attachment to host cells, or by the availability of cellular factors required for viral replication. Therefore, viruses that infect bacteria cannot infect animal or plant cells, and animal viruses generally infect a specific range of cells only, i.e. viruses that infect nerve cells may not necessarily infect the cells of the GI tract. This feature is known as cell **tropism**.

Viral replication

Viral replication consists of specific stages.
  (i) Attachment to host cell and entry. (Since plant cells are surrounded by a thick wall of cellulose, plant viruses rely on mechanical breach of the cell wall, either by an insect vector or by mechanical damage).
 (ii) Replication of viral nucleic acids.
(iii) Synthesis of viral proteins with three sets of functions:
       (a) ensure replication of the genome,
       (b) package the genome into virus particles,
       (c) alter the metabolism of the infected cell so that virus particles are produced.
 (iv) Assembly of viral components.
  (v) Escape from host cells.
This process takes place in three different phases:
  (i) The **initiation** phase introduces the genetic material of the virus into the cell, with attachment, penetration and uncoating of the viral genome.
 (ii) The **replication** phase involves synthesis of DNA, RNA and proteins. In a few cases cellular enzymes replicate the viral genome assisted by viral proteins (e.g. parvovirus), but in the majority, viral proteins are responsible for genome replication with the help of cellular proteins.
(iii) Virus particles are assembled during the release phase and undergo a maturation process before

being released from the cell. Viral proteins are always responsible for this final stage, although host proteins and other factors may be associated. Not all particles released are infectious and particle/infectivity ratios are highly variable, with defective particles produced for numerous reasons. Many infections are abortive.

Information about the reproductive cycle of viruses has been gained from the study of synchronously infected cells, and specific phases have been identified.
  (i) Shortly after infection, for a period of minutes to hours (depending on the virus being studied), only low amounts of parental infectious material can be identified: this is the *eclipse* phase. Genome replication has been initiated but progeny virus has not yet formed.
 (ii) This stage is followed by a *maturation* phase when viral material accumulates exponentially within the cell or surrounding medium.
(iii) After a few hours, cells infected with a lytic virus become metabolically disordered and then die. No further virus is produced, and titres slowly drop.
 (iv) Cells infected with non-lytic viruses can continue to produce viral particles indefinitely.
This reproductive cycle is variable, lasting less than an hour with many bacteriophages, 6–8 hours in Picornaviridae and more than 40 hours in Herpesviridae. Cells infected with poliovirus can yield more than 100 000 copies of virus per infected cell.

Growth characteristics

Different viruses have different modes of reproduction within a host cell – this is known as virus replication and the replication strategy of each virus depends upon the nature of its genome. Viral growth may be described by the overall effect the infection has on the host cell's survival. Not all viruses manifest these growth characteristics and some, such as the Herpesviridae, may demonstrate each growth phase during host infection.

Lytic growth

The virus replicates inside the host cell and then releases virus particles by causing cell lysis. This may be seen microscopically as a 'cytopathic effect' (CPE).

Lysogenic growth

The lytic portion of the cycle is suppressed. Replication produces new virions without killing the host cell. Viral DNA may be incorporated into the host cell DNA and transmitted to the daughter cells. Lysogenic viruses may also have lytic phases.

Latent infections

Latent infections are persistent asymptomatic infection of the host cell by a virus, typical of the Herpesviridae. Appropriate stimulation induces reactivation to lytic growth. Viral DNA may be incorporated into the host cell nucleus and passed on to daughter cells.

Viruses have specific tissue tropism: this property dictates the type of specimen required for diagnosis of a specific virus. Conversely, the system involved in the disease process will direct the differential diagnosis for possible viruses involved. Viruses are commonly implicated in hepatitis, respiratory illnesses, diarrhoea, skin vesicular lesions, aseptic meningitis, pharyngitis and conjunctivitis. An in vivo cytopathic effect (CPE) may be demonstrated by direct examination of biopsy or cytology preparations; these may show nuclear or cytoplasmic inclusion bodies, giant cell formation or cell lysis. In vitro cell culture shows characteristic cellular changes: plaque formation, swelling, granulation/inclusion formation, giant cells, cell lysis, and hemadsorption or hemagglutination. Interferon (IFN) is a protein (peptide) produced by cells after they have been penetrated by viruses. It cannot stop virus replication in that cell, but it is released to adjacent cells and stimulates the production of antiviral factors that prevent infection of neighbouring cells. The IFN peptide is now produced by recombinant technology for use in the treatment of a variety of viral diseases.

Virus classification

Virus classification is helpful in order to make predictions about details of replication, pathogenesis and transmission: this is particularly important when a new virus is identified. As with other microorganisms, viruses are also classified into order, family, subfamily, genus, species and strain/subtype. Families have the suffix -viridae (Herpesviridae, Poxviridae, Retroviridae, Picornaviridae), and genera have the suffix virus (Herpes virus, Hepatitis virus, Lentivirus).

Taxonomic classification is based upon a number of different properties:

(i) morphology: size, shape, enveloped/non-enveloped, tails, spikes,
(ii) physicochemical properties: molecular mass, buoyant density, pH, thermal sensitivity, ionic stability,
(iii) biological properties: host range, transmission, tropism etc.,
(iv) genome: RNA, DNA, segmented sequence, restriction map, modification, etc.,
(v) macromolecules: protein composition and function,
(vi) antigenic properties.

The Baltimore Classification divides viruses into seven (arbitrary) groups (see Table 4.1). By convention, the top strand of coding DNA (5'–3') is (+) sense, and mRNA is (+) sense.

Double-stranded DNA

Double-stranded DNA viruses, e.g. Adenoviruses, Herpesviruses, Poxviruses, Papovaviruses (Polyomavirus). Adeno- and Herpes viruses use host cellular proteins to replicate in the nucleus of their host cell. Poxviruses replicate in the cytoplasm and make their own enzymes for nucleic acid replication.

Table 4.1. Representative viruses grouped by genome structure (ICTV, 1995)

DNA		RNA			
DS-DNA		(−) sense RNA		(+) sense RNA	
Family	Viral members	Family	Viral members	Family	Viral members
Poxvirus	Variola Vaccinia *Molluscum contagiosum*	Orthomyxovirus	Influenza A, B and C	Togavirus	Western and Eastern equine encephalitis **Rubella
Herpesvirus	***Herpes simplex type 1 ***Herpes simplex type 2 Varicella Zoster ***Cytomegalovirus (CMV) Epstein-Barr (EBV) Human Herpesviruses 6, 7, 8	Paramyxovirus	Parainfluenza Mumps Measles Repiratory Syncytial Virus (RSV)	Flavivirus	St. Louis encephalitis Yellow fever Dengue ***Hepatitis C
Adenovirus	Human adenoviruses serotypes 1–48	Bunyavirus	California and La Crosse encephalitis Rift Valley fever Other fever agents Sin nombre and related hantaviruses	Calcivirus	Gastroenteritis-causing calciviruses
Papovavirus	*Human papilloma virus (HPV)	Rhabdovirus	Rabies	Astrovirus	
Polyomaviruses	JC and BK polyomaviruses	Arenavirus	Lymphocytic choriomeningitis Lassa fever agents Other hemorrhagic agents	Coronavirus	SARS
Hepadnavirus	***Hepatitis B	Filovirus	Ebola hemorrhagic fever Marburg hemorrhagic fever	Picornavirus	Enterovirus Polio Coxsackie B Echovirus Enterovirus 68–71, 72 (hepatitis A) Rhinovirus
SS DNA		DS RNA		SS (+) with DNA Intermediate (Reverse transcribing)	
Parvovirus	**B-19	Reovirus	Rotavirus Colorado Tick Fever	Retrovirus	Human T-lymphotrophic virus (HTLV-I and II) ***HIV

* Urogenital pathogen/STD; **prenatal/neonatal pathogen; ***both urogenital pathogen and prenatal/neonatal pathogen
DS, double stranded; SS, single stranded.
Viruses, like bacteria, are divided into genera and species, but the majority are referred to by common names that have been used for some time. For example, the genus Simplexvirus contains herpes simplex virus. Common names are also used for the virus families (poxvirus refers to members of the Poxviridae family).

Single-stranded DNA

Single-stranded (+) sense DNA, e.g. Parvoviruses. Replication takes place in the nucleus, where a (−) strand of DNA is synthesized to serve as a template for the synthesis of (+) strand RNA and DNA.

Double-stranded RNA

Double-stranded RNA, e.g. Reoviruses (rotavirus), Birnaviruses. The double-stranded RNA cannot function as mRNA, and these viruses carry an RNA polymerase to make their mRNA after infecting a cell. Their genome is segmented, and each segment is transcribed separately to produce monocistronic mRNAs.

Single-stranded RNA

Positive (+) sense RNA

Positive (+) sense RNA, e.g. Picornaviruses (Hepatitis A, Foot and Mouth Disease), Coronavirus (SARS), Arteriviruses (Equine Viral Arteritis), Togaviruses, Flavivirus, (Hepatitis C, West Nile Virus, Dengue, Yellow Fever). There are two types.

Non-segmented RNA

- Hepatitis A is a Picornavirus with Polycistronic mRNA, where the genome RNA = mRNA. This means that the naked RNA is infectious and there is no virion-associated polymerase. Translation results in the formation of a polyprotein product, which is then cleaved to form the mature proteins.
- Coronaviruses (e.g. SARS) have a non-segmented (+) RNA that is translated to produce a viral polymerase, which then produces a full-length (−) sense strand. This is used as a template to produce mRNA as an overlapping 'nested set' of monocistronic transcripts, and individual proteins are produced from each subgenomic transcript.

Togaviruses and Flaviviruses

Togaviruses and Flaviviruses have complex transcription; two or more rounds of translation are necessary to produce the genomic RNA, i.e. (+) strands are copied to (−) strands, which are copied to produce more (+) strands.

Negative (−) sense RNA

Negative (−) sense RNA, e.g. Paramyxoviruses (measles, mumps), Orthomyxoviruses (influenza), Rhabdoviruses (vesicular stomatitis, rabies), etc. These viruses have a virion RNA-directed RNA polymerase to copy their (−)RNA into mRNA.

Segmented (Orthomyxovirus)

The (−) sense RNA genome is first transcribed by the virion RNA-dependent RNA polymerase to produce monocistronic mRNA, which also serves as the template for genome replication.

Non-segmented (Rhabdovirus)

Replication also requires a virion RNA-dependent RNA polymerase, and monocistronic mRNAs are produced.

Single-stranded (+) sense RNA with DNA intermediate

Single-stranded (+) sense RNA with DNA intermediate in their life cycle: Retroviruses. Their genome is (+) sense, but unique among viruses, the genome is **diploid**, and serves as a template for reverse transcription instead of as mRNA.

Double-stranded DNA with RNA intermediate

Hepadnaviruses

This group also relies on reverse transcription, but this takes place inside the virus particle on maturation. When the virus infects a new cell, a gap in the genome is first repaired, and this is followed by transcription to RNA.

'*Subviral agents*' are classified separately: this group includes satellites, deltavirus (Hepatitis D), viroids and prions.

Table 4.2.

Virus	Characteristic CPE features	Optimal cell line
Herpesvirus (HSV)	Rapid onset, starts at edges, entire culture affected, rounding, swelling and granularity of infected cells	Fibroblasts
Cytomegalovirus (CMV)	Slow onset, small plaques involved, usually near the tube butt. Rounding, swelling and granularity of infected cells	Fibroblasts
Varicella Zoster Virus (VZV)	Slow onset, elongated granular plaques	Fibroblasts

Laboratory diagnosis of viral disease

Direct examination

Histology

Tissue sections may show characteristic cytopathic changes in infected tissues; these are generally seen as intranuclear or intracytoplasmic inclusions.

Cytology

Characteristic changes may be seen in cellular fluids and smears (bronchoalveolar lavage specimens, cerebrospinal fluid, Papanicolau smears, urine, etc.).

Electron microscopy

Viral particles may be identified by size, location within the cell and presence or absence of envelopes. Although a positive result (visualizing particles or components) confirms the diagnosis, a negative result does not exclude it. Direct detection may also be non-specific, in that more than one virus may have a similar morphology, i.e. the different Herpesviridae may not be distinguishable on the basis of electron microscopy.

Culture

Specimen handling is very important to ensure that the virus can be cultured. Many viruses are labile, and the specimen should be inoculated into culture medium as soon as possible. Specimens must be transported in the correct support medium, on the correct swabs, at the correct temperatures.

Classical tube culture

Classical tube culture is accomplished by inoculating specimens directly over cells that have been grown in monolayers inside culture tubes. The cells are incubated at 37 °C for 1 to 21 days, and reviewed microscopically to detect cytopathic cellular changes (CPE) in specific cell lines. Table 4.2 summarizes the comparative CPEs for several viruses that may be grown in fibroblast cell lines. Since these changes may subtle and not always definitive, positive CPEs are confirmed using immunostains specific for the virus suspected.

Shell vial culture

The *shell vial culture* with immunostaining is a spin amplification culture system that combines enhanced infectivity with fluorescence monoclonal antibody staining for specific identification of viral antigens (Fig. 4.1). The specimen is inoculated into a vial with a coverslip at the bottom, on which permissive cells have been previously grown to near confluence. The specimen is slowly centrifuged onto the cell monolayer, flattening the cells and opening cellular membrane pores that allow more efficient virus infection. After one or more days of incubation, the cells are fixed and stained with antibodies to detect specific viruses. This culture system may be used to detect a number of viruses, but is most important in detecting CMV rapidly and in distinguishing HSV-1 from HSV-2.

Antigen detection systems

Antigen detection systems use enzyme immuno assays (EIAs) designed to detect viral antigens

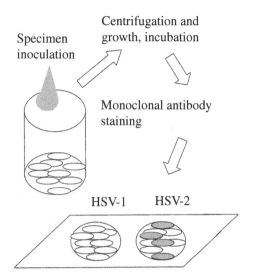

Fig. 4.1. Shell vial culture for virus identification. Schematic diagram illustrating shell vial culture, a spin amplification culture system that combines enhanced infectivity with fluorescent monoclonal antibody staining in order to identify specific viral antigens. This system is important in detecting CMV rapidly and in distinguishing HSV-1 from HSV-2.

present in direct specimens or in cultured specimens. These are often useful for point of care testing for Influenza A and B, Rotavirus, Herpes, Respiratory Syncytial Virus (RSV) etc.

Serologic diagnosis

Serologic diagnosis can be qualitative or quantitative, and is used to test acute and convalescent sera:
 (i) IgM to detect acute infections
 (ii) IgG to assess acute infection, convalescence and past exposures: a fourfold, or greater, rise in titre indicates an acute infection
(iii) Sequential antibody production to key antigens can help in the diagnosis of specific viral infections such as Hepatitis B and Epstein–Barr Virus.
Methods of detection used in serologic diagnosis include:
 (i) immunofluorescent antibody detection (IFA): patient-derived antibodies reacted with virus-infected cells, and antibodies identified using

fluorescent isothiocyanate (FITC) labeled anti-human IgG or IgM antibodies
 (ii) colorimetric or radiometric immunoassays, EIAs or RIAs
(iii) complement fixation for viral antibody titres
(iv) Western blot for HIV diagnosis
 (v) recombinant immuno blot assay (RIBA) for HCV diagnosis.

Molecular diagnostics

The advent of nucleic acid technology has now revolutionized the diagnosis of viral disease, and sophisticated specific test kits for many common viruses have been developed. Both qualitative and quantitative assays are available, including:
 (i) PCR, probe amplification, probe capture assays, ligase chain reaction, and real-time light cycler PCR assays. These are used for a number of viral agents, including human papillomavirus (HPV), human immunodeficiency virus (HIV), HCV and HBV,
 (ii) DNA probes (not amplified),
(iii) Dot blot/Southern blot assay (Human papilloma virus),
(iv) line probe assays (to detect HCV genotypes),

Viruses directly relevant to ART

Viruses directly relevant to ART practice include:
 (i) double-stranded DNA viruses
    Herpes viruses
      Herpes Simplex
      Cytomegalovirus
    Papillomavirus
    Hepatitis B virus (partially double-stranded)
 (ii) single-stranded RNA viruses
    Hepatitis C and D
(iii) retroviruses
    human immunodeficiency virus (HIV) -1 and -2
    human T-cell lymphotrophic virus (HTLV) -I and -II.
This section covers a brief generic description of the virus groups in order to clarify relationships and to

provide an overall perspective for the purpose of comparison. Pathology, consequences and diagnosis for the viruses that have a direct impact upon ART, particularly the sexually transmitted viruses and the blood-borne pathogens, will be discussed in detail in Chapters 7 and 12.

Double-stranded DNA viruses

Herpesvirus

The **Herpesvirus** family is one of the most important virus families in medical practice. They are ubiquitous, infecting virtually everyone, and induce a wide variety of diseases. The viruses enter into a 'latent' phase after recovery from primary infections; various types of stress can then induce the virus to start replicating again, causing symptomatic disease. Eight species of human pathogens in the Herpesvirus family have been identified:

  (i) Herpes Simplex Type 1 (HSV-1): cold sores, but can also cause genital ulcers,
 (ii) Herpes Simplex Type 2 (HSV-2): genital herpes, occasionally oral herpes,
(iii) Varicella-zoster (VZV): chicken pox, shingles,
(iv) Epstein–Barr (EBV): glandular fever, tumours,
 (v) Cytomegalovirus (CMV),
(vi)–(viii) Human Herpes 6, 7, and 8 (HHV 6, 7, 8).

The Herpesvirus genome is a single molecule of linear double-stranded DNA of approximately 120–220 kbp, with terminal repeats at each end of the duplex that allow the molecule to form a circle. HSV-1 and −2 are closely related, overlapping in both structure and in disease pathology; 50% of their DNA sequence is shared. There is very little DNA homology between the other six viruses.

The virion has four structural components:

  (i) core: consists of viral proteins with viral DNA wrapped around them to form an icosahedral capsid, 100 nm in diameter,
 (ii) envelope derived from the host nuclear membrane, containing viral proteins,
(iii) surface projections: peplomers,

(iv) matrix protein in between the capsid and the envelope (tegument = fibrous structure).

The Herpes family

Herpesvirus replication

  (i) Peplomers attach to specific virus receptors on the cell surface of susceptible cells; at least nine different glycoproteins are present.
 (ii) The nucleocapsid enters the host cell through fusion of virus envelope and cell membrane.
(iii) An unidentified host enzyme uncoats the viral DNA.
(iv) Virus core enters the nucleus through a nuclear pore and viral DNA is circularized.
 (v) Viral DNA is transcribed by a host DNA-dependent RNA polymerase, producing 50 different messenger RNAs; the viral genome is transcribed in three blocks sequentially:
    (a) immediate mRNA (alpha): codes for regulatory genes that control transcription,
    (b) delayed early mRNA (beta): codes for enzymes, non-structural regulatory proteins and minor structural proteins,
    (c) late mRNA (gamma): codes for the major structural proteins of the virus.
(vi) Once enough virus structural protein has been made, host cell protein synthesis shuts down and the cell eventually dies. The viral core and capsid assemble in the nucleus, with the structural proteins condensing around viral DNA to form nucleocapsids. The genomic concatomers are cleaved and packaged into pre-assembled capsids.

The viral envelope is acquired from the inner lamella of the nuclear membrane as the nucleocapsid 'buds out' of the nucleus, and particles then assemble in the space between the inner and outer nuclear lamellae before being transported to the cell surface. The proteins in this membrane are almost entirely replaced by viral proteins. Mutations in certain envelope glycoproteins interfere with viral transport. The remaining particles are released when the cell lyses, around 24 hours after infection. The vesicular fluid of active herpetic lesions contains HSV particles in high concentrations.

- Only approximately 25% of viral DNA/protein produced is incorporated into virions – infection is a 'wasteful' process.
- The rest of the DNA/protein accumulates in the cell, which eventually dies. This process produces characteristic nuclear inclusion bodies, which can be seen by electron microscopy.

Viral latency

Certain host cells (nerve cells) can prevent the transcription of delayed early and late genes and the viral genome persists in these as an episome (i.e., not integrated into the host cell DNA). Under these conditions, the virus does not replicate and the cell does not die: the virus instead remains 'latent' within the cell and can be reactivated into active infection under the right circumstances, such as stress, exposure to UV light, or immunocompromise.

As mentioned above, Herpes simplex viruses 1 and 2 are closely related. HSV-1 is ubiquitous, causing disease in over 60% of adult humans worldwide, while HSV-2 is seen primarily as a sexually transmitted pathogen infecting about 20% of adults in the United States.

HSV-1

HSV-1 is acquired primarily during childhood and adolescence and causes oral and ocular lesions. Increasingly, HSV-1 is implicated in causing a significant proportion of newly diagnosed and recurrent genital ulcer disease.

HSV-2

HSV-2 causes genital and anal lesions and may be transmitted to the neonate during parturition. The incidence of genital herpes has increased significantly during the last few decades.

Detailed clinical aspects of Herpes genital ulcer disease are discussed in Chapter 7.

Varicella Zoster virus (VZV)

This virus infects virtually every human, in the form of chicken pox. Although it is mostly a childhood disease (highly contagious!) and is generally mild in healthy children, VZV infections can be severe and even fatal in high-risk groups: neonates, immunocompromised patients and susceptible adults. Recovery from primary infection leads to latency and virus reactivation results in Herpes Zoster (shingles). Shingles can be a painful and debilitating disease: the vesiculopapules are localized with dermatomal distribution, causing a neuronitis that may be associated with protracted pain.

Cytomegalovirus (CMV)

CMV, the largest of the Herpesviruses, is a member of the beta-Herpesviridae subfamily. The complete nucleotide sequence of the virus is known and its expression has been studied in detail: it has the largest genome of all herpesviruses (230 kbp vs. 160 kbp for HSV-1), with an arrangement of unique and inverted repeats, including four genome isomers. Human CMV infection is widespread throughout the world, but is usually asymptomatic or only mildly symptomatic in immunocompetent individuals. Infected persons may excrete virus in urine or saliva for months and the virus can also be found in cervical secretions, semen, feces and milk. CMV is capable of reactivating throughout life to produce asymptomatic shedding or symptomatic disease (particularly in the immunocompromised host). The virus is an important pathogen that may produce severe disease in the newborn when transmitted during pregnancy. The clinical picture of CMV infection, diagnosis, and treatment is described in Chapter 12.

Epstein–Barr Virus (EBV)

Like the other Herpesviruses, EBV is also ubiquitous and worldwide in distribution, with virtually all humans infected by the EBV ($\sim$90% of most populations). The virus causes infectious mononucleosis (glandular fever) and has been strongly associated with nasopharyngeal carcinoma, Burkitt's lymphoma, salivary gland carcinoma, Hodgkin's disease, chronic fatigue syndrome and hairy leukoplakia. The complete nucleotide sequence of the virus is known, and has been shown to have many internal repeats, with numerous genomic variants. Replication/latency has been studied in transformed human cell lines. The virus has two target cells:

- epithelial cells of the oropharynx – virus replication occurs here, but the infection is subclinical;
- human B-lymphocytes, where it results in a nonproductive infection. When B-lymphocytes are infected in vitro, the lymphocytes proliferate rapidly and persistently (immortalization or transformation), instead of releasing progeny virus and lysing. Each transformed lymphocyte has up to several hundred EBV genomes and the early gene products.

The virus causes polyclonal B-cell activation and benign proliferation; the infected B-lymphocytes spread via blood and lymphatics to activate T-lymphocytes and cause foci of lymphoproliferation. This process may be subclinical, or may produce the symptoms of infectious mononucleosis. In the setting of HIV, EBV may cause a malignant clone of immortalized plasma cells to emerge, leading to the development of a primary B-cell lymphoma, usually involving the central nervous system.

No specific antiviral therapy is effective, and no vaccine is yet available.

Human Herpesvirus 6 (HHV-6)

HHV-6 was isolated in 1986, associated with lymphoreticular disorders. It has a tropism for CD4+ lymphocytes and is now recognized as a universal human infection: roseola infantum, or 'fourth disease'. Childhood infection is mild, and adult infection rare but more severe, causing mononucleosis/ hepatitis. This virus is a problem in immunocompromised patients.

Human Herpesvirus-7 (HHV-7)

HHV-7 was first isolated from CD4+ cells in 1990. Its entire genome has been sequenced: it is similar to, but distinct from, HHV-6, with some antigenic cross-reactivity. There is as yet no clear evidence for any relationship to human clinical disease, but it may act as a co-factor in HHV-6 related syndromes.

Human Herpesvirus-8 (HHV-8 Kaposi's sarcoma-related virus)

HHV-8 is correlated with Kaposi's sarcoma in AIDS patients and can also be isolated from primary bone marrow cells (PBMC). This virus contains 'pirated' cellular genes, in an 'oncogenic cluster'. It contains a vGPCR gene (viral G-protein coupled receptor), which acts as a vascular switch, turning on VEGF (vascular endothelial growth factor), which is then responsible for the development of Kaposi's sarcoma. It resembles the Epstein–Barr virus in having a tropism for epithelial and B-cells and may also cause other tumours, e.g. B-cell lymphoma. The virus is normally kept under control by the host's immune system and only becomes a problem during immunosuppression. In non-endemic parts of the world, HHV-8 has been identified in semen of high-risk patients (i.e. AIDS patients with Kaposi's sarcoma), but has not been identified in low-risk populations such as semen donors. However, in high prevalence regions of the world such as Sicily, HHV-8 has been demonstrated in semen even in the absence of HIV infection and Kaposi's sarcoma.

Papillomavirus

Papillomavirus belongs to a different family of double-stranded DNA viruses, the Papovaviruses, which were the first viruses shown to be oncogenic in the laboratory: SV40 virus, one of the most well studied of this family of viruses, is known to cause tumours in mice. The papillomaviruses are spherical, icosahedral, non-enveloped viruses, with a single molecule of circular double-stranded DNA as their genome. There are at least 60 different types of HPV: the target cells are cutaneous and mucosal squamous epithelium, with many of the viral serovars having marked regional tropism (i.e. for hands, feet, laryngeal mucosa, or genital sites).

Several HPV serovars produce genital warts, which are sexually transmitted (see Chapter 9).

Hepatitis viruses

At least six different human pathogenic viruses that cause acute and chronic viral hepatitis have been identified:

HAV = picornavirus, RNA genome,

HBV, HGV = hepadnaviruses, partially double-stranded DNA genome,

HCV, HDV, HEV: RNA genome,

There may be others as yet unidentified.

Hepatitis A and E are mainly spread by the fecal–oral route and do not induce a chronic carrier state. HBV, HCV and HDV produce chronic hepatic infections, and HGV produces no known hepatitis symptoms.

Hepatitis A virus (HAV)

Hepatitis A virus (HAV) is a very small picornavirus (27 nm) with non-segmented single-stranded positive-sense RNA as its genome (representing mRNA). The virus is icosahedral and not enveloped. Its primary target is the lymphoid tissue of the gastrointestinal tract and it is commonly acquired from contaminated food or water. Immunization is readily available by a Hepatitis A vaccine, as well as by passive immunization with gamma globulin. HAV vaccination is given routinely during childhood in some parts of the world.

Hepatitis B virus (HBV)

HBV belongs to the **hepadnavirus** family. It is a 42 nm spherical particle with a lipoprotein envelope composed of hepatitis B surface antigen (HbsAg); the partially double-stranded DNA genome is contained within a 27 nm hexagonal nucleocapsid. The outer shell has virus-specific glycosylated proteins and lipid, so that the shell is equivalent to a viral envelope; removal of this shell by detergents results in loss of infectivity. The complete infectious virion is also known as the 'Dane Particle'. HBV infection can stimulate an acute hepatitis, as well as

produce a chronic syndrome associated with cirrhosis and hepatocellular carcinoma. HBV infections are seen worldwide, but prevalence varies geographically. While the USA, Western Europe and Australia have very low prevalence rates, other population in Africa, South America, South East Asia, Greenland and the Eskimo populations in North America demonstrate prevalence rates of 8% or greater. An effective vaccine is available for HBV and its use globally may help to diminish the burden of human disease with this virus. Features of HBV infection, transmission and diagnosis are described in Chapter 12.

Hepatitis C virus (HCV)

HCV is the predominant agent of post-transfusion Hepatitis (formerly known as 'non-A–non-B hepatitis'). The genes of HCV were characterized by molecular cloning in 1989, as a result of which it was included in the family of Flaviviridae. Although it is less efficiently transmitted than HBV, it is serially transmissible in chimpanzees, inducing hepatitis. HCV has been identified in semen specimens from infected males and is considered to be a blood-borne pathogen. Properties of the virus and its associated disease are described in Chapter 12.

Hepatitis D (delta) virus (HDV)

HDV is a defective single-stranded RNA virus, a 36 nm particle encapsulated by HBsAg: it needs HBV as a helper in order to replicate. HDV uses HBV in order to synthesize a capsid made up of HBsAg and this is used to make up the infective virions for HDV. For this reason, HDV infection is seen only in people also infected with HBV. For example, an individual with chronic HBV infection may be infected with HDV, or an individual may become coinfected with both viruses. HDV viral RNA is complexed with HDV-specific protein, the HDV antigen, without forming the specific morphology of a nucleocapsid: it is thought perhaps to be a viroid.

A **viroid** is a small molecule of single stranded RNA, less than 0.5 kb in size, which can replicate in susceptible cells. The RNA has internal regions that are complementary, and this allows the molecule to self-anneal by internal base pairing. This yields a stable rod-like structure, with complementary sequences at both ends of the molecule, allowing it to form a circle. How they multiply remains unresolved: their genome is too small to code for RNA replicase, and host cells do not have RNA replicase. All viroids identified so far are plant pathogens.

HDV is implicated in causing a fulminant or acute hepatitis when coinfecting with HBV, and often produces a chronic HDV infection in the presence of a previously acquired chronic HBV infection (see Chapter 12, Fig. 12.8). Compared to HBV, the distribution of endemic HDV is much more limited. A more complete discussion of HDV infection may be found in Chapter 12.

Hepatitis E virus (HEV)

Hepatitis E virus (HEV) is enterically transmitted, and is responsible for a 'non-A–non-B' hepatitis. The virus is spherical, non-enveloped, with a single-stranded RNA genome. It has been provisionally classified as a calcivirus, but its genome is substantially different from other calciviruses. HEV has no serological cross-reaction with HAV, HBV, HCV, or HDV and its pathogenesis may be similar to that of HAV. However, a high rate of fulminant and often fatal infection is seen with HEV infection in the pregnant woman.

Hepatitis G virus (HGV)

Hepatitis G virus (HGV) is an enveloped virus without surface projections, slightly pleomorphic, with occasional filamentous forms. The genome consists of circular DNA, which is partially double-stranded and partially single-stranded: neither strand is covalently closed. Its acute disease spectrum is unknown, but it is found with an incidence of 0.3% in cases of acute viral hepatitis, frequently as a co-infection with HCV. It is transmitted via blood-borne transmission. Its role as a sexually transmitted virus is suggested by the relatively high rate of seroprevalence seen in prostitutes. Enzyme immunoassay testing is

not available commercially, but is used for research purposes.

Retroviruses

Prior to the discovery of HIV in the etiology of AIDS, retroviruses were of major interest to experimental oncologists, but of minor importance in medical practice. The AIDS epidemic has brought the retroviruses to the forefront of medical virology, and they have unique features that should be considered in the perspective of assisted reproduction and surgical micromanipulation of oocytes/embryos.

Retroviruses use DNA as an intermediate in their replication: their genome consists of single-stranded RNA, which is reverse transcribed into DNA that integrates into the host cell DNA. This process depends on a virus-associated, virus-specified polymerase, the reverse transcriptase enzyme. Integrating a copy of their genome into the host cell chromosome can result in cell transformation (unrestricted cell division), and they are thus oncogenic in a number of vertebrate species, causing leukemia, sarcoma and mammary carcinoma. The key reverse transcriptase enzyme has three different enzymatic activities.

(i) It uses RNA as a template to synthesize a complementary single-stranded DNA.

(ii) It hydrolyses the RNA primer molecule: this is known as RNA-ase H activity.

(iii) It synthesizes a complementary DNA sequence to form a double-stranded molecule that can be integrated into the host genome.

The enzyme has a further unique feature: it requires a particular cellular tRNA to use as its primer for DNA synthesis.

History of retroviruses

In 1904, Ellerman and Bang observed that a lymphoproliferative disease in chickens could be transmitted by filtrates of cell extracts: this agent was identified as avian myeloblastosis virus (AMV). Paul Ehrlich then proposed the theory of immune surveillance in 1905, which subsequently led to the idea that these infectious agents escaped immune attack by becoming associated with their host cell genome. Peyton Rous (1911) found that sarcomas in chickens could be transmitted by cell filtrates and Rous Sarcoma virus (RSV) was identified. During the 1960s, Howard Temin inhibited retrovirus replication with experiments using actinomycin D, which inhibits DNA synthesis, and he then proposed the concept of reverse transcription. In 1969, Huebner & Todaro proposed the viral oncogene hypothesis and David Baltimore and Howard Temin were awarded the Nobel Prize in 1975 for their work on retroviruses and reverse transcriptase. Human T-cell lymphotrophic virus (HTLV) was identified as the first pathogenic human retrovirus in 1981, and HIV was discovered in 1983.

Retrovirus classification

Two species of virus have been grouped into three subfamilies.
  (i) **Oncornaviruses**: HTLV-I and HTLV-II, have a centrally located nucleoid
 (ii) **Lentiviruses**: HIV-1 and HIV-2, have a cylindrical nucleoid
(iii) **Spumaviruses** – thought to be associated with chronic fatigue syndrome
They have also been grouped according to their morphology by electron microscopy.
  (i) **A-type**: non-enveloped, intracellular immature particles.
 (ii) **B-type**: enveloped, extracellular particles, with spikes (Mouse mammary tumour virus, MMTV).
(iii) **C-type**: similar to B-type particles, but have a central core and barely visible spikes. The majority of mammalian and avian retroviruses are C-type particles: murine leukemia (MuLV), avian leukemia (ALV), HTLV, HIV.
(iv) **D-type**: slightly larger, spikes less prominent: Mason–Pfizer Monkey Virus (MPMV), HIV.
However, molecular genetics has now replaced morphological classification. Comparisons are now made largely on the basis of sequence conservation in their genomes, particularly involving the viral genes that code for **gag, pol**, and **env**.

Retrovirus genetics

Retroviral genetics is very complex! The viruses have an extremely high mutation rate: reverse transcription is apparently error-prone and recombination also occurs during the process. Interactions occur with the host cell DNA, including insertional mutations and transductions.

Retrotransposons are endogenous retrovirus-like genetic elements, which make up 5–10% of the mammalian genome: these can move around to different positions on the DNA.

Transposons are short segments of DNA that can move around within a cell to many different positions on the chromosome. They exist in all organisms, from bacteria to humans, and provide a rapid genetic diversity that acts as a selective pressure for survival of the fittest. They are responsible for the rapid evolutionary changes seen in bacteria (i.e. antibiotic resistance). **IS** is a gene that encodes an enzyme responsible for the movement of the transposon, by inactivating genes into which they land. Composite transposons have also been identified, e.g. antibiotic resistance flanked by 2 IS genes.

An ancient retrotransposon insertion has been reported to be the cause of Fukuyama-type muscular dystrophy, the most common autosomal recessive disorder in Japan (Kobayashi *et al.*, 1998).

Retrovirus pathogenesis

Oncogenes hijack normal control of cell division and cause cell transformation so that the cells continue to divide indefinitely. Normal cells also contain **Onc** sequences, which are genes that are fundamentally important in regulating cell growth. Oncogenes have some form of altered regulation that causes abnormal growth. Due to their ability to insert into the host cell genome, genetically modified retroviruses are under active development as vectors for gene therapy, with the aim of replacing defective genes with 'good' copies.

Human oncornaviruses

Two viruses of the oncornavirus group have been identified in humans: Human T-cell lymphotrophic virus, HTLV-I and HTLV-II. HTLV-I is associated with adult T-cell leukemia (ATL), as well as tropical spastic paralysis (TSP), a Caribbean chronic degenerative neurological disease. In Japan, it has also been found in association with HTLV-I-associated myelopathy: this may be the same disease as TSP. HTLV-II is closely related to HTLV-I, with 65% homology between their genomes. Although very little is known about its pathogenesis and epidemiology, its molecular biology has been described: the genome of both viruses contains four genes: gag, pol, env, and pX, flanked by terminal repeats. It is a cell-associated virus, and is transmitted by cell-to-cell contact: it is infectious for a wide variety of mammalian cells by co-cultivation. However, only infected T-cells are transformed and immortalized. The virus has an extremely long incubation period, in the order of 50 years! Infection is usually acquired at birth and T-lymphocytes of infected persons, found in blood, semen, milk and cervical secretions are the source of infection. Transmission of HTLV-I by blood transfusion is well documented. Details of the pathogenesis and diagnosis of HTLV-I and -II are presented in Chapter 12.

Lentiviruses: human immunodeficiency virus (HIV)

Two species of human lentivirus are well characterized: HIV-1 and HIV-2. Since their discovery, the HIVs have established a worldwide distribution, with the vast burden of human disease focused in sub-Saharan Africa, southern and Southeast Asia and portions of South America. The number of new infections seen each year with these viruses has increased dramatically since the early 1980s. In 1999, new cases were estimated at nearly 4 000 000 in Sub-Saharan Africa alone. Properties of these two viruses, together with details of HIV pathogenesis and diagnosis are described in Chapter 12.

FURTHER READING

Baron, E. J., Chang, R. S., Howard, D. H., Miller, J. N. & Turner, J. A. (eds.)(1994). *Medical Microbiology: A Short Course.* New York: Wiley-Liss.

Bobroski, L., Bagasra, A. U., Patel, D. *et al.* (1998). Localization of human herpesvirus type 8 (HHV-8) in the Kaposi's sarcoma tissues and the semen specimens of HIV-1 infected and uninfected individuals by utilizing *in situ* polymerase chain reaction. *Journal of Reproductive Immunology*, **41**: 149–60.

Calabro, M. L., Fiore, J. R., Favero, A. *et al.* (1999). Detection of human herpesvirus 8 in cervicovaginal secretions and seroprevalence in human immunodeficiency virus type 1-seropositive and -seronegative women. *Journal of Infectious Diseases*, **179**: 1534–7.

Cann, A. J. (1997). *Principles of Molecular Virology*, 2nd edn. Chapter 4. New York: Academic Press.

Cannon, M. J., Dollard, S. C., Black, J. B. *et al.* (2003). Risk factors for Kaposi's sarcoma in men seropositive for both Human Herpesvirus 8 and Human Immunodeficiency Virus. *AIDS*, **17**(2): 215–22.

Diamond, C., Brodie, S. J., Krieger, J. N. *et al.* (1998). Human herpesvirus 8 in the prostate glands of men with Kaposi's sarcoma. *Journal of Virology*, **72**: 6223–7.

Gnann Jr., J. W., Pellett, P. E. & Jaffe, H. W. (2000). Human Herpesvirus 8 and Kaposi's sarcoma in persons infected with human immunodeficiency virus. *Clinical Infectious Diseases*, **30**, Suppl 1: S72–6.

Huang, Y. Q., Li, J. J., Poiesz, B. J., Kaplan, M. H. & Friedman-Kien, A. E. (1997). Detection of the herpesvirus-like DNA sequences in matched specimens of semen and blood from patients with AIDS-related Kaposi's sarcoma by polymerase chain reaction *in situ* hybridization. *American Journal of Pathology*, **150**:147–53.

ICTV (1995). *Virus Taxonomy.* The Sixth Report of the International Committee of Taxonomy of Viruses.

Kelsen, J., Tarp, B. & Obel, N. (1999). Absence of human herpes virus 8 in semen from healthy Danish donors. *Human Reproduction*, **14**: 2274–6.

Kobayashi, K., Nakahori, V., Miyake, M. *et al.* (1998). An ancient retrotransposal insertion causes Fukuyama-type congenital muscular dystrophy. *Nature (London)*, **394**: 388–92.

Leland, D. S. (1996). *Clinical Virology.* Philadelphia, PA: W.B. Saunders Co.

Pellett, P. E., Spira, T. J., Bagasra, O. *et al.* (1999). Multicenter comparison of PCR assays for detection of human herpesvirus 8 DNA in semen. *Journal of Clinical Microbiology*, **37**: 1298–301.

Temesgen, Z. & Wright, A. J. (1999). Antiretrovirals. *Mayo Clinic Proceedings*, **74**: 1284–300.

Viviano, E., Vitale, F., Ajello, F. *et al.* (1997). Human herpesvirus type 8 DNA sequences in biological samples of HIV-positive and negative individuals in Sicily. *AIDS*, **11**: 607–12.

Appendix 4.1: antiviral agents

(Note: all antivirals inhibit specific steps in the process of viral replication; no agent is active against latent or non-replicating viruses.)

Class	Agents	Mode of Action	Indications	Comments
	Amantadine and Rimantadine	Inhibit transmembrane protein M2-mediated conversion of hemagglutinin from native to low pH conformation, resulting in reduced uncoating of viral genome in cellular lysosomes	Influenza A	CNS toxicity common with amantadine and rare with rimantadine
	Zanamivir	Sialic acid analogue; specifically inhibits influenza virus neuraminidase	Influenza A and B	
	Oseltamivir	Pro-drug of sialic acid analogue, GS4071; selective inhibitor of neuraminidase in both influenza A, B	Influenza A, B	Effective for prevention and treatment of influenza
	Acyclovir	Guanosine analogue Inhibits viral DNA synthesis by inhibiting viral DNA polymerase and acting as a DNA chain terminator	Herpes simplex virus 1, 2 Varicella-zoster virus	Human herpesvirus 6 is resistant
	Valacyclovir	Pro-drug of acyclovir; inhibits viral DNA synthesis	Herpes simplex viruses Varicella-zoster virus	Shown to prevent CMV disease in high-risk renal transplant recipients
	Ganciclovir	Acyclic nucleoside analogue of guanine; inhibits DNA polymerase (inhibits cellular more than viral)	Herpesviruses Varicella-zoster virus	Active against herpesvirus 6 FDA approved for CMV retinitis in immunocompromised patients and for patients with advanced HIV ?for prevention of CMV in transplant patients
	Penciclovir	Analogue of acyclic guanine; action similar to acyclovir, but does not act as DNA-chain terminator	Herpes simplex virus 1, 2 Varicella-zoster virus Lesser activity against Epstein–Barr virus	Similar to acyclovir Some activity against HBV Limited activity against CMV
	Famciclovir	Pro-drug of penciclovir	Herpes simplex virus 1, 2 Varicella-zoster virus Lesser activity against Epstein–Barr virus	
	Ribavirin	Purine nucleoside analogue; mechanism of action may be competitive inhibition of host enzymes resulting in reduced intracellular concentrations of guanosine triphosphate and decreased DNA synthesis, inhibition of viral RNA polymerase complex and inhibition of mRNA.	Influenza A, B Respiratory Syncytial virus Hemorrhagic fever Hepatitis A, B, C Lassa fever Hepatitis C virus Others	Broad spectrum against DNA and RNA viruses FDA approved only for serious RSV and in combination with interferon alpha-2b for treatment of chronic hepatitis C Teratogenic, mutagenic, embryotoxic and gonadotoxic in small mammals Contraindicated during pregnancy

Appendix 4.1: *(cont.)*

Class	Agents	Mode of Action	Indications	Comments
	Foscarnet	Inorganic pyrophosphate analogue; non-competitive inhibitor of viral DNA polymerase and reverse transcriptase	Herpes simplex virus 1, 2 Varicella-zoster virus CMV Epstein–Barr virus Influenza A, B HBV HIV	
	Lamivudine	Deoxynucleoside analogue; inhibits DNA polymerase; inhibits HIV reverse transcriptase	Hepatitis B	
	Cidofovir	Acyclic nucleoside phosphonate derivative	Herpes simplex virus 1, 2 Varicella-zoster virus Epstein–Barr virus CMV	Potent Carcinogenic and teratogenic Produces hypospermia in lab animals
Interferons: 3 major classes (interferon-α, interferon-β, and interferon-γ); only interferon-α is approved for viral treatment.	Interferon-alpha 4 commercially available: Alfa-2a Alfa-2b Alfacon-1 Alfa-n3	Glycoproteins with antiviral activity; produced in host in response to inducer. Promotes cell resistance to viruses via production of proteins that inhibit RNA synthesis and enzymes that cleave cellular and viral DNA; inhibits mRNA; cell membrane alterations inhibit release of replicated virions.	Hepatitis B Hepatitis C Interferon-alfa-2b and alfa-n3 approved for treating condyloma acuminatum due to human papillomavirus	
	Trifuridine	Pyrimidine nucleoside	Herpes simplex	Topical use only for ocular herpes infection
Reverse transcriptase inhibitors	Zidovudine Didanosine Zalcitabine Stavudine Lamivudine Abacavir	Block reverse transcriptase activity by competing with natural substrates, incorporated into viral DNA to act as chain terminators in proviral DNA synthesis	HIV	
Non-reverse transcriptase inhibitors	Nevirapine Delavirdine Efavirenz	Bind directly (non-competitively) to reverse transcriptase		
Protease inhibitors	Saquinavir Ritonavir Indinavir Nelfinavir Amprenavir	Inhibit HIV-1 protease	HIV	

FDA: Food and Drug Administration.

FURTHER READING

ANTIVIRAL AGENTS

http://www.doh.gov.ph/ndps/table_of_contents.html
http://www.nlm.nih.gov/medlineplus/druginfo/uspdi/
202668.html
Keating, M. R. (1999). Antiviral agents for non-human immunodeficiency Virus Infections. *Mayo Clinic Proceedings*, **74**,
1266–83.

Physician Desk Reference. (2000). 54th Edn Des Moines, IA: Medical Economics Co.
Temesgen, Z. & Wright, A. J. (1999). Antiretrovirals. *Mayo Clinic
Proceedings*, **74**, 1284–300.
Virk, A., Steckelberg, J. M. (2000). Clinical aspects of antimicrobial resistance. *Mayo Clinic Proceedings*, **75**, 200–
14.

5

Prions

Prion protein

'Prions' (*pro*teinaceous *in*fectious particles) are particles made up of an abnormal glycoprotein that is capable of causing a cell to produce more abnormal protein. The Prion particle is a unique agent, infectious by biological and medical criteria, but different from all known conventional microbes because it contains no elements of nucleic acid genetic material. Prusiner identified and classified prion diseases in 1982, and his work in describing prions as infectious protein particles that cause neurodegenerative disorders (Prusiner, 1991, 1995) gained the Nobel Prize in 1997. All known prion diseases are fatal; they are known as 'spongiform encephalopathies' because they cause the brain to be riddled with holes or 'spongy', with accompanying symptoms of progressive neurological degeneration. The spongiform change occurs without inflammation, inclusion bodies, or apparent immune response.

Prion diseases

Prion diseases, known as **transmissible spongiform encephalopathies, (TSEs)** can be infectious/iatrogenic (5%), inherited (10%), or sporadic ('Classical', 85%).

Animal

The first neurological disease of this kind was described in sheep during the early eighteenth century. Affected sheep rub or 'scrape' their coat against a tree, as if it itches – hence it was given the name 'scrapie' in England. In France, it was known as 'La tremblante' because the animals shake due to ataxia. In 1966, Alper showed that the infectious agent responsible for scrapie in sheep was very UV-resistant, compared with known viruses. This finding led to the suggestion that scrapie might be infectious without the involvement of a nucleic acid. A range of different TSEs has subsequently been identified in animals (Table 5.1).

Human

The human form, Creutzfeldt–Jakob Disease (CJD) was described in Germany and Austria in the 1920s, and is now recognized in different forms (Table 5.2).

Prion structure

Normal cell surface glycoprotein = **PrP^c**
Infectious Prion agent = **PrP^{sc}**
Prion protein = PrP
Prion protein gene = *Prnp*

Prusiner showed the Prion agent PrP^{sc} to be a protease-resistant glycoprotein in brains of scrapie-infected animals, not found in normal animals. The infectious Prion agent PrP^{sc} has now been identified as a conformationally modified isoform of a normal cell-surface glycophosphatidyl inositol-anchored glycoprotein, PrP^c. This protein occurs

Table 5.1. Prion diseases in different animal species

Species	Prion disease	Etiology
Sheep and goats	Scrapie	Infection seen in genetically susceptible sheep
Cows	Bovine spongiform encephalopathy (BSE), 'mad cow disease'. First observed in the UK in 1972, diagnosed in 1986	Acquired from ingestion of prion protein in infected feed supplements. Incubation period 3 to 6 years
Mink	Transmissible mink encephalopathy (TME)	Probably acquired from sheep or cattle
Deer and elk	Chronic wasting disease (CWD)	Origin unknown
Cats	Feline spongiform encephalopathy (FSE)	Acquired by ingestion of BSE-contaminated food products
Ungulates	Exotic ungulate encephalopathy (EUE)	Probably same source as seen in cattle
Rodents, pigs	Experimental scrapie or BSE Can be infected experimentally, but have not been diagnosed with a naturally occurring prion disease, to date	Experimentally induced

Table 5.2. Human prion diseases

Sporadic CJD ('Classical' CJD)	Caused by a somatic mutation or spontaneous conversion of a normal cellular prion protein (PrP^c) to the pathogenic isoform (PrP^{sc}).
Iatrogenic CJD	Linked to receipt of prion contaminated human pituitary-derived hormones, dura mater or transfer of infection via contaminated operating room instrumentation during cranial surgeries.
Kuru	Human infection linked to cannibalism – particularly brain tissues
Familial CJD	Due to germline mutations in a gene on chromosome 20 producing the abnormal PrP^{sc} protein
Fatal familial insomnia (FFI)	Germline mutation in PrP gene
Gerstmann–Sträussler– Scheinker syndrome (GSS)	Germline mutation in PrP gene
New variant CJD	Human equivalent to 'mad cow disease', bovine spongiform encephalopathy (BSE) linked to the consumption of infected high risk bovine derived food products

normally in the brain, cornea, spinal cord, pituitary gland, neural ganglia, spleen, lymphocytes, lung, and muscle of all animals. Its true function is unknown, but it may have a role in copper transport, nerve conduction, cell signalling, regulation of circadian activity and antioxidant reactions. Pathogenic prions are bent, curved, or widened beta-rich oligomers that convert the normal prions by changing their tertiary structure and integrating them into the growing PrP^{sc} aggregate, where it acquires the properties associated with the abnormal protein. The pathogenic prions gain entry to the body through tonsils or Peyer's patches of the small intestine, and they are transported to the brain via the lymphatic system. The PrP gene (*Prnp*) has been cloned, and it is now clear that PrP is host encoded. The *Prnp* gene is identical to *Sinc*, a gene that controls scrapie replication in mice. Prusiner (1995) identified 15 amino acids at the N-terminal end of the PrP protein, and this sequence was used to construct molecular probes to study the sequences of the normal vs. the mutated form of the gene. A point mutation substitutes the amino acid proline for leucine, and this mutation encodes additional copies of an octapeptide repeat towards the 5′ end (Krakauer *et al.*, 1998). The normal protein consists mainly of alpha helices with a spiral backbone, and the new mutated prion protein is predominantly beta sheets with a fully extended backbone. This suggests that the protein undergoes posttranslational modification. It has a molecular weight of 27–30 kD, and may aggregate into 'prion rods', or fibrils. Deposition of these fibrils in neuronal tissues provided early evidence that the diseases were due to prion proteins.

The normal protein; PrP^c is protease sensitive, and dissolves in non-denaturing detergents. Pathogenic PrP^{sc} has quite different properties.

(i) It is relatively protease K-resistant – infectivity is not blocked by treating infective materials with proteases.

(ii) It does not dissolve.

(iii) It is resistant to acid and alkali treatment between pH 2 and 10.

(iv) It has survived two-year immersions in formol saline (Mims & White, 1984).

Replication

The replication of the abnormal prion protein involves recruiting normal PrP^c proteins, and 'flipping' them into a rogue prion-like shape that can infect other cells and animals (Mestel, 1996), in the absence of a nucleic acid template. The resulting PrP^{sc} is a four-helix bundle protein, with four regions of secondary structure (H1–H4). This change starts a chain reaction, and newly converted prions convert other proteins on contact, on the interior of the cell membrane. In cell culture experiments, the conversion occurred inside neuronal cells. PrP^{sc} accumulated in lysosomes, eventually filling them until they lysed and released prions to attack other cells (Prusiner, 1995).

Saborio *et al.* (2001) reproduced prion replication *in vitro*: PrP^{sc} aggregates from a scrapie brain homogenate were disrupted by sonication, and brain homogenates from healthy hamsters were used as a source of PrP^c. In the presence of a minute amount of disrupted PrP^{sc} aggregate as template, a large excess of PrP^c was rapidly converted into protease-resistant PrP^{sc}. Using cycles of incubation-sonication, 97% of

the protease-resistant protein in the sample corresponded to newly converted protein. The investigators describe this procedure as protein-misfolding cyclic amplification (PMCA), conceptually analogous to the PCR procedure for nucleic acid amplification, and propose that it may used as an aid in possible TSE diagnosis to detect low quantities of the abnormal protein before symptoms are apparent.

Transmission

Transmission of a TSE was first discovered in humans with the identification of an elusive and bizarre disease that appeared in New Guinea in the early 1900s. In 1957, Gadjusek and Zigas discovered an epidemic form of the disease in a New Guinea tribe, and this disease, termed 'Kuru', was reported as endemic in a particular district consisting of approximately 8000 individuals, the South Fore. The majority of affected individuals were women and children. Epidemiological studies of the tribes indicated that this tribal group practised ritual mortuary cannibalism in which the women and children consumed the brain of diseased males as a sign of respect, and as a way to acquire some of the diseased tribal member's exceptional qualities. This ingestion of infected neural tissues was later identified as responsible for transmitting the fatal Kuru epidemic. The disease virtually disappeared in New Guinea when cannibalism was terminated, but its study laid the foundation for understanding the pathology and the nature of prion disease.

BSE, the bovine prion, is transmitted via contaminated foodstuffs. Shortly after BSE was recognized, epidemiological studies suggested that the source of infection was meat and bone meal (MBM) supplements fed to the cows as dietary protein supplements. It was originally thought that scrapie was introduced into the MBM supplements when changes in the rendering processes were made less stringent, permitting infective prion survival into the final extracted product. Scrapie had not naturally crossed the species barrier into cows prior to this change in practice, perhaps because large amounts of the protein were required for infection to occur in cows. It is now thought that exotic ungulates in the London Zoo (Nyala or Kudu antelopes from Africa) are more likely to be the source of the bovine infection. The protein would have been introduced into the bovine population when the zoo animals died from TSE and were then introduced into a rendering process for the production of MBM products used in cow feed. BSE infected bovine tissue then re-entered the rendering process, with subsequent amplification of prion in the animal feed MBM supplements, expanding the risk for bovine infection from these supplements. Infected meats or bone meal supplements in animal feeds have allowed BSE to cross species barriers into other animal populations, including large and small cats, mink and additional exotic ungulates at the London Zoo. The first detected case of BSE in Japanese cattle revealed that lipid and protein supplements given to calves in their milk feeds are the probable source of the island nation's outbreak.

Prions are stable in soil and secreted in feces, placenta, or amniotic fluid, and there may be maternal transmission to the embryo or calf. Following a dialysis enrichment procedure, they have also been detected in the urine of scrapie-infected hamsters, BSE-infected cattle and humans suffering from CJD (Shaked *et al.*, 2001). The isoform detected in urine UPrP^{sc} appears to have lower infectivity than brain PrP^{sc}, and may differ in its conformation. Normal PrP$^{c\,is}$ is expressed on blood cells and infectivity can be transmitted via blood products, although the infectious PrP^{sc} agent has not been identified in blood. There are currently no tests sufficiently sensitive to detect infectivity via blood levels of PrP^{sc}. The factors involved in determining whether a prion can cross a species barrier are unknown, but a possible mechanism has been suggested in a yeast model. Prion-like activities have been identified in the yeast *S. cerevisiae*, in the form of two proteins that have non-Mendelian inheritance. These prions can adopt multiple structures and interact with prions from other species (Davenport, 2001).

The first evidence that BSE had crossed the species barrier into humans was seen in 1995 when an adolescent was diagnosed with a new variant CJD (nvCJD). Examination of this and subsequent cases demonstrated that BSE, FSE and nvCJD were all the same disease process crossing species boundaries. As of September 2002, 121 cases of nvCJD had been identified in the UK, 6 in France, 1 in Ireland, and 1 in Italy. Prions have been detected in certain high-risk tissues in infected animals, and consumption of prion-infected tissues is the probable means of transmitting the disease to humans and other animals at risk. High risk materials include brain, spinal cord and eyes, but prion protein has been found in lesser quantities in lymphatic tissues, dura mater, pineal glands, pituitary glands, CSF, placenta, adrenal gland, portions of the intestine, bone marrow, nasal mucosa, liver, lung, pancreas, and thymus. It has been suggested that individuals consuming prion-infected beef products were made more susceptible to infection due to inflammation stimulated by Group A pharyngeal infections. Inflammation enhances the rate of transmission of the prion into the lymphoreticular system, from which it eventually reaches neurons and the central nervous system. Although no prion has been detected in blood, serum or most solid organs, there is a theoretical risk for person-to-person transmitted disease via blood transfusion or tissue transplantation. Of note for the assisted reproduction laboratory, prion proteins have not been detected in the testes, ovary or uteri of infected animals.

Iatrogenic CJD has been described after neurosurgery, corneal and dura mater grafts, and following treatment with human pituitary-derived hormones such as early preparations of gonadotrophins and growth hormones. Because of the very long incubation period, there may be a reservoir of asymptomatic individuals who are infected but do not yet display symptoms of the disease. These may serve as a reservoir of CJD or nvCJD that may be transmitted to patients iatrogenically; therefore, individuals who have ever received human-derived growth hormones, at any time, are excluded from blood or organ donation. The USA also banned blood donations from people who lived in Europe during the height of the BSE crisis, linking the risk of infection to the amount of beef products consumed (proportional to the amount of time spent in the region). All donors who spent more than 3 months cumulative time in Britain or Europe have been eliminated from the donor population in order to address this theoretical risk.

The risk of *in vitro* transmission after attempted 'decontamination' is difficult to evaluate. Assessment has been attempted by mixing infectious particles with cellular products, submitting this to inactivating treatments and then inoculating animals with fractions of the preparation. These protocols have identified some ineffective treatments, for example, soaking in aldehyde. Obviously, application of universal precautions of asepsis and hygiene is essential, especially in anatomy/pathology laboratories and for the re-use of medical devices in neurosurgery or in ophthalmology.

Clinical presentation

Sporadic Creutzfeldt–Jakob disease (CJD)

Sporadic CJD is most frequently diagnosed in patients between the ages of 50–70 years. Initial symptoms are vague and non-specific. Approximately one-third of patients present with fatigue, anorexia and sleep disturbance. Another third suffer confusion and memory loss, and other individuals present with muscle wasting, motor neuron dysfunction and aphasia. Disease progress is sustained, without remission, and is marked by cognitive deficits such as dementia and behavioural abnormalities, the development of myoclonus and the presence of other neurological abnormalities such as pyramidal and cerebellar dysfunction. In the terminal stage of disease, patients lose voluntary muscle control and become mute. The mean time from onset of symptoms until death is 5 months and most patients are dead within 1 year.

New-variant Creutzfeldt–Jakob disease (nvCJD)

In contrast to sporadic CJD, the mean age for onset of symptoms in nvCJD is 29 years, substantially younger than the mean age of 60 for sporadic disease. The clinical manifestations are also quite different when the two groups of patients are compared. Patients with nvCJD are more likely to present with psychiatric manifestations of disease such as depression, social withdrawal, and other behavioural abnormalities. Sensory abnormalities such as paresthesia are also common in this patient population. Survival time is more prolonged for nvCJD with a mean survival time of 14 months, compared with 5 months for the sporadic disease. Each of the patients diagnosed with nvCJD had a history of beef consumption in England during the BSE epidemic.

Pathology

The molecular mechanisms underlying the pathogenesis of the human prion diseases are not understood and there are currently no effective strategies for early diagnosis or treatment of TSEs. Although they are diseases of the central nervous system, the spleen and lymph nodes are involved in early stages of the infection. For the infectious aetiologies such as nvCJD, prions are transported to the lymphoreticular system (LRS) following infection, where they replicate efficiently in the tonsils, spleen, appendix, and lymph nodes. The host fails to mount a classic immune response. The use of transgenic and knockout technology has shown that neither B nor T cells are competent alone for prion replication. It has been suggested that uptake of prions may take place through cellular interaction, perhaps through an immune complex-type interaction. After replication in the LRS, they invade the CNS, probably via the sympathetic peripheral nervous system. So far, PrP^{sc} has not been found in the autonomic nervous system. There is evidence that neurons are involved in spreading the infection along specific pathways to the spinal cord and brain. The first change is abnormal accumulation of PrP^{sc} probably on the surface of neurons. This is followed by release of PrP^{sc} into intercellular spaces, with formation of fibrils (prion rods). The abnormal protein-mediated change in conformation in the host's native PrP^c leads to production of further abnormal PrP^{sc} conformation. Neuronal cells show vacuolization, gliosis, accumulation of the protease-resistant abnormally folded prion isoform, and cell death. The disease has a very long incubation period of more than 10 years in humans, presenting with symptoms of dementia, ataxia and psychiatric symptoms. Once symptoms are recognized, nvCJD and the other prion diseases are fatal within a few months to 2 years.

Genetic disposition, as well as a helper protein (X) appear to be required for establishment of the infection. Rieger *et al.* (1999) suggest that Laminin receptor protein (LRP), a ribosomal protein and cell surface receptor for infectious agents may act as a helper protein. LRP belongs to a family of cell adhesion molecules, and works as a receptor for alphaviruses. It is also associated with the metastatic potential of solid tumours. Genetic predisposition is also suggested by the different rates at which individuals develop nvCJD. Individuals who are homozygous for methionine at codon 129 of the PrP^c gene (40% of the population) have been shown to be at greatest risk for the early development of symptomatic disease. The first case of nvCJD has been detected in a heterozygous individual; although the onset of disease may be slower in this genetic population, it is not eliminated. Individuals with other amino acids at codon 129 (methionine/valine or valine/valine) are also susceptible to nvCJD, but the incubation period is longer.

Diagnosis

Due to the potential danger of transmitting prions from infected but asymptomatic individuals, as well as the risk associated with in using any human or animal-derived products used in transfusion or blood and urine pharmaceutical products, research into a preclinical test for the mutated prion has attracted significant commercial interest. The standard experimental method used to test for TSE infectivity involves inoculating a sample of infected material (neuronal tissue) into the brain of a laboratory

mouse and then monitoring the animal. Because such tests can take up to 12 months to yield a result, the development of assays for rapid detection is a high research priority. Western blotting or enzyme-linked immunosorbent assay (ELISA) techniques are quicker and more economical, but they are less sensitive, and it is not clear whether they can be used to identify animals incubating the disease. These assays involve digesting infected tissue with a protease, and then identifying the protease-resistant prion with the use of antibodies. To date (2003), the European Commission (EC) has approved three such tests: the Bio-Rad test developed by the Commisariat à l'Energie Atomique (CEA) in France; Prionics-Check developed by Prionics AG in Switzerland; and the Enfer test system developed by Enfer Technology in Ireland. New regulations in Europe require that brain tissue from slaughtered cattle be tested using one of these approved tests before the animals can be sold as beef. Testing became mandatory on January 1 2001 for all 'at risk' animals and as of July 1 2001, based on fact that the incubation period for BSE ranges from 4–6 years, all cows aged over 30 months have to be tested. However, the tests are based upon immunological reagents, and it is apparently difficult to develop reagents that reliably differentiate between the two isoforms. Veterinary authorities across the EC have reported hundreds of false positives using these tests. A new approach was developed by Paramithiotis *et al.* (2003), who found that hydrophobic PrP tyrosine residues that are sequestered, and thus 'hidden' in native PrP^c become exposed to solvent during the conformational conversion to Prp^{Sc}. This observation suggested that a conserved tripepetide, Tyr–Tyr–Arg might become accessible to antibodies raised against synthetic peptides containing this sequence. Polyclonal and monoclonal antibodies raised against this repeat motif recognized the pathological isoform but not the normal PrP^c, as assessed by immunoprecipitation, plate capture immunoassay and flow cytometry. Many of the polyclonal antibodies were cross-reactive with PrP^{Sc} from mice, hamsters, sheep, cattle and humans. The antibodies also recognized misfolded but protease-sensitive PrP, a molecular species that has recently been identified as characteristic of certain prion strains, early prion infection and interspecies prion transmission. The authors suggest that this protease-sensitive prion may represent a transient intermediate between normal structure and the abnormal aggregated isoform that is protease resistant. This new approach, using antibodies against conformation-selective exposure of peptide sequences, may provide tools for diagnostics, research and therapies in the future. Non-immunological tests are also being investigated, including the use of plasminogen, which sticks to rogue but not normal protein (Fischer *et al.*, 2000). Miele *et al.* (2001) reported that EDRF protein, an erythroid-specific marker, may act as a diagnostic marker for infection in cattle; this possibility is a subject of further ongoing research.

For the diagnosis of human disease, CSF may be tested for the detection of 14-3-3 protein, which appears to act as a marker of neuronal cell death. This assay detects the beta isoform of the protein using antibody-based technologies (ELISA or Western blot). Although detection of the 14-3-3 beta isoform is very sensitive in the evaluation of dementia, including Alzheimer's disease, patients with HSV encephalitis may produce some false positive results. Tissue diagnosis of CJD demonstrates characteristic spongiform changes in the brain. In sporadic CJD, amyloid plaques may be seen in the brain tissue, while in nvCJD the amyloid plaques may demonstrate surrounding vacuolization of the tissue in a 'daisy-like' pattern. Immunostaining of these prion-protein filled plaques confirms the diagnosis. There is no test approved for the routine screening of asymptomatic humans for this disease.

Further diagnostic tests remain under development, and there are encouraging reports regarding the use of antibody therapy in mice (White, 2003). Continued research in this area will hopefully, in due course, result in reliable diagnostic tests and perhaps a potential cure for the diseases. In the meantime, every ART laboratory should have an awareness of the potential dangers when using blood-derived products and when considering re-use of instruments. Hormones used in fertility treatments have been derived both from urine and from culture techniques that utilize serum supplements, and serum supplements are also used in embryo culture systems. Although the risk of prion transmission in ART may be very small, the highest possible levels of safety must be maintained by continued care and vigilance, both by manufacturers of pharmaceuticals and supplies, and by healthcare personnel involved in their use.

REFERENCES

www.prionics.ch

Davenport, R. J. (2001). Getting yeast prions to bridge the species gap. *Science*, **291**: 1881.

Fischer, M. B., Roecki, C., Parizek, H. P. S. & Aguzzi, A. (2000). Binding of disease-associated prion protein to plasminogen. *Nature (London)*, **408**: 479–83.

Gadjusek, D. C. & Zigas, V. (1957), Degenerative disease of the central nervous system in New Guinea: the endemic occurrence of 'kuru' in the native population, *New England Journal of Medicine*, **257**, 974–8.

Krakauer, D. C., de Zanotto, P. M. & Pagel, M. (1998). Prion's progress: patterns and rates of molecular evolution in relation to spongiform disease. *Journal of Molecular Evolution*, **47**: 133–45.

Mestel, R. (1996). Putting prions to the test. *Science*, **273**: 184–9.

Miele, G., Manson, J. & Clinton, M. (2001). A novel erythroid-specific marker of transmissible spongiform encephalopathies. *Nature Medicine*, **7** (3): 361–3.

Mims, C. A. & White, D. C. (1984). *Viral Pathogenesis and Immunology*. Boston: Blackwell Scientific Publications.

Paramithiotis, E., Pinard, M., Lawton, T. *et al.* (2003). A prion protein epitope selective for the pathologically misfolded conformation. *Nature Medicine*, **9**(7): 893–9.

Prusiner, S. B. (1991). Molecular biology of prion diseases. *Science*, **252**: 1515–21.

Prusiner, S. B. (1995). Prion diseases. *Scientific American*, **272**(1): 48–56.

Rieger, R., Lasmezas, C. I. & Weiss, S. (1999). Role of the 37 kDa laminin receptor precursor in the life cycle of prions. *Transfusion Clinique et Biologique*, **6**(1): 7–16.

Saborio, G. P., Permanne, B. & Soto, C. (2001). Sensitive detection of pathological prion protein by cyclic amplification of protein misfolding. *Nature*, **411**: 810–13.

Shaked, G. M., Shaked, Y., Jaruv-Inbal, A., Halimi, M., Avraham, I. & Gabizon, R. (2001). A protease-resistant prion protein isoform is present in urine of animals and humans affected with prion diseases. *Journal of Biological Chemistry*, **276**(34): 1479–82.

White, A. R. (2003). Monoclonal antibodies inhibit prion replication and delay the development of prion disease. *Nature*, **422**: 80–3.

FURTHER READING

Aguzzi, A. (2001). Blood simple prion diagnostics. *Nature Medicine*, **7**(3): 289–90.

Aguzzi, A. & Brandber, S. (1999). Shrinking prions: new folds to old questions. *Nature Medicine*, **5**(5): 486.

Bonetta, L. (2001). Scientists race to develop a blood test for vCJD. *Nature Medicine*, **7**(3): 261, 361–3.

Brown, P. (1997). The risk of bovine spongiform encephalopathy ('mad cow disease') to human health. *Journal of the American Medical Association*, **278**: 1008–11.

Buckley, C. D., Rainger, G. E., Bradfield, P. F., Nash, G. B. & Simmons, D. L. (1998). Cell adhesion: more than just glue. *Molecular Membrane Biology*, **15**(4): 167–76.

Cashman, N. R. (1997). A prion primer. *Canadian Medical Journal Association*, **157**(10): 1381–6.

Cohen, F. E., Pan, K., Huang, Z., Baldwin, M., Fletterick, R. J. & Prusiner, S. B. (1994). Structural clues to prion replication. *Science*, **264**: 530–1.

Darbord, J. C. (1998). Inactivation of prions in daily medical practice. *Nature Medicine*, **4**(10): 1125.

Gadjusek, D. C. (1977). Unconventional viruses and the origin and disappearance of Kuru. *Science*, **197**, 943–60.

Gadjusek, D. C., Gibbs, C. J. & Alpers, M. (1966). Experimental transmission of a kuru-like syndrome to chimpanzees. *Nature*, **209**: 794.

Ironside, J. W. (1998). Prion diseases in man. *Journal of Pathology*, **186**(3): 227–34.

Johnson, R. T. & Gibbs, G. J. (1998). Creutzfeldt–Jakob disease and related transmissible spongiform encephalopathies. *New England Journal of Medicine*, **339**: 1994–2004.

Kermann, E. (1998). Creutzfeld–Jacob disease (CJD) and assisted reproductive technology (ART) *Human Reproduction*, **13** (7): 1777.

La Bella V., Collinge, J., Pocchiari, M. & Piccoli, F. (2002). Variant Creutzfeld–Jakob disease in an Italian woman. *The Lancet*, **360**: 997–8.

Lewis, R. (2001). Portals for prions? Investigators look at potential pathway for prions. *The Scientist*, **15**: 21–3.

Lindenbaum, S. (1979). *Kuru Sorcery*. Mountain View, CA: Mayfield Publishing Co.

Masison, D. C., Maddelein, M. L. & Wickner, R. B. (1997). The prion model for [URE3] of yeast: spontaneous generation and requirements for propagation. *Proceedings of the National Academy of Sciences, USA*, **94**: 12503–8.

Oesch, B. (1985). A celllular gene encodes scrapie PrP 27–30 protein. *Cell*, **40**: 735–46.

Parker Jr, J. C. & Snyder, J. W. (1999). Prion infections in Creutzfeldt–Jakob disease and its variants. *Annals of Clinical and Laboratory Science*, **29**(2): 112–16.

Pattison, J. (1998). The emergence of bovine spongiform encephalopathy and related disease. *Emerging Infectious Diseases*, **4**(3): 390–4.

Priola, S. A. (1999). Prion protein and species barriers in the transmissible spongiform encephalopathies. *Biomedicine and Pharmacotherapeutics*, **53**: 27–33.

Prusiner, S. B. (1997). Prion diseases and the BSE crisis. *Science*, **278**: 245–51.

Prusiner, S. B. (1998). Prions. *Proceedings of the National Academy of Sciences*. USA **10**(95): 13363–83.

Reichl, H., Balen, A. & Jansen, C. A. M. (2002). Prion transmission in blood and urine: what are the implications for recombinant and urinary-derived gonadotrophins? *Human Reproduction*, **17**(10): 2501–8.

Safar, J., Wille, H., Itri, V. *et al*. (1998). Eight prion strains have PrP(Sc) molecules with different conformations. *Nature Medicine*, **4**(10): 1157–65.

Scully, R. E., Mark, E. J., McNeely, W. F. & McNeely, B. U. (eds.) (1993). Case records of the Massachusetts General Hospital. *New England Journal of Medicine*, **328**: 1259–66.

Serpell, L., Sunde, M. & Blake, C. C. M (1997). The molecular basis of amyloidosis. *Cellular and Molecular Life Sciences*, **53**: 871–87.

Silar, P. & Daboussi, M. J. (1999). Non-conventional infectious elements in filamentous fungi. *Trends in Genetics*, **15**(4): 141–5.

Steelman, V. M. (1994). Creutzfeldt–Jakob Disease: recommendations for infection control. *American Journal of Infection Control*, **22**: 312–18.

Tan, L., Williams, M. A., Kahn, M. K., Champion, H. C. & Nielsen, N. H. (1999). Risk of transmission of bovine spongiform encephalopathy to humans in the United States. *Journal of the American Medical Association*, **281**: 2330–9.

Taylor, K. L., Cheng, N., Williams, R. W., Steven, A. C. & Wickner, R. B. (1999). Prion domain initiation of amyloid formation in vitro from native Ure2p. *Science*, **283**: 1339–43.

Wadman M. (1999). Fear of BSE could hit US blood banks. *Nature*, **397**: 376.

Wickner, R. B. (1994). Evidence for a prion analog in *S. cerevisiae*: the [URE3] non-Mendelian genetic element as an altered URE2 protein. *Science*, **264**, 566–9.

Woolley, I. (1998). Transmissible spongiform encephalopathy and new-variant Creutzfeldt–Jakob Disease. *Clinical Microbiology News*, **20**: 165–8.

World Health Organization. Report of a WHO consultation on medicinal and other products in relation to human and animal transmissible spongiform encephalopathies. WHO/EMC/ZOO/97.3 Available at http://www.who.int/emc/ diseases/bse/tse_9703.html#a17.

6

Parasitology

Introduction

Although all species of microorganisms discussed so far can be described as 'parasites', the term traditionally refers to parasitic protozoa, helminths (worms) and arthropods.

Parasites are divided into two classes.

Unicellular: protozoans (Kingdom Protista); four phyla (see Table 6.1a).

Multicellular: helminths – flatworms (flukes and tapeworms) and roundworms

  Arthropods – have chitinous exoskeletons with jointed appendages (lice, mites, ticks, etc.).

Classification of parasites is based upon taxonomic groups and the body site infected. Diagnosis of parasite infections may be made by fecal examination for ova and parasites, antigen detection systems, serologic tests and examination of thick and thin blood films. Molecular techniques for the detection and identification of parasitic infections are also under development.

Terminology

Parasite life cycles and their interrelationship with hosts are described by specific terms:

host: an organism that harbours or nourishes another parasite,

  definitive host: harbours the adult or sexual form of the parasite,

  intermediate host: harbours larval or asexual stages of the parasite,

  reservoir host: a non-human host that can maintain the infection in nature in the absence of human hosts.

parasitism: the parasite benefits at the expense of the host.

  endoparasite: lives inside the host, e.g. intestinal parasites, cause infection,

  ectoparasite: lives on the surface of the host, e.g. pubic lice, cause infestation.

symbiosis: close association of two species that are dependent on one another.

commensalism: there is benefit to one organism but no significant effect on the other, e.g. intestinal protozoa that have no pathologic effect on the host, such as *Entamoeba coli*.

schizogony (merogony): asexual multiplication of *Apicomplexa* (intracellular blood parasites); multiple intracellular nuclear divisions precede cytoplasmic division.

sporogony: sexual reproduction of *Apicomplexa*; spores and sporozoites are produced.

adult: the sexually mature stage of helminths and arthropods.

larva: immature stages of helminths and arthropods.

vector: an arthropod that transmits an infection.

  mechanical vector: transmits disease mechanically, through contamination via its body parts or feces, e.g. houseflies contaminating food with typhoid bacilli.

  biological vector: is essential in the life cycle of the parasite for development to infectious stages, e.g. malaria parasites in mosquitoes.

Table 6.1a. Classification of parasites

Unicellular Protozoa Kingdom: Protista		Multicellular Helminths Phylum: Nemathelminthes	
	Organisms		Organisms
Phylum: Sarcomastigophora	*Acanthamoeba spp.*	**Class :**	*Ancylostoma braziliense*
Subphylum: Sarcodina	*Blastocystis hominis*	**Nematoda**	*Ancylostoma caninum*
Class: Lobosea	*Entamobea coli*	(roundworms)	*Ancylostoma duodenale*
(amoeba)	*Entamoeba gingivalis*		*Angiostrongylus cantonensis*
	Entamoeba hartmanni		*Angiostrongylus costaricensis*
	*Entamoeba histolytica***		*Anisakis* spp.
	Entamoeba polecki		*Ascaris lumbricoides*
	Endolimax nama		*Brugia malayi*
	Iodamoeba butschlii		*Capillaria hepatica*
	Naegleria fowleri		*Capillaria philippinensis*
			Dirofilaria immitis
Phylum: Sarcomastigophora	*Chilomastix mesnili*		*Dracunulus medinensis*
Subphylum: Mastigophora	*Dientamoeba fragilis*		*Enterobius vermicularis***
Class: Zoomastigophorea	*Enteromonas hominis*		*Loa loa*
(flagellates)	*Giardia lamblia***		*Mansonella ozzardi*
	Trichomonas hominis		*Mansonella perstans*
	*Trichomona vaginalis***		*Mansonella streptocerca*
	Trichomonas tenax		*Necator americanus*
			Onchocerca volvulus
Order: Kinetoplastida	*Leishmania braziliensis* complex		*Strongyloides stercoralis*
(hemoflagellates)	*Leishmania donovani* complex		*Trichinella spiralis*
	Leishmania mexicana complex		*Trichuris trichiura*
	Leishmania tropica complex		*Toxocara canis*
	Trypanosoma brucei rhodiense		*Toxocara cati*
	Trypanosoma brucei gambiense		*Wucheria bancrofti*
	Trypanosoma cruzi		
	Trypanosoma rangeli		
Phylum: Ciliophora		**Class:**	*Diphyllobothrium latum*
Class:		**Cestoda**	*Dipylidium caninum*
Kinetofragminophorea	*Balantidium coli*	(tapeworms)	*Echinococcus granulosus*
(ciliates)			*Echinococcus multilocularis*
			Hymenolepis diminuta
			Hymenolepis nana
			Taenia saginata
			Taenia solium
Phylum: Apicomplexa	*Babesia*	**Class: Digenea**	*Clonorchis sinensis*
Class: Sporozoea	*Plasmodium falciparum*	(trematodes, the flukes)	*Fasciola hepatica*
	Plasmodium malariae		*Fasciolopsis buski*
	Plasmodium ovale		*Heterophyes heterophyes*
	Plasmodium vivax		*Metagonimus yokogawai*
			Paragonimus mexicanus
			Paragonimus westermani

	Unicellular Protozoa Kingdom: Protista		Multicellular Helminths Phylum: Nemathelminthes
	Organisms		Organisms
Phylum: Apicomplexa	*Cryptosporidium parvum*		*Schistosoma haematobium*
Class: Sporozoea	*Cyclospora cayetanensis*		*Schistosoma japonicum*
Subclass: Coccidia	*Isospora belli*		*Schistosoma mansoni*
	Sarcocystis hominis		
	Sarcocystis suihominis		
	Sarcocystis lindemanni		
	*Toxoplasma gondii***		
	Note: *Pneumocystis carinii* is now classified as an atypical fungus		
Phylum: Microspora	*Brachiola vesicularum*		
Subclass: Microsporida	*Enterocytozoon bieneusi*		
	Encephalitozoon cuniculi		
	Encephalitozoon hellem		
	Encephalitozoon intestinalis (formerly *Septata intestinalis*)		
	Nosema connori		
	Pleistophora spp.		
	Trachipleistophora anthropopthera		
	Trachipleistophora hominis		
	Vittaforma corneae (formerly *Nosema corneum*)		
	Microsporidium africanum (not yet described)		

*Urogenital pathogen/STD **prenatal /neonatal pathogen; ***both urogenital pathogen and prenatal/neonatal pathogen
****enteritis (homosexual/proctitis)

Table 6.1b. Arthropod parasites

	Phylum: Arthropoda	
Class: Arachnida	Class: Insecta	Class: Crustacea
Mites *Sarcoptes scabei**	(flies, mosquitoes, bugs, lice, fleas)	Copepods (water fleas)
Scorpions	Diplopoda (millipedes)	
Spiders	Chilopoda (centipedes)	
Ticks	Suckling lice *Phthirus pubis**	

*Ectoparasite.

Tables 6.1a and b outlines the basic classification of parasites, with a list of common parasites within each class. Those that are relevant to reproductive medicine are indicated with asterisks.

Unicellular: protozoa

Protozoa are unicellular eukaryotes, i.e. single-cell organisms: their cells contain a nucleus, nuclear membrane, organelles, multiple chromosomes and mitotic structures during reproduction. Protozoa have no cell wall, but are instead surrounded by a cell membrane that encloses the cytoplasm. Some species are encased in shells, and some can form highly resistant cysts. They are **heterotrophic**, obtaining food by ingesting organic matter via a process of endocytosis and digesting it within the cell. The majority reproduce asexually by simple binary fission, by multiple fissions or by longitudinal or transverse binary fission. Some have specialized modes of sexual reproduction. At least 30 species of protozoa infect humans, many of them found worldwide. Increased travel and immigration has spread the prevalence of parasitic protozoal infections that are still common in many countries. Protozoal infections are transmitted through ingestion or inhalation of the infective stage, by self-inoculation or via an arthropod vector. A few protozoa are transmitted via sexual contact.

Classification of protozoa

Protozoa are grouped into four phyla, based on their form of locomotion.

(i) Phylum: **Sarcomastigophora**
    Subphylum: **Sarcodinia**
        Class: **Lobosea** (the amoeba)
The Lobosea use pseudopodia for movement, and reproduce asexually.

(ii) Phylum: **Sarcomastigophora**
    Subphylum: **Mastigophorea** (sometimes referred to as a superclass for the flagellates; includes *Giardia*)
        Class: **Zoomastigophorea** (flagellates)
           Order: **Kinetoplastida** (includes the Trypanosomes and *Leishmania* spp.)
The Zoomastigophora have one or more flagellae, which are used for locomotion; they reproduce asexually.

(iii) Phylum: **Ciliophora**
    Class: **Kinetofragminophorea** (the ciliates)

The Kinetofragminophorea move by means of cilia. Reproduction may be asexual, and the organisms may also exchange nuclear material during conjugation.

(iv) Phylum: **Apicomplexa**
    Class: **Sporozoa** (includes malaria organisms and *Babesia*)
        Subclass: **Coccidia**
Sporozoa are generally non-motile, intracellular parasites that have several organelles organized into an 'apical complex'. Reproduction involves both sexual and asexual cycles.

(v) Phylum: **Microspora**
    Subclass: **Microsporidia**
Microsporidia have only recently been recognized as tissue parasites in immunocompromised patients, and are known to cause intestinal disease in HIV-positive patients. At least ten genera have been identified, but many organisms have not yet been classified. They are characterized by a unique hypodermic needle-like infection apparatus contained within their spores. The taxonomy of microsporidia will be amended significantly in the near future, on the basis of nucleotide sequence data.

Lobosea (amoeba)

Sarcodinia (subphylum); **Lobosea** (class); **Amoebida** (order). Amoeba move by using cytoplasmic protrusions known as pseudopods. These organisms cause both intestinal and tissue infections in humans and can also live in the human body as commensals.

Intestinal pathogenic amoeba and commensals in the oral/GI tract

Entamoeba histolytica, the organism responsible for amoebic dysentery (bloody diarrhoea), is a typical Sarcodine. *E. histolytica* infection is prevalent in the tropics and subtropics, and may cause infection in dogs, cats, rats, humans and other primates. It can be transmitted sexually by male homosexuals, and is a leading cause of 'gay bowel syndrome'. In 2–8% of cases, the colon wall is invaded and invasive trophozoites enter the circulation. These can cause an amoebic liver abscess if carried to the liver.

All other amoeba found in human feces are non-pathogenic commensals.

Entamoeba hartmanni	minor species of *E. histolytica*, not pathogenic
Entamoeba coli	non-pathogenic commensal
Entamoeba. gingivalis	found in human mouth, associated with poor hygiene
Endolimax nana	non-pathogenic commensal
Entamoeba polecki	found in pigs and monkeys; seen occasionally in humans, and may cause disease linked to high parasite burden
Iodamoeba butschlii	non-pathogenic commensal
Blastocystis hominis	commensal with probable pathogenicity linked to very high parasite burden; reproduces both asexually and by sporulation.

Transmission

Intestinal amoeba are acquired via contaminated food or water.

Life cycle

Amoeba usually exist in two stages: the trophozoite, a motile feeding stage that reproduces and the cyst, a non-feeding immotile stage that is infectious. The cyst is surrounded by a tough protective wall that makes it resistant to harsh environmental conditions. When cysts are ingested, the cyst wall breaks down in the small intestine (excystation), allowing trophozoites to develop, colonize the lumen and begin to reproduce. Some trophozoites will transform into cysts, which are excreted in the stool.

Diagnosis

Amoeba are identified on the basis of: (i) size and shape of the cyst (ii) shape of the cyst nucleus and numbers of nuclei present (iii) intracellular structures (iv) type of motility exhibited by the trophozoite. For example, the *E. histolytica* cyst is 10–20 μm in size, has one, two or four nuclei, and has a cigar-shaped chromatoid body; the trophozoite also

is 10–20 μm, is progressively motile and contains red blood cells that have been ingested. *Entamoeba hartmanii* is a commensal that can be confused with *E. histolytica* because the cyst stage also has one, two or four nuclei and a cigar-shaped chromatoid body, but differs in that both the cyst and trophozoite are <10 μm, and the trophozoite exhibits a sluggish motility. It contains ingested bacteria instead of erythrocytes. Identification of amoeba is based on wet preparations of feces (necessary for observation of trophozoite motility) and a permanent trichrome stain of fecal material to study nuclear and intracellular structure.

Treatment

Treatment of *E. histolytica* depends on the site of infection; all positive cases should be treated. Iodoquinol, paromomycin and metronidazole, alone or in combination, are used to treat *E. histolytica* colonization. Emetine is used for treatment of amoebic liver abscesses.

Tissue amoeba

Naegleria fowleri and *Acanthamoeba* spp. are free-living amoeba. They are found in stagnant water, and are opportunistic human pathogens.

Naegleria is an amoeboflagellate, alternating from an amoeboid form to a flagellated form in the free-living state. Only the amoeboid stage (the trophozoite) is found in host tissues. *Naegleria fowleri* is usually acquired from swimming in small lakes and ponds. The organism can survive chlorination, and infection has been reported from drinking unfiltered, chlorinated tap water. It enters the nasal mucosa, migrates along the olfactory nerves, and invades the brain within a few days. Primary amoebic meningoencephalitis (PAM) is rapidly progressive and usually fatal, with diagnosis made at autopsy.

Acanthamoeba (at least six species) causes granulomatous amoebic encephalitis (GAE), a chronic form of meningoencephalitis in humans, usually in immunocompromised individuals. Infection occurs via inhalation of contaminated aerosols or dust, or through broken skin or mucous membranes. The organism has been found in lungs, vagina, skin lesions, eyes, ears and nasal and sinus passages. It may also cause keratitis, usually from contaminated contact lens solutions or from wearing contact lenses while swimming in contaminated waters. Species of *Acanthamoeba* are resistant to chlorination. Both trophozoites and cysts of *Acanthamoeba* are recovered from tissue biopsies of skin, corneal scraping or brain. The cyst has a double-walled wrinkled appearance when seen in tissue, and tissue trophozoites, rarely seen in the motile state, have pseudopodia.

The related amoeba *Balamuthia mandrillaris* is another agent of GAE in immunocompromised individuals, mainly those with AIDS. It has also been found in healthy children and in many primates, as well as horses and sheep.

Treatment

Acanthamoeba spp. vary in their sensitivity to antimicrobials. Amphotericin B is used for *Naegleria* amoebic meningoencephalitis; azoles, in combination with fluocytosine for amoebic encephalitis (*Acanthamoeba* or *Balamuthia*); propamidine for *Acanthamoeba* keratitis.

Sarcomastigophora (flagellates)

Sarcomastigophora (phylum); **Zoomastigophorea** (class); **Mastigophora** (subclass) use specialized whip-like flagella for motility, and reproduce asexually. Flagellates inhabit the gastrointestinal tract, the urogenital tract, blood and other tissues in humans. *Giardia lamblia*, *Dientamoeba fragilis* and some *Trichomonas* species are intestinal pathogens; *Trichomonas vaginalis* is a urogenital pathogen, discussed in detail in Chapter 8.

Giardia lamblia

G. lamblia, also known as *G. intestinalis*, causes traveller's diarrhea worldwide (giardiasis), with a higher prevalence in crowded areas with poor sanitation.

Transmission

Infection results from ingestion of cysts transmitted by infected food or water, feces, flies and fomites.

Life cycle

The cyst stage of *G. lamblia* is infective and the trophozoites multiply asexually in the small intestine via binary fission. Infective cysts are passed in feces.

Diagnosis

G. lamblia is differentiated from non-pathogenic flagellates that may be found in the intestinal tract by physical appearance of both the cyst and the trophozoite, using direct preparations from feces and trichrome-stained permanent slides.

Treatment

Furazolidone and quinacrine are approved by the FDA for treating giardiasis. Albendazole and metronidazole are also used (not FDA approved).

Dientamoeba fragilis

D. fragilis also causes diarrhea. It is more common in children, and prevalence may be higher in institutionalized individuals. Although it has no observable flagella, this parasite is included with the Sarcomastigophora flagellates.

Transmission

The mode of infection is uncertain but is probably hand-to-mouth from fecal contamination or via direct contact with an infected individual.

Life cycle

D. fragilis is found in crypts of the colonic mucosa; when seen in feces it moves by pseudopodia, and may be confused with amoeba. The infective trophozoite (no cyst stage) multiplies asexually in the caecum via binary fission. Trophozoites are passed in faces.

Diagnosis

Fecal examination reveals motile trophozoites or trophozoites on trichome-stained permanent slides.

Treatment

Iodoquinol, tetracycline, and paromomycin are effective in treating dientamoeba infections.

Intestinal commensal flagellates

Trichomonas hominis, Trichomonas tenax, Retortamonas intestinalis, Chilomastix mesnili and *Enteromonas hominis* are intestinal commensal flagellates that may be confused with the pathogens. *T. tenax* is a mouth commensal that occasionally (rarely) produces disease in respiratory sites. *T. hominis* and *T. tenax* may sometimes be found together in the oropharynx.

Trichomonas vaginalis

The flagellate *Trichomonas vaginalis* is the only pathogenic protozoan that infects the vagina and the urethra, causing vaginitis and non-specific urethritis. Although women usually exhibit symptoms, males tend to be asymptomatic carriers. The parasite is sexually transmitted, usually via intercourse. There is no cyst formation, and it must pass from individual to individual to remain alive. The trophozoite stage of *T. vaginalis* is both the infective and the diagnostic stage; diagnosis is based on physical appearance and characteristic jerky motility of the trophozoites found in urine, urethral discharge, or vaginal discharge. *T. vaginalis* infection may also be observed on the Papanicolaou smear (see Chapter 8 for details).

Treatment

Metronidazole

Systemic flagellates

Systemic flagellates, or hemoflagellates, belong to the order **Kinetoplastida**. These flagellates require an arthropod as an intermediate host, and use blood as their means of transport from the portal of entry. They are found in tissue other than the intestine and undergo metamorphosis from non-motile to motile forms, exhibiting different morphology in different locations. Two intermediate forms are usually found in the vectors. Prototypes of this group include *Leishmania* and *Trypanosoma*.

Leishmania spp.

The genus *Leishmania* has four species complexes that are pathogenic:
  L. tropica or Old World
  L. mexicana or New World
  L. braziliensis
  L. donovani.

Clinical manifestations

- *L. tropica* complex and *L. mexicana* are responsible for cutaneous infections (Oriental Sore, Baghdad boil, Delhi boil).
- *L. braziliensis* invades skin lesions and may spread to the lymphatics causing chronic mucosal ulceration leading to disfigurement (New World leishmaniasis, espundia, uta), and cutaneous leishmaniasis when cell mediated immunity is compromised.
- *L. donovani* causes visceral leishmaniasis with invasion of macrophages in the bone marrow, liver and spleen (Kala-Azar, Black fever, Dumdum fever).

Transmission

All species of *Leishmania* that infect humans are zoonotic with dogs, rodents or foxes as the usual hosts. The organisms are spread from the animal host by the bite of a sandfly (*Phlebotomus*).

Life cycle

A promastigote, the infective form, migrates to the sandfly's salivary glands and is regurgitated when the sandfly bites a human. The promastigotes invade the wound site and are taken up by macrophages where the promastigote converts to an amastigote (the diagnostic form). The amastigotes multiply in macrophages. Depending on the species, amastigotes may: (i) be restricted to macrophages in skin lesions (ii) spread to the lymphatics or (iii) invade the bone marrow, liver and spleen macrophages.

Diagnosis

The parasites are identified when amastigotes (referred to as Donovan bodies) are identified in macrophages.

Treatment

L. tropica is treated with local heat and antimony; antimony and amphotericin B are used for *L. braziliensis*, and antimony and pentamidine for *L. donovani*. Ketoconazole, paromomycin, Sodium Stb (not FDA approved) and meglumine (not FDA approved) are also used to treat leishmaniasis.

Trypanosoma spp.

Trypanosomes are systemic flagellates, found in the blood at one stage during their life cycle.

(i) *Trypanosoma brucei rhodesiense* causes East African (Rhodesian) sleeping sickness, and *T. brucei gambiense* causes West African (Gambian) sleeping sickness.

Transmission

Both subspecies are spread by the tsetse fly (*Glossina*).

Life cycle

The fly bites an infected individual and ingests trypomastigotes (infective form), which develop into epimastigotes in the gut of the fly. The infective trypomastigotes develop and move to the fly's salivary glands. When the insect bites a human the trypomastigotes are deposited and first multiply in the peripheral blood, then later multiply in lymph nodes and the central nervous system.

Clinical manifestation

Sleeping sickness is a chronic relentless disease that eventually affects the central nervous system resulting in coma and death.

Diagnosis

The trypomastigote can be demonstrated on a human blood, plasma or CSF smear or in tissue biopsies from lymph nodes or CNS tissue.

Treatment

Treatment of trypanosomiasis depends on the disease phase. In general, pentamidine or suramin are used to treat early stages of African trypanosomiasis without CNS involvement. The late stage is treated with melarsoprol or tryparsamide. Elfornithine (DFMO-ornidyl) is used for early and late stages of *T. brucei* without CNS involvement; melarsoprol or suramin for early stages of *T. brucei gambiense* and *T. brucei rhodesiense* without CNS involvement.

(ii) *Trypanosoma cruzi*, found in Central and South America, causes Chagas' disease. The life cycle and the insect vector differ from those of trypanosomes that cause sleeping sickness.

Transmission

T. cruzi is transmitted by the *Triatoma*, which is referred to as the 'kissing' bug or the reduviid bug. The reduviid bug lives in houses made of mud, sticks, and thatch and feeds on warm-blooded hosts at night. The insect is attracted to mucous membranes (e.g. conjunctiva of the eye). The parasite is maintained in animal reservoirs, including armadillos, dogs, cats, opossums and rodents.

Life cycle

When the reduviid bug bites an infected human it ingests trypomastigotes, which are converted to epimastigotes in the gut of the bug. The epimastigotes multiply and develop into the infective form, the trypomastigotes, which are passed in the bug's feces. When the bug bites the next individual, it fecally contaminates the wound. The trypomastigotes from the feces are usually rubbed into the wound in response to itching from the bite. Trypomastigotes can invade various tissues (heart muscle, CNS) in humans, where they develop into amastigotes within macrophages.

Clinical manifestation

In adults, Chagas' disease may result in an enlarged heart, oesophagus and colon. Sudden death is usually due to an enlarged flabby heart. In children the disease is manifested by periorbital edema (Romana's sign), cardiac ganglia destruction, megacolon, dilation of the oesophagus, destruction of cardiac ganglia and rapid death. *T. cruzi* crosses the placenta and can cause prenatal infection.

Diagnosis

Amastigotes can be found in heart muscle, liver, or CNS macrophages; they are round or oval, with a prominent nucleus and a dark staining, bar-shaped kinetoplast (modified mitochondrion). Trypomastigotes are occasionally found in blood and diagnosis may be made from stained blood smears. Serologic tests are useful in chronic infections on a human blood, plasma or cerebrospinal fluid (CSF) smear, or in tissue biopsies from lymph nodes or CNS tissues.

Treatment

T. cruzi can be treated with benznidzole or nifurtimox for acute or early stage infection, but neither are approved by FDA for this purpose.

Non-pathogenic trypanosomes may be found in humans, e.g. *Trypanosoma rangelii* has been identified in humans in both Central America and South America. These trypanosomes may confuse diagnosis of pathogens.

Ciliophora (ciliates)

Ciliophora (phylum); **Kinetograminophorea** (class) are the ciliates, organisms that move by means of cilia and have two different kinds of nuclei. These protozoa multiply asexually by binary fission and sexually reproduce by conjugation with exchange of micronuclei.

Balantidium coli

The only ciliate pathogenic for humans is *Balantidium coli*, a swine parasite.

Clinical manifestation

Balantidium coli is the largest parasitic protozoon (60 μm × 40 μm); it invades the intestinal tract to produce intestinal lesions and cause severe dysentery. There have been reports of *B. coli* in vaginal infections, probably due to fecal contamination of the vagina.

Transmission

Spread by flies, via contaminated food, water or fomites (i.e. exposed to pig feces).

Life cycle

The ingested cyst stage passes to the small intestine where it excysts, and trophozoites multiply asexually in the large intestine. Both cysts and trophozoites are found in feces or intestinal mucosa.

Diagnosis

The organism is easily recognized in feces due to its size, the presence of cilia and the presence of two nuclei in both the cyst and trophozoite stages.

Treatment

Iodoquinol, metronidazole or tetracycline.

Apicomplexa (sporozoa)

Apicomplexa (phylum); **Sporozoea** (class) are intracellular parasites of blood and other tissues. Classic pathogens and parasites such as malaria are in this group, and some members have recently been recognized as opportunists. These protozoa have no apparent organelles of locomotion, have a life cycle that includes both asexual (schizogony) and sexual (gametocyte production and sporogony) reproduction and usually carry out their life cycle in two hosts. They have organelles organized into an 'apical complex' that functions in the penetration of cells. *Plasmodium, Piroplasma and Toxoplasma* species belong to this group.

Plasmodium

Plasmodium species cause malaria, which is endemic in tropical and subtropical areas worldwide. There are four species of *Plasmodium* that cause malaria:

P. vivax is the most widespread, found in temperate climates as well as tropical and subtropical regions.

P. ovale is most frequently reported from West Africa, but is also found sporadically in other parts of tropical Africa, South America, and Asia.

P. malariae and *P. falciparum* are found in tropical and subtropical areas.

Transmission

The mode of disease transmission and parasite life cycle is the same for all four species. The female *Anopheles* mosquito is the biologic vector and definitive host. The mosquito carrying *Plasmodium* parasites introduces infective sporozoites in its saliva when it bites a human host. Malaria can also be transmitted via contaminated needles and blood transfusions.

Life cycle

Sporozoites enter the circulation, reach the liver within 30–60 minutes and each sporozoite becomes a cryptozoite that reproduces asexually, forming many merozoites. The merozoites attach to receptors on erythrocytes and are endocytosed. In the red blood cells the organisms feed on hemoglobin, and the merozoites mature through the trophozoite (ring form) stage to become schizonts within 36–72 hours. Each schizont produces 6–24 merozoites. When the schizont is mature, the red blood cell (RBC) ruptures and releases the merozoites, which invade new RBCs. This cycle continues with the rupture of red blood cells, and symptoms appear when toxic materials are released from the lysed red cells. Later in the malarial infection, some merozoites will develop into male sex cells (microgametes) and female sex cells (macrogametes). When the female *Anopheles* mosquito takes in a blood meal from an infected individual, she ingests gametocytes and the sexual cycle begins. The gametes unite in the stomach of the mosquito and form a motile zygote that encysts on the mosquito's stomach wall. After further maturation the cyst ruptures and releases many sporozoites that migrate to the mosquito's salivary glands, to be deposited when the mosquito bites the next person.

Clinical manifestation

Paroxysms that accompany red blood cell lysis are partly due to an allergic response to released parasitic antigens; they are characterized by 10–15-minute periods of shaking and chills followed by a high fever. These symptoms may last from 2–20 hours. *P. malariae* can invade only older red blood cells while *P. vivax* and *P. ovale* primarily infect immature reticulocytes. *P. falciparum* can invade both reticulocytes and old red blood cells and can also change red blood cell membranes. These differences result in different pathologies, with complications associated with *P. malariae* and *P. falciparum* infections. Since there are only small populations of young blood cells at any one time, infections with *P. vivax* and *P. ovale* are not as severe as infections with the other species. *P. malariae* may lead to a nephrotic syndrome due to circulating complexes of malarial antigen and human antibodies on the basement membrane of the glomerulus. Infection with *P. falciparum* is the most serious, since it usually results in complications including renal failure from tubular necrosis and damage due to adhesion of the parasites to endothelial cells in the brain, visceral organs and placenta. Cerebral damage results from decreased blood flow to the brain: this infection may be fatal.

Diagnosis

Diagnosis of malaria depends on demonstrating and identifying trophozoites, schizonts or gametocytes in peripheral blood. Species of *Plasmodium* are differentiated based on the time required for sporozoites to develop to the schizont stage, the number of new merozoites produced, the morphology of the trophozoites, the appearance of the gametocytes for some species, and the morphology of the infected red blood cells.

Treatment

Chloroquine is used in combination with pyrimethamine for *P. vivax*, *P. malariae* and *P. ovale* prophylaxis, and, when sensitive, in combination with proguanil for *P. falciparum*. Chloroquineresistant *P. falciparum* strains (CRPF) are now widespread in South America, India, Southeast Asia and Africa. Mefloquine or doxycycline is recommended for CRPF prophylaxis, and atovaquone with proguanil (malarone), or artemisinin, artemether and artesunate for multi-drug resistant *P. falciparum*. Quinine plus doxycycline is used for *P. falciparum* resistant to chloroquine, doxycycline for *P. malariae* prophylaxis (add quinine for treatment), and primaquine (after chloroquine has been given) for *P. vivax* and *P. ovale*.

Piroplasma

Piroplasma (subclass) includes the genus **Babesia**, an intraerythrocytic parasite. *Babesia* species infect cattle and other animals, and occasionally cause human infection, usually in individuals who have been splenectomized. *Babesia microti*, endemic in southern New England, infects people with intact spleens.

Transmission

Babesiosis is transmitted by the hard tick, *Ixodes dammini*, which also carries Lyme disease. Rodents serve as reservoir hosts. Infection can also be transmitted transplacentally and via transfusion.

Life cycle

The *Babesia* life cycle involves two hosts, the tick *Ixodes dammini* and the white-footed mouse *Peromyscus leucopus*. The organisms multiply in red blood cells in the human intermediate host.

Clinical manifestations

Clinical symptoms resemble malaria, with nonsynchronous fever, chills, sweats, anorexia, and myalgia. Hemolytic anemia may result if cell hemolyis is prolonged. Spleen and liver disease are possible complications and, in severe cases, there may be renal failure, respiratory syndrome and intravascular coagulation.

Diagnosis

Diagnosis depends on identification of the parasites in blood. *Babesia*, like *Plasmodium*, is found inside red blood cells, but unlike *Plasmodium* species, *Babesia* may be observed outside cells. Trophozoites of *Babesia microti* tend to lie inside the cells in pairs at an acute angle or as a tetrad in a 'Maltese cross' formation. *Babesia* may be confused with the ring form of *Plasmodium falciparum*.

Treatment

Clindamycin, azithromycin or atovaquone in combination with quinine is used for treatment. Chloroquine relieves symptoms, but does not reduce the parasitemia.

Coccidia

Coccidia (subclass) includes *Toxoplasma gondii*, *Sarcocystis* spp., *Cyclospora* spp. and *Isospora belli*. In these parasites, schizogony occurs in nucleated cells of many species of mammals and birds, and sporogony occurs in the intestinal mucosa of the definitive host. Infective oocysts pass into the feces and infection occurs when a host ingests the oocyst.

Toxoplasma gondii

Toxoplasma gondii causes toxoplasmosis.

Transmission

T. gondii undergoes schizogony in all nucleated cells in the majority of animals and birds; the house cat is the usual definitive host. The cat becomes infected either transplacentally, or by eating infected small animals that contain tissue oocysts. Animals or humans become infected by ingesting infective sporozoite-containing oocysts present in cat feces, via ingestion of food or water that has been contaminated or by accidental hand-to-mouth transmission (e.g. from the litter box). The parasite may also be transmitted via blood transfusions and organ transplants, as well as by ingesting raw meat that contains bradyzoites, especially from pigs, cows, sheep and rabbits.

Life cycle

Both schizogony and sporogony occur in the intestinal mucosa of the cat, and infective oocysts are viable for up to one year in soil. When oocysts are ingested or inhaled, sporozoites are released and penetrate the intestinal wall. They travel in the bloodstream and divide mitotically in tissue as trophozoites called tachyzoites. Infected cells lyse and release the tachyzoites, which in turn infect more cells. In the late or chronic stage of the disease, cyst-like structures known as bradyzoites form in the brain and other tissues. These cysts can remain viable for extended periods of time, held in check by the host's immune system.

Clinical manifestation

The infection is usually asymptomatic, but may be symptomatic in the early stages, resembling infectious mononucleosis or other viral illnesses. Toxoplasma infection is most serious in the pregnant woman, as tachyzoites in maternal circulation cross the placenta to cause congenital toxoplasmosis, with possible mental retardation or blindness later in the child's life.

Transmission via organ transplantation is serious, since the immunocompromised recipient will be unable to respond to the infection. Toxoplasmosis is also severe in the setting of HIV infection, and its presence as a symptomatic disease may be diagnostic for AIDS.

Diagnosis

The disease is diagnosed by serology and in tissue biopsies. Serologic methods include latex agglutination tests, fluorescent antibody methods, ELISA or the Sabin–Feldman dye test in tissue biopsy smears. Bradyzoites are PAS (periodic acid-Schiff) positive and positive by Wright's Giemsa Staining in BAL (bronchoalveolar lavage) and sputum specimens.

Treatment

Atovaquone in combination with pyrimethamine, pyrimethamine with either clindamycin or spiramycin, and spiramycin for acute infections in pregnant women.

Sarcocystis

Sarcocystis species (*S. hominis*, a cattle parasite, and *S. suihominis*, a pig parasite) have a life cycle similar to that of *T. gondii*.

Transmission

Dogs, cats or humans can become definitive hosts if they eat uncooked meat of the intermediate host (beef or pork) containing sarcocysts. Humans can become accidental intermediate hosts if they ingest oocysts that form sarcocysts in muscles.

Life cycle

Sarcocysts release bradyzoites that invade intestinal cells and undergo gametogony to produce infective oocysts. When pigs or cattle ingest oocysts from fecally contaminated food, sporozoites are released and reach muscle tissue, where they form sarcocysts.

Clinical manifestation

Immunocompromised hosts may have severe diarrhea, fever and weight loss when infected.

Diagnosis

Distinctive oocysts with two sporocysts, each with four mature sporozoites can be identified in feces.

Treatment

There is no treatment for *Sarcoystis* spp. tissue disease; antidiarrheal treatment is used for accidental ingestion.

Isospora belli

Humans are the only definitive host for *Isospora belli*. The infection occurs commonly in South America and Southeast Asia, and has been reported as a cause of diarrhea in AIDS patients.

Transmission

I. belli is directly transmitted via sporulated oocysts in fecally contaminated water and food (no intermediate host).

Life cycle

Both schizogony and sporogony occur in the cytoplasm of epithelial cells in the small intestine. Two spherical sporoblasts develop within the oocyst, and after being passed in feces, these mature into sporocysts, each containing four infective sporozoites.

Clinical manifestation

Infection is mild, with symptoms including anorexia, nausea, abdominal pain and diarrhea. Malabsorption is a potential problem with this infection.

Diagnosis

I. belli is diagnosed by identifying the immature oocyst, containing 1–2 immature sporoblasts, in feces. Oocysts are recovered using the zinc sulfate flotation method and are stained with iodine.

Treatment

Sulfadiazine combined with pyrimethamine; TMP/SMX (trimethoprim/sulfamethoxazole).

Cryptosporidia

Cryptosporidium parvum is an opportunist that causes gastrointestinal infection in both normal and immunocompromised patients. The infection occurs worldwide, and there are probably many mammalian reservoir hosts. It has been associated with outbreaks of diarrhea in day-care centres and in community-wide outbreaks traced to contaminated drinking water supplies.

Transmission

The infection is acquired by the ingestion of oocysts from the feces of infected humans or animals. Human infection with *C. parvum* was first reported in 1976, and although it was originally thought to infect only immunocompromised patients, it is now recognized as an emerging pathogen. An outbreak in Georgia in 1987 affected 13 000 individuals, and the source of infection was identified as the county's public water supply. A large waterborne outbreak in Milwaukee (1993) affected over 400 000 people with clinically significant gastrointestinal symptoms in both immunocompetent and immunocompromised individuals. Other outbreaks (1993 and 1996) were associated with drinking unpasteurized apple cider (the apples were probably contaminated from oocysts in the soil) and an outbreak in 1995 was linked to chicken salad that may have been contaminated by a food handler in a home day-care centre.

Life cycle

The parasite reproduces both sexually and asexually in humans; the asexual cycle is initiated when a human ingests the infective oocyst. Both trophozoites and schizonts attach to the intestinal wall, and eight merozoites develop within the schizont.

Following maturation, a new schizontic cycle or a sexual cycle is initiated in the mucosa of the intestine. Microgametocytes and macrogametocytes unite and form mature gametes that merge to form an oocyte, which then develops into an oocyst. The oocyst is autoreinfective, since both the sexual and asexual stages occur in humans.

Clinical manifestation

Infection causes an acute diarrhea, lasting 1–2 weeks, but is self-limiting in individuals with a normal immune system. Immunocompromised patients often develop chronic diarrhea with *C. parvum* infection, and patients with AIDS have developed respiratory cryptosporidiosis – this disease serves as an AIDS-defining illness.

Diagnosis

Mature oocysts (containing four sporoblasts) can be identified in feces. The parasite is very small (4–6 μm oocyst), and flotation techniques for feces, followed by phase-contrast microscopy are helpful for identification. Acid-fast smears of fecal material are also useful. These non-specific assays have now been replaced by techniques that use monoclonal antibodies, such as enzyme immunoassays or direct fluorescence staining of cryptosporidium in stools.

Treatment

The majority of *C. parvum* infections are self-limiting in immunocompetent hosts and require no treatment. In the immunocompromised host, illness may be prolonged and may not respond to therapy. Treatment under these conditions is generally attempted with atovaquone and paromomycin. Spiramycin has been used experimentally.

Cyclospora

Cyclospora cayetanensis (formerly referred to as cyanobacterium-like body, or coccidian-like body, CLB) is very similar in appearance to *Cryptosporidia*, with oocysts that are larger.

Transmission

The parasite is transmitted via contaminated food or water. There have been several outbreaks in the United States since 1990: an outbreak in a Chicago hospital was due to contaminated drinking water from a rooftop reservoir, and later outbreaks were associated with raspberries imported from Guatemala, as well as with contaminated vegetables (fresh basil, green onions and Mesclun lettuce).

Life cycle

The complete life cycle for *Cyclospora* has not been determined, but probably includes birds that shed this organism in their guano. This fecal matter contaminates food products or water supplies that are ingested by humans to initiate infection. Oocysts require 1–2 weeks to sporulate and become infectious.

Clinical manifestation

The organism causes a self-limiting diarrhea that lasts from 3–4 days with possible relapses occurring over a 2–3 week period. It can cause chronic infection in AIDS patients.

Diagnosis

Immature oocysts 8–10 μm in size containing immature sporoblasts are seen in feces. A modified acid-fast stain may be used, but the affinity of the oocysts for the stain is highly variable within the same specimen.

Treatment

C. cayetanensis infection is usually self-limited in a competent host, and antidiarrheals may be used. Treatment with sulfadiazine and pyrimethamine, or TMP/SMX is only required in immunocompromised patients with symptoms persisting more than 10 to 14 days.

Microsporidia

Microsporidia are very small (1–2.5 μm) obligate intracellular tissue parasites that until recently were rarely seen in humans. The majority of human infections occur in immunocompromised individuals, in particular as a complication of AIDS.

Genera of microsporidia

There are ten genera:

Brachiola vesicularum	*Pleistophora* spp.
Enterocytozoon bieneusi	*Vittaforma corneae* (formerly
Enterocytozoon cuniculi	*Nosema corneum*)
Encephalitozoon hellem	*Trachipleistophora hominis*
Encephalitozoon	*Trachipleistophora*
(Septata) intestinalis	*anthropopthera*
	Nosema connori
Microsporidium africanum ('catch-all' for species not yet	
fully described)	

Transmission

Infection is acquired by ingestion of spores from fecally contaminated material, and may also occur by inhalation of spores.

Life cycle

Microsporidia inject infective contents from a spore into the host cell via a small polar tube. The organism multiplies in the host cell by merogony (binary fission) or schizogony (multiple fission) and sporogony (sexual reproduction). *E. bieneusi* releases thick-walled spores into the intestine, which are passed in the stool.

Clinical manifestation

Microsporidia have been found in eyes, lungs, kidney, heart, liver, adrenal cortex and the central nervous system. They have also been found in association with other infections, including tuberculosis, leprosy, malaria, schistosomiasis and Chagas' disease. *E. bieneusi* is found most often in AIDS patients, and can also cause a self-limiting diarrhea in immunocompetent patients. *Encephalitozoon*

cuniculi and *E. hellum* are most frequently associated with eye infection and these diseases are considered AIDS-defining illnesses.

Diagnosis

Microsporidial disease is diagnosed via histology using acid-fast and PAS (Periodic Acid Schiff) stains or electron microscopy. Modified trichome stained thin fecal smears may reveal spores, but positive controls are necessary.

Treatment

Microsporidial infections are often refractory to the currently available therapies. Albendazole is the treatment of choice for symptomatic disease, but it is not often curative.

Multicellular parasites: Helminths and arthropods

Metazoan helminths are multicellular worms, classified as roundworms (*Nemathelminthes*) or flatworms (*Platyhelminthes*); both phyla include human pathogens. Some insect species of arthropods are human ectoparasites.

Nemathelminthes (phylum) Nematoda (class)

The nematode class includes free-living genera as well as some that are host dependent. These worms have a cylindrical non-segmented body and species vary in size from a few millimetres to more than 1 metre in length. They have a mouth, complete digestive, excretory and nervous systems, but no vascular system or respiratory tract. The sexes are separate; males are smaller and more slender, and females have characteristic ova. Most roundworms generally have only one host and generally do not multiply in humans, the definitive host. Tissue nematodes require an intermediate host. Females produce from hundreds to millions of offspring and those with a more complex life cycle (requiring several hosts) produce the largest numbers of offspring. Either fertilized eggs or larvae may be infective, depending on the species: usually the filariform or third larval stage

Table 6.2. Intestinal roundworms

Roundworm	Common name
Enterobius vermicularis	Pinworm
Trichuris trichiura	Rectal whipworm (third most common intestinal worm)
Necator americanus	Hookworm
Ancylostoma duodenale	Hookworm
Ascaris lumbricoides	Large intestinal roundworm
Strongyloides stercoralis	Threadworm
Trichinella spiralis	Mealy pork infestation
Dracunculus medinensis	Guinea worm
Angiostrongylus cantonensis	Rat lungworm
Anisakis	Sushi parasite
Capillaria philipinensis	Sushi parasite

is infective. They may be transmitted via ingestion of eggs or larvae or via an insect vector, and cause intestinal infections as well as blood and other tissue infections. Disease correlates with the number of organisms ingested (worm load), nutritional status and age of the host and duration of the infection. Pathogenicity of nematodes may be due to:

(i) migration of adult or larvae through tissues (e.g. lungs),
(ii) piercing of the intestinal wall,
(iii) anemia from bloodsucking,
(iv) allergic and non-specific host responses to parasite secretions and excretions, and to degenerating parasite material.

Migrating roundworms cause blood or tissue eosinophilia.

Table 6.2 lists the common intestinal roundworms.

Enterobius

Enterobius vermicularis, 'pinworm' or 'seatworm infection' is found worldwide, associated with crowded conditions, and infects children 5–10 years of age.

Transmission

Infection is acquired by ingesting eggs that are distributed in air and in the house, and is usually transmitted hand-to-mouth.

Life cycle

The ingested eggs hatch in the small intestine, where the larvae mature and develop into adults that live in the colon. The gravid female migrates to the perianal region at night and lays eggs, then re-enters the intestine where more larvae hatch, introducing an autoinfection. Occasionally females are observed in the vagina or the appendix.

Clinical manifestation

Patients may be asymptomatic, but usually have loss of appetite, abdominal pain, loss of sleep, nausea, vomiting, vulval irritation and anal pruritus due to migration of the female to the anal area.

Diagnosis

Eggs and adults are usually recovered from the perianal region using a cellophane tape preparation taken early in the morning when the patient first wakes. The adult female or characteristic ova are seen; ova are 55 μm × 25 μm, thick-walled with the shell flattened on one side, usually embryonated.

Treatment

Mebendazole or pyrantel pamoate.

Trichuris

Trichuris trichiura (whipworm) is prevalent in warm climates and in areas of poor sanitation.

Transmission

Infective eggs containing larvae are ingested.

Life cycle

The larvae hatch in the small intestine and penetrate the intestinal villi, where they develop, move back to the lumen and progress to the cecum to mature. The adults live in the colon, with the anterior portion of the worm attached by a spearlike projection. The adult female releases undeveloped eggs in feces; the eggs require approximately one month in the soil to embryonate and become infective.

Clinical manifestation

Light infections of *T. trichiura* rarely cause symptoms. Heavy infections (500–5000 worms) may result in bleeding, weight loss, abdominal pain (colitis) vomiting, chronic diarrhea (possibly blood tinged) and inflammation from the worms threading themselves through the mucosa. Rectal prolapse, an emergency condition, may occur in undernourished children, and a diet inadequate in iron and protein may result in hypochromic anemia. Chronic infections can stunt growth.

Diagnosis

Depends on demonstrating characteristic eggs in the feces: 50 μm × 25 μm, yellowish to brown, barrel-shaped shell with polar plugs, containing an undeveloped unicellular embryo.

Treatment

Albendazole or mebendazole

Ascaris

Ascaris lumbricoides or 'large intestinal roundworm' is the largest of the intestinal nematodes, reaching 15–35 centimetres in length; it is responsible for the majority of intestinal nematode infections, affecting more than one billion individuals worldwide. Like *T. trichiura*, it is prevalent in warm climates and areas of poor sanitation. *A. lumbricoides* and *T. trichiura* require the same soil conditions and therefore often co-exist.

Transmission

Infective eggs containing larvae are ingested.

Life cycle

Once ingested, the larvae hatch out of the eggs in the small intestine, penetrate the intestinal wall to enter the circulation, and migrate to the liver and then to the lungs. In the lungs the larvae break out of lung capillaries into the alveoli, travel to the bronchioles, and are coughed up to the pharynx, swallowed and returned to the intestine where they mature to adults. The female passes undeveloped eggs in the feces, and the eggs require approximately one month in the soil to embryonate and become infective.

Clinical manifestation

Intestinal infection with a light worm load may be asymptomatic, but with an increasing worm burden symptoms appear, including abdominal pain, loss of appetite and colicky pains due to the presence of the adult in the intestine. Complications include intestinal blockage or appendix obstruction from migrating adults; children with heavy worm burdens can develop malnutrition.

Migrating adult worms may perforate the bowel wall and cause peritonitis or they may ascend through the bile duct and invade the liver causing hepatitis and abscess formation. The tissue phase (larva migrating through the lung) may cause a pneumonia known as Loeffler's syndrome, characterized by allergic asthma, edema, pneumonitis and eosinophilic infiltration.

Diagnosis

Characteristic eggs are found in feces. Eggs may be fertile or infertile: fertilized eggs are yellowish brown with a mammilated albuminous covering and contain an undeveloped unicellular embryo. Non-fertilized eggs have a heavy albuminous coating, a thin shell and an amorphous mass of protoplasm. Adult worms are large and white with a tapered anterior; the male has a curved tail. Adults may exit via the nose, mouth or anus.

Treatment

Albendazole or mebendazole; pyrantel pamoate is an alternative treatment. Symptoms occurring during the severe pulmonary stage may be alleviated with corticosteroid treatment. Nasogastric suction or surgery, along with antimicrobials may be used for intestinal obstruction by the adult worms.

Hookworm

The adult phases of *Necator americanus* (New World hookworm) and *Ancylostoma duodenale* (Old World hookworm) can be distinguished: *N. americanus* has cutting plates and *A. duodenale* has teeth. Hookworm, which infects nearly a quarter of the world's population, is associated with poor sanitation in agrarian regions. Like *Ascaris* and *Trichuris*, they are found in warm, sandy soil conditions.

Transmission

Hookworm is acquired when filariform larvae from the soil penetrate human skin.

Life cycle

The larvae enter the bloodstream and lymphatics, migrating to alveoli in the lung. They travel to the bronchioles, are coughed up to the pharynx, swallowed and returned to the small intestine where the larvae mature into adults. The female releases eggs that can be found in human feces. In warm soil, embryos develop rapidly (2 days) into rhabditiform larvae, molt twice and develop into infective filariform larvae (third stage).

Clinical manifestation

A small red itchy papule (ground itch) develops at the site of larval penetration. Large numbers of larvae in the lungs may cause bronchitis or mild pneumonia. Symptoms are more severe on reinfection, when coughing, wheezing, headache and bloody sputum may be seen. The majority of symptoms are associated with the adult worm, especially when there is a heavy worm burden, and include diarrhea, fever, nausea, vomiting and blood loss (up to 0.03–0.2 ml per worm/per day). Hemorrhages may occur at the site of attachment. Microcytic hypochromic anemia may develop with chronic infections, and mental and physical development may be delayed in children.

Diagnosis

Eggs found in feces are indistinguishable for the two species of hookworm, characterized by a thin, colorless shell containing an embryo at the 4–8-cell cleavage stage. The adult is rarely seen in stool, but rhabditiform larvae may be observed and must be distinguished from *Strongyloides stercoralis*.

Treatment

Mebendazole or pyrantel pamoate, together with iron replacement therapy. Thiabendazole ointment is used for cutaneous larva migrans.

Strongyloides stercoralis

Strongyloides stercoralis (threadworm), like hookworm, is found in warm, subtropical and tropical areas. *S. stercoralis* has a complicated life cycle: it can exist in a free-living state, or the parthenogenic female can live as a parasite and develop homogenically.

Transmission

Direct infection occurs when rhabditiform larvae (first stage) develop in the intestine from fertile eggs, are passed in the stool, develop into filariform larvae in the soil, and penetrate human skin.

Life cycle

The larvae enter the circulation, reach the lungs, break out of lung capillaries, migrate up the bronchial tree over the epiglottis and enter the digestive tract to mature to the adult stage. *S. stercoralis* can also develop indirectly (heterogenic). The rhabditiform larvae develop to free-living non-parasitic adults, and lay eggs that develop to rhabditiform larvae. These then develop to infective filariform larvae that can penetrate human skin. Autoinfection occurs when rhabditiform larvae develop to the infective stage in the intestine.

Clinical manifestation

Unlike hookworm, there is no papule at the site of penetration. Symptoms with *S. stercoralis* infection correlate with the developmental stage of the parasite. Larval migration causes pulmonary and cutaneous symptoms: pneumonia is the primary pulmonary symptom in the immunocompetent host, and there may be recurring allergic skin manifestations, including redness and itchiness. Intestinal symptoms include sharp, stabbing abdominal pain, chronic diarrhea, constipation, vomiting, and weight loss. In severe infections (disseminated strongyloidiasis or hyperinfection) a large number of filariform larvae develop in the intestine and migrate to the heart, liver and central nervous system causing a fulminating, often fatal infection. Heavy infections may also result in anemia, enteropathy due to protein loss, and edematous congested bowel. Patients with AIDS or those on chronic high dose steroid therapy (usually for chronic obstructive pulmonary disease) can develop a superinfection syndrome with autoreinfection cycle. Infection in immunocompromised patients with hyperinfection may be fatal, due to bacterial infection secondary to the spread of larvae and intestinal leakage.

Diagnosis

In feces, *S. stercoralis* is identified by recovering representative rhabditiform larvae: 275 μm × 16 μm with short buccal cavity, hourglass-shaped esophagus and prominent genital primordium. These larvae must be differentiated from hookworm larvae in feces; *S. stercoralis* eggs cannot be distinguished from hookworm eggs, although the eggs of *S. stercoralis* are rarely shed in feces. The female adult (2.5 mm) is rarely seen in stool; the male has not been identified. Duodenal aspirates may also yield larvae or eggs resembling those of hookworm. In cases of disseminated strongyloidiasis, filariform larvae

(500 μm long with a notched tail and an esophageal-intestinal ratio of 1:1) may be found in sputum. ELISA is used to diagnose *S. stercoralis* infection serologically.

Treatment

Ivermectin, albendazole. Thiabendazole may be used, but it is not always effective.

Trichinella spiralis

Trichinella spiralis is a tissue roundworm that causes trichinosis; carnivorous mammals are the primary hosts for this parasite, which is found worldwide.

Transmission

T. spiralis is transmitted to humans via the ingestion of undercooked meat (pork, bear, deer, walrus, etc.), containing encysted infective larval forms in muscle.

Life cycle

The larvae are released from the tissue capsule in the intestine and rapidly mature to the adult stage. The female produces live-borne larvae that penetrate the intestinal wall and enter the circulation to be carried to all parts of the body; the larvae encyst in striated muscle in humans.

Clinical manifestation

During the intestinal phase the first week following infection, patients may be symptom free or may have inflammation and edema of the small intestine causing nausea, vomiting, diarrhea, abdominal pain, headache and fever. During migration and encapsulation phases symptoms are common and may include high fever, periorbital edema, muscular pain or soreness, headache, pleural pain and general weakness. The larvae encapsulate in striated muscle of the face and diaphragm within 3 weeks of migration, and calcify within 18 months. In tissue other than muscle, the larvae promote an inflammatory reaction and are absorbed. A heavy infection may be fatal during the migration phase.

Diagnosis

Adults or larvae of *T. spiralis* are difficult to find in stool, and diagnosis of trichinosis is based on identification of encysted coiled larvae in biopsied muscle. X-rays may reveal calcified larvae. Serology (ELISA) is indicated 3–4 weeks after infection if there is a history of eating undercooked pork or bear and the patient has eosinophilia with the classic symptom of periorbital edema.

Treatment

Rest, anti-pyretics and analgesics are recommended for self-limiting or non-life-threatening infections. Life-threatening infections are treated with prednisone and albendazole. Thiabendazole is also used, but its effectiveness has not been documented. Patients are also given steroids to decrease the inflammmation and allergic response associated with the parasite's migratory phase of infection.

Dracunculus medinensis

Dracunculus medinensis (guinea worm or 'fiery serpent of the Israelites'), the largest adult nematode that is parasitic for humans (the female is up to 1 metre long) is found in the Middle East, Africa and India.

Transmission

The worm has an intermediate host, the copepod *Cyclops* spp. (water flea) and infection is acquired by drinking water containing infected copepods.

Life cycle

D. medinensis larvae are released in the intestinal cavity, penetrate the intestinal wall and migrate to deep connective tissue. About a year after infection, the large mature gravid female migrates and appears subcutaneously, usually in the legs, where it produces a painful blister in the skin overlying the worm's anterior end. Cool water stimulates the female to expose her uterus, the blister ruptures and larvae are released into the water. If the water contains copepods, the larvae are ingested by the fleas and develop to the infective larval stage.

Clinical manifestation

An infected individual has blister-like inflammatory papules that ulcerate on contact with water. Other symptoms include nausea, vomiting, urticaria and difficulty in breathing just before the worm exposes her uterus. The painful ulcer may be disabling, and if the worm is broken, this can cause a severe inflammatory reaction and secondary bacterial infections. Infected copepods can easily be filtered from drinking water, and this measure is being used in efforts to eradicate dracunculiasis worldwide.

Treatment

Gradual removal of the worm by gentle traction takes several days. Mebendazole is used for treatment, as well as removal of the adult worm from the skin, aspirin for pain, and measures to prevent secondary infection.

Zoonotic infections

Zoonotic infections occur when parasites that live in animals infect people. The infection is accidental and humans are not part of the normal life cycle.

Cutaneous larval migrans

Cutaneous larval migrans or 'creeping eruption' is a zoonotic infection that humans acquire from cat or dog hookworm. It is common in areas with large pet populations, but is prevalent in the Southern USA, Central and South America, Africa and Asia. Individuals who come into contact with soil that contains pet-contaminated feces are at risk. Small children are at particular risk because of their play habits (e.g. playgrounds and close contact with pets).

Transmission

Cutaneous larval migrans is acquired when the filariform larvae of the dog or cat hookworm (*Ancylostoma braziliense* or *Ancylostoma caninum*) penetrate the skin.

Life cycle

The hookworm filariform larvae are unable to complete their life cycle after penetrating the skin, and the worms continue to burrow under the skin.

Clinical manifestation

Symptoms of cutaneous larval migrans include an allergic response to the worm under the skin, characterized by red, itchy tracks (creeping eruptions), usually found on the legs.

Treatment

Ivermectin and albendazole.

Visceral larval migrans

Visceral larval migrans (VLM) is also referred to as toxocariasis. This zoonotic infection is acquired from dog and cat roundworms (*Toxocara canis*, *Toxocara cati*), and is found worldwide. Individuals who come into contact with soil that contains pet-contaminated feces are at risk. Infection in children is often associated with exposure to puppies.

Transmission

Visceral larval migrans is acquired from ingestion of infective stage larvae of developed roundworm eggs from soil.

Life cycle

The roundworm larvae migrate to the intestines where they hatch, penetrate the gut and leave the abdominal cavity to invade the liver, lungs, eye or brain, causing symptoms and pathology.

Clinical manifestation

Symptoms of the infection are associated with larval migration in human tissues, and clinical manifestation is characterized by eosinophilia, elevated isohemagglutinins, hepatomegaly and pulmonary inflammation. Cough, fever and often a history of seizures are associated with VML. The larvae may also encyst in the eye, causing ocular larval migrans that mimics retinoblastoma, a malignant tumour.

Treatment

Ivermectin and albendazole.

Other zoonotic infections

Other infections caused by zoonotic roundworms are considered according to their geographic distribution.

Angiostrongylus cantonensis and *Angiostrongylus costaricensis* are rat lungworms found in the Far East and in Costa Rica. *A. cantonensis* causes eosinophilic meningoencephalitis, and the adult worms of *A. costaricensis* lay eggs in the mesenteric arteries near the cecum, causing granulomas and abdominal inflammation. The rat is the normal animal host for this nematode. Snails or prawns are intermediate hosts for *A. cantonensis*, and *A. costaricensis* is acquired by eating unwashed vegetables contaminated with mucous secretions from the slug intermediate host. Mebendazole is the usual treatment.

Anisakis spp., roundworms of fish (e.g. herring) and marine animals are found in Japan and the Netherlands, causing intestinal infections when humans acquire the infective stage larvae. Eosinophilic granulomas form around the migrating larvae in the wall of the small intestine or stomach, causing abdominal pain. Mebendazole is the usual treatment.

Infective filarial larvae of **Dirofilaria** spp., filariae of dogs, foxes and raccoons, are found worldwide, and are spread to humans by mosquito bites. Acquiring the infective filarial larvae causes tropical eosinophilia or eosinophilic lung, characterized by high eosinophilia, high levels of IgE and a chronic cough from pulmonary infiltrates. Albendazole is the usual treatment.

Capillaria phillippinensis is a fish nematode. Infection occurs in humans when they ingest raw infected fish. Adult worms multiply in the human intestine, causing a blockage that can lead to a malabsorption syndrome characterized by persistent and extreme diarrhea. Secondary infection or cardiac failure can lead to death. Infection with *C. phillippinensis* is treated with mebendazole.

Gnathostoma spp. are found in the Far East. Dogs and cats are the normal hosts, and humans acquire the infection when they ingest larvae from raw infected fish or from poultice and leech treatments. Acute visceral larval migrans is followed by intermittent chronic subcutaneous swellings, and later, central nervous system invasion.

Gongylonema pulchrum, the pig nematode, is found worldwide. Human infection is due to accidental ingestion of an infected roach or dung beetle. Symptoms result from worms migrating in facial subcutaneous tissues.

Thelazia spp. have several mammals as their normal host, and the adult forms live in the conjunctival sac or tear duct. Contact with infected roaches or flies can lead to infections that cause eye irritation.

Filarial parasites

Filarioidea (superfamily) are slender tissue roundworms transmitted by an arthropod as intermediate host. They have complex life cycles; adult female filariae produce living embryos (microfilariae) that migrate to skin, lymphatics or blood, depending on the species. In some species, microfilariae are more prevalent in peripheral blood at certain times of the day or evening, coinciding with the feeding pattern of the intermediate arthropod host species. *Wucheria bancrofti, Brugia malayi, Loa loa,* and *Onchocerca volvulus* are human parasites that must be distinguished from the non-pathogenic species, *Mansonella*.

Wucheria bancrofti causes elephantiasis, referred to as Bancroftian filariasis.

Transmission

The parasite is transmitted by mosquitoes (*Culex, Aedes, Anopheles*) in tropical and subtropical regions.

Life cycle

Infective filariform larvae enter the skin via a mosquito bite, larvae migrate to the lymphatics and develop into adult worms. Female worms produce diagnostic microfilariae that live in the blood, and the mosquito ingests these with its blood meal. The microfilariae develop to infective filariform stage in the arthropod intermediate host.

Clinical manifestation

The adult worms elicit an immune response in the lymphatic system, with cellular reactions, hyperplasia and edema. A very strong granulomatous reaction produces a layer of fibrous tissue around dead worms, blocking small lymphatics with development of collateral lymphatics. During this time, patients may experience fever, headache, chills, local swelling, redness, lymphangitis in male and female genitalia and the extremities. Elephantiasis, which is deforming and debilitating, occurs in less than 10% of patients, usually after years of infection; it is due to chronic obstruction of the lymphatics with fibrosis and proliferation of dermal and connective tissue, i.e. the enlarged areas become hard and leathery. 'Filaria fevers' are seen in endemic areas, characterized by recurrent acute lymphangitis and adenolymphangitis without microfilariae. Tropical eosinophilia or Weingarten's syndrome, which is similar to asthma, is characterized by high eosinophilia without microfilariae.

Diagnosis

W. bancrofti is diagnosed on smears from blood taken between 10 pm and 2 am, correlating with the arthropod's feeding pattern. Microfilariae are sheathed and nuclei do not extend to the tip of the tail.

Treatment

Diethylcarbamazine and ivermectin kill microfilariae.

Brugia malayi, like *Wucheria bancrofti*, causes elephantiasis, referred to as Malayan filariasis in the Far East: Korea, China and the Philippines. The life cycle is the same as that of *W. bancrofti* and the vector is the *Mansonia* and *Anopheles* mosquito. The clinical picture resembles that of *W. bancrofti*, but Malayan filariasis is more often asymptomatic. *B. malayi* is also diagnosed on smears from blood taken between 10 pm and 2 am, correlating with the arthropod's feeding pattern. Nuclei are not continuous and there are two nuclei at the tip; *B. malayi* has a sheath.

Treatment

Diethylcarbamazine, albendazole, ivermectin

Loa loa

Loa loa (eyeworm) is transmitted by mango flies (*Chrysops*) in the African equatorial rain forest.

Life cycle

Typical filarial worm life cycle: adults migrate through subcutaneous tissue and occasionally cross the eye under the conjuctival membrane.

Clinical manifestation

Migrating worms cause a temporary inflammatory reaction, with the appearance of painful itchy swellings (Calibar swellings) that last about a week at one body site and then appear at another site. Dead adults induce a granulomatous reaction, with possible proteinuria and endomyocardial fibrosis. Infection is more serious in visitors to endemic areas than it is for natives.

Diagnosis

May be made based on Calibar swellings and on demonstrating the worm in the conjunctiva of the eye. Smears are made from blood taken around noon. *Loa loa* is sheathed and has a continuous row of nuclei at the tip.

Treatment

Diethylcarbazine (DEC) is used for treatment and prophylaxis.

Onchocerca volvulus

Onchocerca volvulus causes onchocercosis or river blindness, referred to as 'blinding filarial'. The parasite is found in Africa, Central America and South America. Infection with this organism is the leading cause of acquired blindness in parts of Africa.

Transmission

The vector is the black fly (*Simulium*).

Life cycle

Typical filarial worm life cycle with adults residing in subcutaneous tissue.

Clinical manifestation

Adult worms are encapsulated in fibrous tumors in subcutaneous tissue. An inflammatory and granulomatous reaction around the worm creates nodules up to 25 mm in size that appear anywhere in the body. Microfilariae can collect in the cornea and iris, causing keratitis and atrophy of the iris, leading to blindness.

Diagnosis

The nodules are diagnostic. A snip of skin placed in saline can reveal microfilarie as confirmation. Microfilariae do not have a sheath, and nuclei do not extend to the tip of the tail.

Treatment

Ivermectin

Adult worms may also be surgically excised from subcutaneous tissue.

Mansonella species

Mansonella species are human parasites; they do not induce pathology, but do produce microfilariae in the blood and must be distinguished from pathogens.

Mansonella perstans is found in Central and South America and in Africa; *Mansonella ozzardi* in Central and South America. Both produce microfilariae in the blood that have no sheath; the nuclei of *M. perstans* extend to the tail tip, and the nuclei of *M. ozzardi* do not extend to the tail tip.

M. streptocerca is found in tropical Africa. It produces microfilariae in skin, and must be differentiated from parasites that cause pathology. *M. streptocerca* is unsheathed, nuclei extend to the tip of the tail and it has a 'shepherd's crook'.

Treatment

M. perstans is treated with mebendazole; DEC is used for *M. streptocerca*.

Platyhelminthes

Platyhelminthes (phylum) are multicellular leaf-like flatworms, diagnosed by their ova. There are four classes, two of which are medically important: the class *Cestoda* includes the tapeworms, which have flat segmented bodies and the class *Digenea* includes the trematodes or flukes, which are leaf-shaped with flattened non-segmented bodies. With the exception of the blood flukes the platyhelminthes are hermaphroditic.

Cestodes (tapeworms)

Cestoda is referred to as 'tapeworm' because of its long ribbon-like appearance, ranging from a few millimetres to more than 20 metres in length. Adult tapeworms are linear with flat proglottids and rectangular segments. The anterior end of the worm has a modified segment, the scolex, and a chain of proglottids (head and neck) called strobila. The head may be adapted for attachment. These worms do not have a body cavity, have no respiratory or blood vascular system, and internal organs are embedded in parenchyma tissue. Adult tapeworms live in the intestinal tract of the vertebrate host and larval stages inhabit an intermediate host. They rely on the tegument (external surface) to release enzymes, absorb nutrients (via specialized microvilli) and release waste products. Proglottids also serve as male and female reproductive organs in these hermaphrodites. The proglottids near the terminal end contain the uterus filled with fertilized eggs: the embryo or first stage larvae within the eggs is called an onchosphere or hexacanth with six hooklets that facilitate entry into the intestinal mucosa of the intermediate host. Significant pathogens include *Hymenolepis nana, Hymenolepis diminuta, Taenia saginata, Taenia solium, Diphyllobothrium latum, Dipylidium caninum, Echinococcus granulosus* and *Echinococcus multicularis*. Humans ingest the larval stage (cysticercus, cysticercoid, plerocercoid) in raw or undercooked meat or fish; infection can also be acquired from raw vegetables contaminated with animal feces. Diagnosis is based on identification of representative eggs in feces.

Hymenolepis nana

Hymenolepis nana, the dwarf tapeworm is found in subtropical and tropical regions. It is common in the Southeastern part of the USA and is the most prevalent tapeworm infection in that country. It causes intestinal infection in children and individuals who are institutionalized and living in close quarters.

Transmission

Humans are infected when they accidentally ingest eggs found in mouse or rat fecal material. Although an intermediate host is not required, the *Hymenolepis* spp. are found in the house mouse – fleas and beetles can serve as transport hosts. Cysticercoid larvae can develop in these insects and infect humans or rodents if accidentally ingested.

Life cycle

Ingested eggs hatch in the small intestine, an onchosphere invades intestinal villi and the cysticercoid larva forms and emerges into the lumen. The scolex evaginates and attaches to the mucosa to mature and adults in the intestine release infective embryonated eggs from gravid proglottids as they disintegrate. Autoinfection occurs when the embryonated eggs of *H. nana* hatch in the gastrointestinal tract to form invasive onchospheres to repeat the cycle.

Clinical manifestation

Light infections are usually asymptomatic. Heavy infections may cause abdominal pain, diarrhea, intestinal enteritis, headache, irritability, dizziness and anorexia.

Diagnosis

Eggs in feces are 30×50 μm, spherical to oval and greyish in color. The hexacanth embryo is contained within an inner membrane and there are 2 polar thickenings (with 4–8 polar filaments radiating from the thickenings) between the inner membrane and the egg wall. The adult worm found in the intestine is 40 mm long with a small scolex, 4 suckers and a rostellum with spines.

Treatment

Praziquantel

Hymenolepis diminuta

Hymenolepis diminuta is the rat tapeworm: it is a zoonotic cestode infection found worldwide, but is less common than *H. nana*.

Transmission

The adult lives in the intestine of the rat and a flea or beetle is required as intermediate host. Humans accidentally ingest a flea or brain beetle that is infected with the cysticercoid larva.

Life cycle

As with *H. nana*, the hexacanth embryo is released into the intestine and forms a cysticercoid larva that moves to the lumen of the intestine, attaches and matures. Adults in the intestine release embryonated infected eggs in the feces.

Clinical manifestation

Infection produces mild symptoms, and tapeworms are often spontaneously lost.

Diagnosis

Eggs in the feces are oval, 50–75 μm, straw or grey in color and have an inner membrane with inconspicuous polar thickenings, but no filaments. The adult is 20–60 centimetres long.

Treatment

Praziquantel

Taenia saginata and *Taenia solium*

Taenia saginata (beef tapeworm) and *Taenia solium*, pork tapeworm, cause taeniasis; *T. solium* also can cause cysticercosis, a larval tissue infection.

Transmission

Humans serve as the definitive host for *Taenia* when they ingest undercooked pork or beef containing the cysticercus, which has developed in the cow or pig. Infection of the human as the intermediate host of the pork tapeworm (cysticercosis) results from ingestion of the eggs from the stool of a human definitive host for the adult worm. As the intermediate host, the human becomes infested with the larval form of the organism that encysts in tissues all over the body.

Life cycle

The scolex attaches to the intestinal mucosa and larvae mature to the adult stage in the small intestine. The adult releases free eggs or gravid proglottids in the feces. The cow, pig or human intermediate host ingests the eggs, the onchosphere hatches and penetrates the intestinal wall and is carried via blood to tissue. The onchosphere develops in tissue to the infective cysticercus. *T. solium* larvae can develop in human tissue as well as in pig tissue.

Clinical manifestation

The majority of infected individuals are asymptomatic, but may have vague abdominal pains, indigestion and loss of appetite. Eosinophilia is moderate. Motile proglottids that break off in the intestinal tract may migrate out of the anus. If *T. solium* eggs are accidentally ingested or released from a proglottid in the intestinal tract, the eggs hatch in the intestine and larvae migrate to form cysticercus bladders in any organ or the nervous system; the patient may develop cysticercosis or neurocysticercois (NCC). This infection can be fatal if the racemose form, an aberrant cluster of larval cysticercosis from migration, develop in brain tissue. Symptoms include headache, vomiting, papilledema and epilepsy.

Diagnosis

Taeniasis is diagnosed by identifying representative eggs in feces. Eggs of *T. saginata* and *T. solium* cannot be distinguished in feces – both are yellowish-brown and embryonated with a 6-hooked onchosphere (hexacanth embryo). The overall diameter is 35–45 μm, with a thick wall and radial striations. Proglottids and scolices may be found in feces. The gravid proglottid for *T. solium* has 7–13 uterine branches on each side of the uterine trunk and the gravid proglottid for *T. saginata* has 15–20 branches. The *T. solium* scolex has a rostellum with a double row of 25–30 hooklets and *T. saginata's* scolex has 4 suckers.

Treatment

Niclosamide or praziquantel (including *T. solium* cysticercosis); albendazole for *T. solium* cysticercosis.

Diphyllobothrium latum

Diphyllobothrium latum, the broadfish tapeworm, is an intestinal parasite that is found worldwide in populations where pickled or raw freshwater fish is consumed.

Transmission

Infection is acquired when fish containing plerocercoid larvae is ingested in raw or undercooked fish.

Life cycle

Plerocercoid larva scolices are released in the intestine and develop into adults. Unembryonated operculated eggs are passed in human feces, but must reach water to mature. The first intermediate host, the copepod, ingests the larval stage (coracidium) that develops into a procercoid larva. Fish, the second intermediate host, ingest the infected copepod, and larvae invade the flesh after leaving the fish intestines. A plerocercoid larva (scolex with little tissue) develops in the fish flesh.

Clinical manifestation

Symptoms of infection include vague abdominal pain, indigestion, loss of appetite, weight loss and weakness. The organism competes for vitamin B12, so that long-term infection can lead to megaloblastic anemia and eventually can cause CNS disturbances. Although there is only one adult, it grows to 20 metres and can cause intestinal obstruction.

Diagnosis

Eggs, proglottids and scolices may be seen in feces. Eggs are oval, 60–80 μm × 40–50 μm with an inconspicuous operculum and a small knob at the opposite end to the operculum. The eggs are unembryonated when passed and do not have shoulders – this allows them to be distinguished from the fluke eggs of *Paragonimus westermani*. Proglottids, rarely found in feces, are wider than they are long, rosette-shaped or with a coiled uterus. The scolex is 2–3 mm long, elongated with dorsal and ventral sucking grooves.

Treatment

Praziquantel, niclosamide

Diphyllobothrium or *Spirometa* spp.

Diphyllobothrium or *Spirometa* spp. are cestodes of dogs, cats and other mammals that cause sparginosis. The parasite is found in Far East freshwater areas, commonly in Southeast Asia.

Transmission

Humans ingest a copepod containing the infective procercoid larvae when they ingest reptiles or amphibians or when plerocercoid larva invade after raw tissue from the second intermediate host is used as a poultice (e.g. for eye infections).

Clinical manifestation

Migration of larvae cause subcutaneous nodules that are itchy and painful. Internal abscesses or cysts may appear, and eyes can also be affected by invading larvae.

Diagnosis

Laboratory diagnosis is based on identifying small (up to 40 mm) worms that are white and ribbon-like with a rudimentary scolex.

Treatment

Similar to that for *D. latum* (praziquantel, niclosamide).

Dipylidium caninum (zoonotic cestode infection)

Dipylidium caninum is a cestode of dogs and cats, found worldwide. Humans are an accidental host, with infection occurring mostly in children. Larvae mature to the adult stage in dog, cat or human intestine.

Transmission

Humans accidentally ingest cysticercoid larva in infected dog or cat fleas, the intermediate host.

Clinical manifestation

Infected individuals are usually asymptomatic, but mild gastrointestinal disturbances may occur. The tapeworms are often lost spontaneously.

Diagnosis

Fecal examination shows eggs, 20–40 μm in size in packets of 15–25, resembling *Taenia* eggs. Proglottids are pumpkin seed-shaped with twin genitalia, two genital pores on each side of the proglottid.

Treatment

Praziquantel

Echinococcus granulosus (zoonotic cestode infection)

Echinococcus granulosus causes echinococcosis (hydatid cyst, hydatid disease and hydatidosis). Domestic dogs are the definitive host for the adult tapeworm, and infection occurs primarily in sheep-raising areas where domestic dogs are used for herding. Humans are accidental hosts.

Transmission

Humans acquire the infection when they are in close contact with an infected dog and ingest eggs containing the infective hexacanth embryo.

Life cycle

The adult lives in canine intestines and releases eggs into the soil; sheep and other herbivores ingest eggs containing the infective hexacanth embryo. Eggs hatch in the intestine, and the hexacanth embryo burrows into the mucosa to enter the blood vessels and is carried to the liver. The embryos are usually trapped in the liver, but some may disseminate in the circulation and lodge in other organs. The embryo develops into a hydatid cyst, and when a dog eats infected viscera of the herbivore, the cyst is digested in the canine intestine. Each scolex in the cyst develops into an adult tapeworm and eggs are released in feces. When a human ingests infective eggs, by close contact with a dog or herbivore intermediate host, the life cycle does not complete its normal development.

Clinical manifestations

The larval form causes pathology in human tissues, usually the liver. The embryo develops a central cavity-like structure that is lined with germinal membrane, the hydatid cyst. Hydatid cysts develop slowly, usually about 1 cm/year. The clinical picture varies according to the organ or organs affected and the size of the hydatid cyst is determined by the organ in which it develops. Symptoms can be due to the space occupying mass, or because of leakage, rupture, or secondary bacterial infection. In the liver, symptoms develop when the cyst reaches a significant size and causes jaundice or portal hypertension. In the lungs, symptoms such as coughing, shortness of breath and chest pain appear after the cyst becomes large. In bone, a limiting membrane does not develop and the cysts are able to fill the marrow to eventually erode the bone. Pressure from the increasing size of the cyst may cause necrosis of surrounding tissue. Cyst rupture frees germinal epithelium that may serve as a new source of infection, and a large amount of foreign protein is liberated that may induce an anaphylactic response.

Diagnosis

Several methods are used for diagnosis, including serology (indirect hemagglutination and ELISA), X-ray examination, ultrasound or computerized tomography (CT) detection of cysts or calcified cysts in organs, and biopsy. Although scolices, brood capsules, hydatid or daughter cysts can be detected on biopsy, this is not recommended as leaking of cyst fluid after biopsy can cause anaphylactic reactions.

Treatment

Albendazole

Echinococcus multilocularis (zoonotic cestode infection)

Echinococcus multilocularis, which causes alveolar hydatid disease, resembles *Echinococcus granulosus* in its morphology and life cycle. The intermediate hosts are rodents, and the definitive host is usually a fox, but dogs and cats can also become infected by eating infected rodents. The largest number of human infections is reported from Alaska (from sled dogs), the Soviet Union, and northern Japan.

Transmission

Humans may be infected by ingesting raw plants contaminated with feces of infected foxes, dogs, or cats.

Life cycle

Similar to that of *E. granulosus* in a canine host. In humans, eggs hatch and develop into cysts that bud externally (alveolar cysts).

Clinical manifestation

Cysts in humans produce aggressively growing, tumour-like masses in the liver (alveolar hydatid disease). The cyst is not sharply defined from surrounding tissues; it has a very thin, laminated membrane, with cavities separated from each other by connective tissue. In humans the cyst is usually sterile and may undergo central necrosis and even calcification with continuing growth at the periphery. Cysts can spread and produce metastases by direct extension or through the blood or lymphatics to the lungs and brain. Since it is found most frequently in the liver, the infection may be mistakenly diagnosed as liver cancer in places where diagnostic facilities are limited.

Treatment

Albendazole, mebendazole or praziquantel; radical surgery if possible.

Trematodes (flukes)

Platyhelminthes (phylum); *Digenea* (class) include the flukes or trematodes found primarily in the Orient, Africa and South America. The trematodes range in size from a few millimetres to several centimeters in length. With the exception of the schistosomes or blood flukes, which are cylindrical, they are dorsoventrally flattened, non-segmented and leaf-shaped with oral and ventral suckers. Their digestive system is simple, consisting of an oral cavity, which opens in the centre of the oral sucker and a blind intestinal tract that ends in one or two sacs without an anal opening. Like the cestodes, the tegument is metabolically active, absorbing nutrients and releasing waste products. Adults live in human organs (lung, intestine, blood, liver) where they complete sexual reproduction. The class produces large numbers of ova that must reach water to mature. All flukes have one or two intermediate hosts (e.g. snail, mussels or crabs). With the exception of schistosomes (blood flukes), all are hermaphroditic, and their ova are operculated, with a lid-like structure.

Intestinal and lung flukes

Life cycle

All flukes have the same life cycle, with one or two intermediate hosts; the first intermediate host is the snail. Eggs from human feces, urine or sputum mature to the miracidium or first larval stage when they reach water. The ciliated miracidium within the egg may be ingested by a snail, or is released from the egg and penetrates the snail. Sporocysts (undifferentiated germinal tissue) develop and reproduce asexually within the snail, with release of many rediae containing the sporocysts. Rediae develop and produce the second larval stage, cercariae, which are released into the water. Schistosome cercariae are infective and directly penetrate human skin, but hermaphrodite cercariae secrete a thick wall and encyst as metacercaria. Depending on the species, the metacercariae attach to aquatic vegetation or invade the flesh of aquatic animals (fish, crab or crayfish). Humans ingest infective metacercaria in raw or undercooked aquatic animals or on aquatic vegetations. The metacercariae are digested in the intestinal tract, are excysted and then migrate to their target tissue. Following penetration, schistosome cercaria become schistosomules that enter the bloodstream and migrate to vessels at a target site, where they develop to mature male and female flukes.

Digenea organisms are categorized by site of infection.

Fasciolopsis buski, Metagonimus yokogawai and *Heterophyes heterophyes* are intestinal flukes.

Fasciola hepatica and *Clonorchis sinensis* are liver flukes.

Paragonimus westermani is the lung fluke.

Schistosoma mansoni, S. haematobium and *S. japonicum*, the blood flukes, are the most common.

Fasciolopsis buski

Fasciolopsis buski is referred to as 'the giant intestinal fluke', a parasite endemic in the Far East. Pigs and dogs are reservoir hosts.

Transmission

Humans acquire the infection by ingesting infective metacercariae on freshwater vegetation, including bamboo shoots and water chestnuts.

Clinical manifestation

Adults live in the duodenum of the small intestine or bile duct, causing mechanical and toxic damage.

The fluke can cause mucosal ulceration and inflammation, diarrhea, anorexia, edema, ascites, nausea, vomiting and intestinal obstruction in heavy infection. A heavy infection, characterized by marked eosinophilia, may be fatal.

Diagnosis

Laboratory diagnosis depends on identifying adults and/or eggs in feces. The adult fluke is flattened (2–7 cm long), lacking the cephalic cone seen in *F. hepatica*. Adults are not usually seen, except in purged specimens. Eggs are yellowish-brown (130 μm × 80 μm), unembryonated when passed and have a small, inconspicuous operculum. Eggs cannot be distinguished from those of *F. hepatica*.

Treatment

Praziquantel or triclobendazole and niclosamide

Metagonimus yokogawi and *Heterophyes heterophyes*

Metagonimus yokogawi and *Heterophyes heterophyes* are intestinal flukes found in the Middle East and Far East.

Transmission

Humans acquire the infection by ingesting the metacercaria in undercooked or raw fish.

Clinical manifestation

Adults live in the small intestine.

There are few clinical symptoms, unless the patient has a heavy worm load. A heavy parasite burden can cause diarrhea, colic and stools with large amounts of mucus.

Diagnosis

Vase or flask-shaped (28–30 μm long, 15–16μm wide) eggs are identified in feces. The eggs are operculated with inconspicuous shoulders and have a small terminal knob. Eggs resemble each other and resemble *Clonorchis sinensis*. Adults are small (1–2 mm) and delicate.

Treatment

Praziquantel

Fasciola hepatica causes liver rot. The parasite is found in sheep- and cattle-raising areas with sheep as the natural host for *F. hepatica*, with humans serving as accidental hosts.

Transmission

Humans acquire the infection by ingesting metacercaria on raw water vegetation, especially watercress.

Clinical manifestation

The larvae reach the liver by migrating through the intestinal wall and peritoneal cavity. Adults live in the biliary passages and the gallbladder.

Light infections are usually asymptomatic. Tissue damage during migration through the liver may cause an inflammatory reaction, secondary infections and fibrosis of liver ducts. Heavy infections with *F. hepatica* may result in hepatomegaly, cirrhosis, liver obstruction with jaundice, diarrhea and abdominal pain.

Diagnosis

Adults are 3 centimetres long with a prominent cephalic cone. The unembryonated eggs are operculated, and cannot be distinguished from those of *F. buski*.

Treatment

Bithionol

Clonorchis sinensis

Clonorchis sinensis is the Oriental or Chinese liver fluke (previously named *Opisthorchis*). This parasite is limited to the Far East, where dogs and cats are reservoir hosts.

Transmission

Humans acquire the infection from ingesting the metacercaria in raw, undercooked or pickled fish.

Clinical manifestation

The immature fluke migrates to the liver and adults live in the bile ducts.

Few, if any, clinical symptoms are noted with light infections. Heavy or repeated infections may result in inflammation with fever, diarrhea, and pain. Fibrotic changes and obstruction of the bile duct may occur. Chronic cases with a heavy worm burden from repeated infections may have serious consequences, including hepatic complications, and rarely, pancreatitis, cholangitis, bile duct stones and cholangiocarcinoma.

Diagnosis

Eggs are identified in stool or duodenal aspirate. They are 15–16 μm $\times$ 29–35 μm, embryonated when passed, flask-shaped and operculated with prominent shoulders at the operculum and a knob at the opposite end.

Treatment

Praziquantel

Paragonimus westermani

Paragonimus westermani is the lung fluke found in the Orient (also seen in Africa and South America) that causes pulmonary distomiasis and may infect other tissues (e.g. brain, skin, liver). The parasite usually infects tigers, leopards, dogs and foxes.

Transmission

Humans acquire the infection by ingesting metacercaria in raw, pickled or undercooked freshwater crabs or crayfish.

Clinical manifestation

Metacercaria excyst in the intestine and burrow through the intestinal wall and diaphragm to enter the lung.

Migration causes few symptoms, but lung habitation induces a non-specific inflammatory response with persistent cough, chest pain and hemoptysis. Chronic bronchitis and increasing fibrosis may result. Both clinical symptoms and chest radiographs may resemble tuberculosis with patchy infiltrates and calcification in the lungs.

Diagnosis

Adult flukes, which are reddish brown and 1 centimetre long, live within capsules in the bronchioles. Eggs are identified in bloody sputum (or in feces if coughed up and subsequently swallowed). The unembryonated eggs are broadly oval, 80–120 μm $\times$ 50–60 μm with a flattened operculum, slight shoulders, and a thickening of the shell at the end opposite the operculum. Eggs are similar to those of

D. latum, but may be distinguished by the presence of shouldered operculae and the absence of the abopercular knob.

Treatment

Praziquantel, triclobendazole

Schistosoma species – the blood flukes

Schistosoma species are found worldwide and rank second only to malaria in terms of worldwide parasitic infections. *Schistosoma mansoni, or* Manson's blood fluke, is found in Africa and Central and South America; *S. japonicum*, the Oriental blood fluke, is found in the Far East and *S. haematobium*, the bladder fluke, is endemic in the Middle East and in Africa. Adult schistosomes live in the colon, rectum and bladder, (depending on the species), with the female residing in an involuted chamber (gynecophoral canal) that extends the length of the male. These flukes are cylindrical rather than dorsoventrally shaped and the eggs are not operculated.

Life cycle

The life cycle differs from that of other flukes. Embryonated eggs are passed in feces or urine, miracidia hatch in fresh water and penetrate the first intermediate host, the snail. Sporocysts, then cercaria are produced over a six-week period. Cercariae migrate from the snail into water and those that encounter human skin will shed their forked tails, secrete enzymes and begin penetration. Now referred to as a schistosomule, they enter the bloodstream and migrate through vessels to the appropriate site to develop to adult male or female schistosomes. Paired adults of *Schistosoma mansoni* live in liver sinuses and venules of the large intestine, *S. japonicum* lives in liver sinuses and venules of the small intestine and *S. haematobium* lives in veins surrounding the bladder.

Clinical manifestation

Symptoms of infection are related to the species and to the fluke's life cycle. Cercarial penetration may cause a local dermatitis, including redness, rash and irritation that last approximately 3 days. Larval migration causes generalized symptoms that last up to a month and may resemble typhoid, including fever, malaise, myalgia and hepatosplenomegaly. Adults acquire host antigens on their surface that decrease the host immune response, and therefore cause little inflammatory damage. Egg production and migration through tissues causes acute damage. The adult female dilates the vein in order to lay eggs; the vein contracts, and with the secretion of enzymes, the eggs penetrate vessel walls and tissues. Eggs make their way to the lumen of the intestine or bladder and egg spines cause tissue trauma to vessel walls during the early acute stage of infections. Hematuria may be seen with *S. haematobium* infection and diarrhea may be noted with *S. mansoni* or *S. japonicum* infections. In chronic cases, eggs remain in the tissue and induce granuloma formation that results in fibrotic changes and thickening. Scarring of veins, ascites, pain, hypertension, anemia, splenomegaly and hepatomegaly may also accompany infection. Infection with *S. japonicum* is more serious than infection with *S. mansoni* due to greater egg production by this species. Microscopic bleeding into the urine is seen during the acute phase of urinary schistosomiasis. Dysuria, urine retention and urinary tract infections are noted during the chronic phase. Nephrotic syndrome may occur in *S. mansoni* and *S. haematobium* infection and cancer of the bladder has been associated with *S. haematobium* infection.

Diagnosis

S. mansoni and *S. japonicum* diagnosis is based on identification of characteristic eggs in feces or rectal biopsy; *S. haematobium* eggs are recovered from concentrated urine (collected between 12 pm and 2 pm). Eggs of *S. mansoni* are 115–175 μm × 45–75 μm, elongated with prominent lateral spine. Eggs of

S. japonicum (60–95 μm × 40–60 μm) are found with a small, curved rudimentary spine. *S. haematobium* eggs are elonged, 110–170 × 40–70 μm with a terminal spine. Other diagnostic methods include serology and ELISA.

Treatment

Praziquantel for all species; metrifonate for *S. haematobium*.

Schistosome zoonosis

Schistosome dermatitis or Swimmer's itch is found worldwide and occurs when cercaria of flukes, birds or other mammals penetrate humans. Foreign proteins elicit a tissue response characterized by small papules (3–5 mm in diameter), edema, erythema, and intense itching. Symptoms last about one week and disappear when the cercaria die and degenerate.

Arthropods

Arthropods can be a necessary part of the life cycle of human parasites: ticks, mites, fleas, venomous spiders and scorpions can act as direct agents of human disease. This large phylum contains over 80% of all animal life, and directly causes or transmits over 80% of all diseases. They may be ectoparasites (lice, mites), or act as mechanical or biological vectors of disease (ticks, mosquitoes). Their bites can inject toxins or venoms and cause delayed or immediate hypersensitivity reactions (including anaphylaxis). Myiasis is caused by larvae of non-blood-sucking flies that invade tissue.

Arthropoda includes segmented invertebrates with chitinous exoskeletons and bilaterally paired jointed appendages. The head is adapted for sensory input and for chewing, and they have either a single lens or compound eyes. The body cavity is filled with a blood-like substance and they have respiratory, digestive, excretory and nervous systems. Most *Insecta* and all *Arachnida* undergo metamorphosis. Incomplete metamorphosis has three stages:

(i) egg,
(ii) nymph-miniature adult that will molt to become a mature adult (nymphal form after each molt is an instar),
(iii) Imago, the sexually mature adult.

Complete metamorphosis has four stages: egg, larva, pupa (enclosed in a case), adult.

There are five classes of arthropods, but three contain those that are medically important:

(a) Insecta
(b) Arachnida
(c) Crustacea

Insecta

Insecta have a body that is divided into head, thorax, and abdomen. They have one pair of antennae and often eyes, three pairs of legs, and often have wings on the thorax. Medically important insects include *Diptera* (flies and mosquitoes), *Anoplura* (lice), and *Siphonaptera* (fleas).

Pubic lice

Phthirus pubis or *Pediculosis pubis* infestation is prevalent in situations of crowding or poor personal hygiene, caused by an ectoparasite, the crab louse or pubic louse. They usually infest pubic hair, but may also be found in other areas of coarse body hair, including eyebrows, eyelashes, axillary and leg hair.

Transmission

Infestations are usually acquired by close contact, sharing of clothing or sexual contact.

Life cycle

The pubic louse is oval in shape, about 2 mm in diameter, with clawlike legs and rounded body – like a miniature crab. The insects glue their nits to the hair shafts, nymphs hatch from the eggs and mature to adults in about one month. Both nymphs and adults feed on blood.

Clinical manifestation

Hemorrhagic papules or macules develop at the site of bites, pruritus and excoriation are common.

Diagnosis

Adult crabs or nits are seen in the pubic hair or on clothing. Nits are oval and usually yellow to white.

Treatment

Infestations can be treated with topical lindane or 1% permethrin. Treatment should be repeated after 10 days to ensure elimination.

Arachnida

Arachnida have four pairs of legs in the adult stage. The body is divided into cephalothorax and abdomen, which may be fused. They have no distinct head and no antennae, and undergo simple metamorphosis. This group includes spiders, scorpions, ticks and mites. Of medical importance are *Acarina* (ticks and mites), *Ixodidae* (hard ticks), *Argasidae* (soft ticks), and *Sarcoptidae* (mites).

Scabies

Scabies is caused by the mite species, *Sarcoptes scabei*. Scabies may be a genital infection, and can be sexually transmitted.

Sarcoptes scabei is an ectoparasite, found worldwide with a higher prevalence associated with crowded conditions and poor hygiene.

Transmission

The infestation is acquired by direct contact with infested skin or with contaminated clothing or bedding.

Life cycle

Adult mites burrow in the superficial layers of the epidermis; females are about 0.5mm in diameter, males are much smaller. The female deposits eggs in the burrows, and these hatch in 3 to 4 days. Newly hatched larvae also burrow in the skin and mature to adults within 4 days. The mite's secretions cause allergic reaction in the skin.

Clinical manifestation

Areas commonly affected include interdigital webs, genitalia, umbilicus, areolae, axillary folds, extensor areas over the elbows and knees and the flexor areas of the wrists. Initial lesions are intensely pruritic small red papules or vesicles and excoriation with secondary bacterial infection is common. Infestations may resolve spontaneously, but some become chronic and may persist for years.

Diagnosis

Close inspection of the skin with a hand lens may reveal the characteristic burrows and diagnosis can be confirmed by examining skin lesion scrapings for mites or eggs.

Treatment

Topical permethrin cream (5%) provides effective treatment.

Crustacea

Crustacea are aquatic forms that have an external skeleton of shell and breathe via gills. The majority develop by incomplete metamorphosis, but some species undergo complete metamorphosis. The class includes crabs, water fleas, lobsters, shrimp, barnacles and wood lice. Some are medically important as the intermediate hosts of human parasites (e.g. copepods).

FURTHER READING

Alberts, B., Johson, A., Lewis, J., Raff, M., Roberts, K. & Walter, P. (2002). *Molecular Biology of the Cell*, 4th edn. New York: Garland Science, New York.

Ash, L. B. & Orihel T. C. (1997). *Atlas of Human Parasitology*, 4th edn. Chicago, IL: ACP Press.

Baron, E. J., Chang, R. S., Howard, D. H., Miller, J. N. & Turner J. A. (1994). *Medical Microbiology: A Short Course*. New York: Wiley-Liss Inc.

Bogitsh, B. J. & Cheng, T. C. (1998). *Human Parasitology*, 2nd edn. New York: Academic Press.

de la Maza, L. M., Pezzlo, M. T. & Baron, E. J. (1997). *Color Atlas of Diagnostic Microbiology*. St. Louis: Mosby Publishers.

Delost, M. D. (1997). *Introduction to Diagnostic Microbiology*. · St. Louis: Mosby Publishers.

Forbes, B. A., Sahm, D. F. & Weissfeld, A. S. (1998). *Bailey & Scott's Diagnostic Microbiology*, 10th edn. St. Louis: Mosby Publishers.

Leventhal, R. & Cheadle, R. F. (1989). *Medical Parasitology. A Self-Instructional Text*, 3rd edn. Philadelphia: F. A. Davis Publishing Company.

Leventhal, R. & Cheadle, R. F. (1996). *Medical Parasitology. A Self-Instructional Text*, 4th edn. F. A. Davis Publishing Company, Philadelphia.

Leventhal, R. & Cheadle, R. F. (2002). *Medical Parasitology. A Self-Instructional Text*, 5th edn. Philadelphia: F. A. Davis Publishing Company.

Markell, V. J. (1992). *Medical Parasitology*, Philadelphia, PA: W.B. Saunders Company.

Morello, J. A., Mizer, H. E., Wilson, M. E. & Granato, P. A. (1998). *Microbiology in Patient Care*, 6th edn. New York: McGraw-Hill.

Neva, F. A. & Brown, H. W. (1994). *Basic Clinical Parasitology*, 6th edn. Norwalk, CT: Appleton & Lange.

Roberts, L. S. & Janovy, J. Jr. (1996). *Foundations of Parasitology*. Dubuque, IA: William C. Brown Publishers.

Schaechter, M., Medoff, G. & Schlessinger, D. (1989). *Mechanisms of Microbial Disease*. Philadelphia, PA: Williams & Wilkins.

Zeibig, E. A. (1997). *Clinical Parasitology: A Practical Approach*. Philadelphia, PA: W. B. Saunders Company.

Appendix 6.1. antiparasitic agents

Actions are directed against various metabolic pathways, including energy metabolism, cell wall synthesis, protein synthesis, membrane function, nucleic acid synthesis, cofactor synthesis. Some agents selectively affect the neuromuscular systems of helminths

Agent	Mode of action	Indications	Limitations/comments
Albendazole (Albenza)	Prevents glucose absorption by binding to free γ-tubulin; inhibits polymerization of tubulin and the microtubule-dependent uptake of glucose	*Ancyclostoma braziliense* cutaneous larva migrans *Angiostrongylus cantonensis* *Angiostrongylus costaricensis* *Ascaris lumbricoides* *Brugia malayi* *Brugia timori* *Echinococcus multilocularis*[a] *Giardia lamblia* *Gnathostoma spinigerum* *Microsporida (Enterocytozoon and Encephalitozoon)* *Necator americanus* and *Ancylostoma duodenale* *Taenia solium cysticercosis* *Trichostrongylus orientalis* *Trichuris trichiura* *Wucheria bancrofti* *Strongyloides stercoralis* *Trichinella spiralis*	Avoid use in pregnant women FDA approved only for cysticercosis and hydatid disease [a] Radical surgery indicated, when possible
Amphotericin B	See Appendix to Chapter 3	*Naegleria* amebic meningoencephalitis Leishmaniasis	Liposomal amphotericin B is FDA-approved for visceral leishmaniasis
Antimony (Sodium Stb)	Inhibits sulfhydryl enzymes and phosphofructokinase	Mucocutaneous leishmaniasis caused by *Leishmania braziliensis* Visceral leishmaniasis *Leishmania donovani, L. chagasi* *L. infantum*	

Drug	Mechanism of action	Organism/Disease	Notes
Artemisinin, artemether and artesunate	Possibly acts by inducing oxidant stress	*Plasmodium falciparum*	Not FDA approved; Not available in US; Avoid use in pregnant women; Especially if multidrug resistant
Atovaquone (Mepron)	Action not fully understood against *Pneumocystis carinii*; In *Plasmodium* species, may inhibit enzymes linked to mitochondrial electron transport; ultimately blocks synthesis of ATP and nucleic acids.	*Babesia microti*[a]; *Cryptosporidium parvum*[b]; *Plasmodium falciparum*[c]; *Toxoplasma gondii*[d]	[a]In combination with quinine and/or clindamycin and/or azith romycin; [b]In combination with paromomycin; [c]For prophylaxis and treatment; in combination with proguanil; [d]In combination with pyrimethamine
Azithromycin	See Appendix 2.3	*Babesia microti*	Not FDA approved; In combination with quinine and/or clindamycin and/or atovaquone
Azoles (iatraconazole, ketoconazole, fluconazole)	See Appendix to Chapter 3	Amebic encephalitis (Acanthamoeba or Balamthia)	In combination with flucytosine
Benznidzole	Causes oxidative stress	*Trypanosoma cruzi*, acute or early infection	Not FDA approved; Not available in US
Bithionol		*Fasciola hepatica*	Not FDA approved
Chloroquine – a cinchona alkaloid	Precise mechanism is not known; collects in lysosomes and interferes with pigment formation; the ferriproto porphyrin IX–chloroquine complex is highly toxic to the parasite	*Plasmodium*; *P. vivax, P. ovale, P. malariae*[a]; *P. falciparum*[b]	[a]In combination with pyrimethamine; [b]When sensitive (only in Mexico, Central America, the Caribbean and parts of the Middle East); in combination with proguanil for prophylaxis
Clindamycin	See Appendix 2.3	*Plasmodium*; *Babesia*; *Toxoplasma*	Not FDA approved
DEC (diethylcarbamazine)	Causes hyperpolarization of muscle membrane	*Loa loa*; *Brugia malayi*; *Mansonella streptocerca*; *Toxocara canis*	Not FDA approved
Diloxanide furoate		Amebiasis	Not for use in pregnancy

(cont.)

Appendix 6.1. (*cont.*)

Agent	Mode of action	Indications	Limitations/comments
Doxycycline	See Appendix 3 to Chapter 2	*Plasmodium malaria*[a]	Not for use in pregnancy; Not for use in children <8 years of age [a]Prophylaxis or combined with quinine for treatment
Elfornithine (DFMO-Ornidyl)	Inhibit protein synthesis, mainly in the trophozoite stage	*Trypanosoma brucei gambiense*, early and late stages	Not for use in pregnancy Not for use in lactating women
Emetine		Amebic liver abscess	Not for use in pregnancy, or <5 years of age
Furazolidone	See Appendix 2.3	*Giardia lamblia*	
Halofantrine	Collects in the lysosomes and interferes with pigment formation; the FP-chloroquine complex is highly toxic to the parasite	*Plasmodium falciparum* *P. vivax*	Not for use in pregnancy Not for use in children <1 year of age, Not for use in individuals with cardiac disease, including prolonged QT wave Do not repeat treatment due to toxicity
Iodoquinol	Physician's Desk Reference (PDR) does not include mode of action	*Dientamoeba fragilis* *Entamoeba histolytica* colonization *Balantidium coli*	Not for use in iodine sensitive patients
Ivermectin	Produces paralysis in helminths; appears to open chloride-sensitive channels or intensifies γ-aminobutyric acid (GABA)-mediated neurotransmission in nematodes, causing immobilization	*Strongyloides stercoralis* *Ancylostoma braziliense* cutaneous larva migrans *Wucheria bancrofti* *Brugia malayi* *Brugia timori* *Onchocerca volvulus* *Mansonella streptocerca* Lice Scabies	Broad spectrum; very potent Not for use in pregnancy Not for use in children <5 years of age FDA approved only for onchocerciasis and strongyloidiasis
Ketoconazole	See Appendix to Chapter 3	Leishmaniasis	
Malarone (atovaquone and proguanil combination)		*Plasmodium falciparum*	Prophylaxis

Drug	Mechanism	Indication/Organisms	Notes
Mebendazole	Prevents glucose absorption by binding to free γ-tubulin; inhibits polymerization of tubulin and the microtubule-dependent uptake of glucose	Angiostrongylus cantonensis Angiostrongylus costaricensis Ascaris lumbricoides Balantidium coli Capillaria philippinensis Echinococcus Enterobius vermicularis Trichostrongylus orientalis Trichuris trichiura Dracunculus medinensis Mansonella perstans Trichinella spiralis[a] Hookworm	Not for use during pregnancy, especially during first trimester of pregnancy [a]Add prednisone
Mefloquine	Exact mechanism is not known (PDR); Collects in lysosomes and interferes with pigment formation; the FP-chloroquine complex is highly toxic to the parasite	Plasmodium falciparum	When resistant to chloroquine Not for use in patients with cardiac conduction defects or arrhythmias or for patients receiving beta-adrenergic blockers for these conditions; Not for use in children <3 months of age Not for use in patients with seizures or psychiatric disorders Avoid during pregnancy, if possible (increased risk of stillbirth)
Meglumine		Leishmaniasis	Not FDA approved
Melarsoprol		Trypanosoma brucei gambiense, T. brucei rhodesiense, early hemolymphatic stage without CNS involvement	Do not use during pregnancy Available from Center for Disease Control and Prevention (CDC) Service
Metrifonate		Schistosoma haematobium	Not FDA approved Avoid during pregnancy, if possible
Metronidazole	See Appendix 2.3	Trichomonas vaginalis Giardia lambia[a] Dracunculus medinensis	[a]Not FDA approved for giardiasis
Niclosamide	Inhibits mitcochondrial conversion of ADP to ATP	Tapeworms Diphyllobothrium latum Taenia solium	No longer available in US

(cont.)

Appendix 6.1. (cont.)

Agent	Mode of action	Indications	Limitations/comments
Nifurtimox	Causes oxidative stress	*Trypanosoma cruzi*, acute or early stage infections	Not FDA approved
Paromomycin	An oral aminoglycoside See Appendix 2.3	*Cryptosporidium* *Dientamoeba fragilis* *Entamoeba histolytica* colonization *Giardia lamblia* Leishmaniasis	NOT FDA approved for all indications Secondary drug for amoebiasis and in pregnant women in whom giardiasis is not severe enough to require metronidazole. Available from CDC
Pemethrin (topical)		*Pediculus capitis* *Phthirus pubis* *Sarcoptes scabiei*	
Pentamidine	Not known; may bind to DNA	Leishmaniasis African trypanosomiasis (early without CNS involvement)	Not FDA approved
Praziquantel	Appears to interfere with calcium homeostasis and cause flaccid paralysis in adult flukes. Host immune response is necessary for antihelmintic effects in schistosome infections – disrupting surface membrane of parasite may cause antigens to be exposed to the action of the host immune system.	*Diphyllobothrium latum* *Dipylidium caninum* *Echinococcus* Flukes: *Clonorchis sinensis* *Fasciolopsis buski* *Heterophyes heterophyes* *Metagonimus yokogawai* *Ophisthorchis viverrini* *Nanophyetus salmincola* *Paragonimus uestermani* *Schistosoma haematobium* *Schistosoma mansoni* *Schistosoma japonicum* *Schistosoma mekongi* *Hymenolepis nana* *Hymenolepis diminuta* *Taenia saginata* *Taenia solium* cysticercosis *Taenia solium*	

Drug	Mechanism	Organism/Use	Notes
Primaquine (cinchona alkaloid)	Interferes with mitochondrial function	*Plasmodium vivax* *Plasmodium ovale*	Not for use in pregnancy Not for use in children <1 year of age Not for use in patients with glucose 6-phosphate dehydrogenase (G6PD) deficiency After chloroquine has been given
Proguanil	Interferes with synthesis of folic acid	*Plasmodium falciparum*	Not FDA approved Available outside US as combination with atovaquone
Propamidine		*Acanthamoeba* keratitis	In combination with polymyxin B, neomycin, gramicidin and topical polyhexamethylene biguanide
Pyrantel pamoate	Cholinergic agonist that acts on acetylcholine receptors producing muscle contraction, or causes neuromuscular blockage by interaction with nicotine receptors, leading to paralysis	Ascariasis, hookworm and pinworm alternative treatment[a] *E.vermicularis*	[a]Albendazole and mebendazole are used primarily for ascaris and hookworm
Pyrimethamine	Folic acid antagonist	*Toxoplasma gondii* acute infection and any infection, including ocular infection, in immunocompromised patients[a] Malaria	[a]Not for use during first trimester of pregnancy [a]Used with clindamycin or sulfdiazine
Quinacrine	Collects in the lysosomes and interferes with pigment formation; the FP-chloroquine complex is highly toxic to the parasite	*Giardia lamblia*	Not for use during pregnancy Not for use in patients with psoriasis
Quinine (a cinchona alkaloid)	Collects in the lysosomes and interferes with pigment formation; the FP-chloroquine complex is highly toxic to the parasite; may function by disrupting lysosome membrane	*Babesia microti*[a] *Plasmodium falciparum* resistant to chloroquine[b]	[a]In combination with clindamycin [b]In combination with doxycycline, clindamycin or mefoquine
Sodium Stb		Cutaneous leishmaniasis (*Leishmania major, L. tropica, L. aethiopica, L. braziliensis*)	Not FDA approved

(cont.)

Appendix 6.1. (*cont.*)

Agent	Mode of action	Indications	Limitations/comments
Spiramycin		*Toxoplasma gondii* acute infection in pregnant women	Available from FDA
Sulfadiazine		*Toxoplasma gondii* congenital infection Malaria Isosporiasis[a] Cyclosporiasis[a]	[a]Not for use during first trimester of pregnancy Not for use in newborns (except for treatment of congenital toxoplasmosis) [a]Combined with pyrimethamine or trimethoprim
Suramin	Inhibits glycolytic enzymes	*Trypanosoma brucei gambiense*, *T. brucei rhodesiense* early hemolymphatic stage without CNS involvement	Available from CDC
Tetracycline	See Appendix 3, Chapter 2	*Balantidium coli* Malaria	Not for use in pregnancy Not for use in children <8 years of age
Thiabendazole	Similar to mebendazole. Prevents glucose absorption by binding to free γ-tubulin; inhibits polymerization of tubulin and the microtubule-dependent uptake of glucose	*Angiostrongylus cantonensis* *Angiostrongylus costaricensis* *Ascaris lumbricoides* Strongyloidiasis, Cutaneous larval migrans	Not for use in pregnancy
Triclabendazole		Fascioliasis Paragonimiasis	Not FDA approved
TMP/SMX	Trimethoprim/sulfamethoxazole; interferes with folic acid production	*Cyclospora cayetanensis* *Isospora belli*	Not FDA approved Not for use in patients with allergy to sulfa

FURTHER READING

ANTIPARASITIC AGENTS

http://www.doh.gov.ph/ndps/table of contents2.htm

http://www.nlm.nih.gov/medlineplus/druginfo/uspdi/
202668.html

http://www.usadrug.com/IMCAccess/ConsDrugs/
Atovaquonecd.shtml

http://www.icp.ucl.ac.be/~opperd/parasites/chagas4.htm

http//www.vet.purdue.edu/depts/bms/courses/chmrx/
parahd.html

Bogitsh, B. J. & Cheng, T. C. (1998). 2nd Edn. *Human Parasitology*. New York: Academic Press.

Kasten, M. J.(1999). Clindamycin, metronidazole, and chloramphenicol, *Mayo Clinic Proceedings*, **74**, 825–33.

Rosenblatt, J. E. (1999). Antiparasitic agents. *Mayo Clinic Proceedings*, **74**, 1161–75.

Wood, J. J., Liu, L. X. & Weller, P. F. (1996). Review article: drug therapy and antiparasitic drugs, *New England Journal of Medicine*, **334(18)**, 1178–84.

Part II

Infections in reproductive medicine

7

Genital ulcer diseases

Genital ulcer disease is linked to an increased risk of HIV transmission in both homo- and heterosexual practice, and therefore the 1990s has seen its emergence as a very important sexually transmitted disease process. Whereas syphilis has been known for centuries to cause significant disease in the sexual contacts and offspring of infected patients, other agents producing soft ulcers such as chancroid and herpes simplex have now increased in prevalence. The incidence of genital ulcer disease caused by syphilis plummeted in developed countries following the availability of penicillin, and the other diseases have increased in significance. Some of these diseases can be managed by antibiotic treatment, but others such as herpes simplex virus (HSV) persist for life as a latent infection with the potential for intermittent reactivation to active disease. Education targeted towards limiting the spread of these agents and the identification of treatment modalities has become an integral part of curbing the HIV epidemic worldwide.

Five different microbial agents are commonly associated with genital ulcer disease:

(i) Herpes simplex viruses (HSV-1 and HSV-2)

(ii) *Treponema pallidum:* syphilis

(iii) *Haemophilus ducreyi:* chancroid

(iv) Invasive serovars of *Chlamydia trachomatis,* causing lymphogranuloma venereum (LGV)

(v) *Calymmatobacterium granulomatis,* causing Donovanosis

The prevalence of the different types of disease varies dramatically in different populations. In developed countries such as the United States, the United Kingdom and Europe, the majority of cases of genital ulcer disease are caused by herpes simplex viruses, with only a small proportion of cases due to the other agents. In Africa, chancroid and HSV are the most common diseases; Donovanosis is the disease most frequently seen in Australia and Papua New Guinea.

This diverse group of pathogens all present with the formation of ulcers as a primary symptom. The ulcerative lesions occur primarily in the genitals, but any body site may be involved, particularly those that come into contact with infectious genital fluids (genitalia, hands, lips, face and oral mucosa). The ulcerative lesions produced by each pathogen can be distinguished by clinical features such as appearance, tenderness, propensity to bleed, presence or absence of vesicles, chronicity, and intermittent recurrence of symptoms (Table 7.1). In the sections that follow, each agent will be discussed in detail with emphasis on a description of the agent, its epidemiology, life cycle, transmission, clinical presentation, diagnosis and treatment.

Herpes simplex virus infection

Herpes simplex viruses (HSV-1 and HSV-2)

Primary infection by HSV occurs by direct or indirect contact with herpetic lesions, through a break in mucous membranes (mouth, throat, nose, eye, genitals). The initial infection is usually asymptomatic, although there may be minor local vesicular lesions.

Table 7.1. Differential characteristics of genital ulcers

Etiology	Description of lesions	Pain	Number	Bleeding	Texture	Direct microscopy
HSV-1 and -2	Shallow red and weeping ulcers, preceded by vesicular lesions	Yes	Multiple, often clustering with satellite lesions surrounding the parent lesion	None	Soft	Tzank cells with multiple intranuclear inclusions
Syphilis (1°) (*T. pallidum*)	Sharply demarcated firm-based ulcerative papule	No	Usually single	None	Firm	Spirochetes
Syphilis (2°)	Lesions may be macular, papular, maculopapular, and pustular. Lesions on the skin, palms and soles are often pigmented and dry while those on mucous membranes are wet	No	Usually multiple	None	Firm	Spirochetes abound in lesions
Chancroid (*H. ducreyi*)	Excavated papule with sharply demarcated edges and a moist soft base. Often purulent	Yes	One or more	None	Soft	Gram-negative rods like 'schools of fish' or chains
Donovanosis (*Calymmatobacterium granulomatis*)	Beefy, vascular, rolled edges,	No	Usually single	Yes	Firm	Intracellular bacteria with bipolar staining 'safety pin like'
LGV (*Chlamydia trachomatis*)	Inconspicuous	No	Usually single, usually not noticed	None	Soft	Intracellular cytoplasmic vacuole with gram negative bacilli

Epithelial cells at the site of inoculation are the primary targets for infection and viraemia can spread via blood and lymphatics to the secondary targets, neurons of the dorsal root sensory ganglia, brain and meninges. The skin around the oral and genital orifices, the oral cavity, the cornea, vagina, cervix, anal canal and urethra are the most common sites for herpetic lesions. *Herpetic whitlow*, common among healthcare personnel, is a special type of herpetic infection of the skin that causes a painful finger lesion. Herpes virus *meningitis* is severe but self-limiting, without sequelae. In contrast, Herpes simplex viral *encephalitis* is a very severe disease, with high mortality and permanent residual damage – the temporal lobes are the main sites of infection. *Neonatal* HSV infection is acquired through contact with HSV in the birth canal. This infection, which can be severe, is preventable. Mortality is very high (>50%) and CNS sequelae are common. Prompt treatment reduces mortality and abdominal delivery to avoid contact with HSV infection in the birth canal is recommended.

Epidemiology

HSV-1 and HSV-2 are closely related viral strains in the family Herpesviridae. Because the two viruses overlap both in structure and in disease pathology, they must be discussed together when considering genital ulcer disease. HSV-1 is ubiquitous, is spread by casual contact and through salivary exchange, and has classically been viewed as the oral herpes. It does indeed account for the majority of primary and secondary HSV cases that occur 'above the belt', causing recurrent herpes of the head, neck and hands. HSV-2 is only rarely responsible for recurrent disease in these locations.

HSV-1 also causes an increasingly significant proportion of newly diagnosed genital ulcer disease. Studies performed in the United Kingdom, Japan, and the United States have demonstrated that HSV-1 accounts for 40% or more of all first episodes of symptomatic herpes genitalis. This trend may be due to several factors, including changes in sexual behaviour with an increased emphasis on oral genital contact. HSV-1 transmission during childhood

may also be decreasing in frequency, leaving a large proportion of young adults susceptible to primary infection during subsequent sexual maturity. Primary infection with HSV-1 in children is generally seen as oropharyngeal disease, but young adults are at increased risk of acquiring and transmitting HSV-1 as a sexually transmitted disease. In contrast to the primary disease, recurrent disease is commonly due to HSV-2, which causes an estimated 90–95% of all recurrent herpes genitalis. This strain is more likely to recur in the genital site and to recur with greater frequency and wider disease manifestations. HSV-1 will recur on an average of 0–3 times during the first year of genital infection, whereas HSV-2 recurs from 0 to >10 times during this same period. Both viruses show site specificity: in nongenital locations, HSV-2 is much less likely to recur than HSV-1. Overall, HSV-2 probably accounts for less than 10% of all cases of primary oral herpes.

Many cases of herpes genitalis are asymptomatic or minimally symptomatic, whether caused by HSV-1 or HSV-2: the infected individual may not recognize that he or she is infected. Although infection with one of the simplex viruses may impart immunity to infection with the other virus, this immunity is incomplete. Serologic prevalence studies of HSV-1 and HSV-2 indicate that many patients have antibodies to both viruses. The protective effect of HSV-1 antibodies may contribute to producing a less symptomatic or asymptomatic primary disease following infection with HSV-2.

Life cycle

HSV-1 and HSV-2 are obligate intracellular parasites, requiring a host cell to carry out their own reproduction or replication. HSV invades an epithelial cell nucleus, where the host cell is commandeered to produce more viral particles at the expense of the cell's own function. Viral DNA is transcribed into mRNA in the nucleus, for translation into viral proteins on ribosomes in the cell cytoplasm. These proteins are then either inserted into the nuclear membrane or are transported into the nucleus to produce the viral protein coat, the capsid. Viral genomic DNA in the nucleus is enclosed into the completed viral capsid, which is then enrobed in the cell's nuclear membrane, now containing viral proteins. These membrane-coated viral capsids are known as *virions* and represent the infective viral particle. Particles may leave the cell during a lytic phase of infection in which the host cell is destroyed, or the virus may travel along sensory nerves to enter dorsal root ganglia, where host cell and viral genomic DNA survive together in a quiescent (latent) phase of infection. Stress, febrile illness, menstruation, and other situations of host immune compromise can induce viral reactivation and cause further active lytic phase viral infection. The propensity of the virus to reactivate or come out of latency to produce active disease depends first on the type of HSV (HSV-1 or HSV-2) and also upon the anatomic location of the nerve in which the virus has become latent. Reactivation is site specific, with HSV-1 producing more numerous and clinically aggressive head and neck disease, while HSV-2 is more likely to recur with greater frequency and with greater symptomatology in the genital region. It is this propensity for reactivation that has given the herpes simplex viruses a reputation as 'the gift that keeps giving'.

Transmission

Both herpes simplex viruses may be transmitted by several different modes. Salivary spread is the primary mode of transmission for HSV-1, and this virus has classically been viewed as a childhood illness, with a large proportion of infections seen during the first several years of life. This trend in disease transmission has decreased substantially in many parts of the world, where over 70% of adolescents may still be susceptible (seronegative) to HSV-1. HSV-1 is now increasingly seen as a sexually transmitted disease, either through transfer of HSV-1 from the oral site of one individual to the genitals of another via direct contact or through fomites, or it may be transmitted as a true STD via genital–genital contact. Similarly, HSV-2 may be transmitted either via sexual contact or, less commonly, via contaminated oral secretions. Vertical transmission is also an important mode of viral transfer. Pregnant women may transfer virus to the fetus *in utero* leading to congenital HSV infection, or the neonate may be infected by contact with infected genital secretions during parturition. Vertical transmission is most likely when the pregnant woman has primary symptoms of an acute infection with HSV. Similarly, transmission to the neonate is seen most efficiently during the mother's primary infection or when birth coincides with an active herpetic outbreak in the mother.

Clinical presentation

The clinical presentation of HSV infection depends upon the site of inoculation and also upon whether the illness is primary or reactivation disease. In the generic sense, HSV causes blistering lesions with an acute inflammatory response. Lesions are initially tense and fluid-filled, but rapidly rupture with minor pressure to produce shallow, painful ulcerative lesions.

In the head and neck region, symptomatic primary disease presents most commonly as ulcerative pharyngitis, with lesions on the posterior pharynx; they may also occur in any site in the mouth including gums, tongue and tonsillar tissues as well as other facial locations including the skin and eyes. Infection may be transferred via infected saliva onto the hands and inoculated into other body sites including the genitals. Although HSV-1 is the predominant simplex virus producing disease in the head and neck region, HSV-2 is also occasionally seen, and primary disease caused by both viruses is indistinguishable without diagnostic testing.

Similarly, the clinical presentation of primary herpes genitalis is identical for both HSV-1 and HSV-2. Primary disease is commonly bilateral, with many vesicular lesions present. The parent lesions become surrounded by several smaller satellite lesions that coalesce to form large soft fluid-filled blisters. These blisters are easily disrupted with even minor trauma, such as rubbing against clothing, leaving shallow, painful red ulcers. Lesions may be pruritic or produce a burning sensation. Primary genital disease may also be accompanied by extra-genital disease such as herpes oralis, herpetic whitlow or herpes ocularis in about 10% of all cases of primary herpes genitalis. These extragenital manifestations may represent autoinoculation from genital to non-genital sites or may arise from oral-genital or hand-genital contact as a sexually transmitted disease.

Recurrence in the head and neck region, commonly seen as the ubiquitous cold sore or fever blister, is almost exclusively HSV-1. These lesions occur either on the lip, at the mucocutaneous junction of the lip with the face or in perioral facial skin. Reactivation may occur in the same site each time, or may occur at various different sites around the mouth representing reactivation from different neuronal sites of latency. Recurrent reactivation disease is reported in 33% of young men and 28% of young women surveyed in North America. This population of patients with recurrent infections serves as a reservoir of virus to infect susceptible hosts. Autoinoculation into new sites within the same host may occur, but does not happen as often as is seen during the primary infection. HSV-1 mediated reactivation may occur one or more times each year, with intermittent symptomatic disease reported in some individuals persisting for decades. Overall, the frequency and severity of symptoms appears to decrease with time. Primary HSV-2 rarely leads to reactivation disease in the head and neck region. If reactivation should occur, it is usually only once, and within the first year following primary infection. Reactivation disease in the hands may be caused either by HSV-1 or HSV-2, with HSV-1 having the predisposition to reactivate more commonly than HSV-2.

The natural history of genital herpes has been well studied. Recurrent disease is primarily due to HSV-2, with only 5% of all cases of reactivation disease being caused by HSV-1. HSV-2 is the more aggressive of the viruses when it comes to genital reactivation. The frequency and severity of infection with HSV-2 does diminish with time, although asymptomatic shedding may be seen for years. If HSV-1 recurs in the genital site, the frequency is seldom more than once or twice and is usually not detected after the first year of infection.

Laboratory diagnosis

Diagnostic tests currently available may be divided into several categories:
  (i) direct examination of cellular materials and infected tissues;
 (ii) antigen detection assays;
(iii) culture techniques;
(iv) serology;
 (v) molecular diagnostic tests.
The choice of test selected for diagnosis depends upon whether the patient is symptomatic or asymptomatic and upon the required sensitivity and specificity.

Acute illness with fresh, unbroken blisters presents several testing options, and direct detection assays are helpful for a rapid diagnosis. Virus infected epithelial cells demonstrate multiple nuclei with characteristic intranuclear inclusions: these are known as 'Tzank cells', and they can be identified on Wright's or Pap stained smear preparations. Demonstration of Tzank cells is probably the most common point of care test used to make the diagnosis of HSV infection (Fig. 7.1). Positive identification confirms infection with a Herpes virus, but is not specific

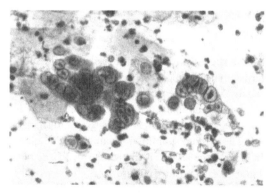

Fig. 7.1. HSV Tzank cells in a Pap smear preparation. HSV infection may be detected on Pap smears and skin scrapings by identifying the typical multinucleate cells with large intranuclear inclusions. These inclusions are surrounded by a pale staining halo, which is ringed by host cellular DNA at the periphery of the nucleus. An acute inflammatory exudate can also be seen in this slide, a common finding both in acute infections and in reactivation disease.

for Herpes simplex and cannot differentiate between HSV-1 and HSV-2 infections. The sensitivity of direct detection using the Tzank smear is low, about 40% compared to culture.

Direct fluorescence antibody or *indirect peroxidase staining* of direct specimens will help in the speciation of the Herpes simplex viruses, but these techniques are not usually performed in the physician office. Similar to the Tzank preparation, the sensitivity of these direct tests is low at 31–80% (depending on the specimen source) compared to culture.

When *biopsy* material is available, immunohistochemical staining or electron microscopic demonstration of HSV infected cells in tissues may be used for diagnosis. The sensitivity of electron microscopy compared to culture for cases of HSV genitalis is quite low (43–60%), making this an undesirable diagnostic assay.

Several products for *antigenic detection* of HSV are commercially available. These assays have the benefit of a potentially rapid turn-around time (3–5 hours); their sensitivity compared to culture ranges from 35–93% depending upon the product. The Herp-Check assay (Dupont) demonstrates a range of sensitivity from 59–99% with the highest sensitivities seen in symptomatic cases.

Culture

Culture is generally still considered the gold standard for the diagnosis of acute (currently symptomatic) herpes infections, and must be performed if in vitro susceptibility testing is required. Culture is most effective if swabs or scrapings from fresh blistering lesions are submitted for analysis. The older the lesions, the less likely that virus will be isolated. Higher rates of positive culture are seen for primary disease than for subsequent reactivation. Specimens should be collected into antibiotic-containing transport medium and delivered to the laboratory on wet ice. If not processed immediately, specimens should be refrigerated until cultured. Tube culture in one of several cell lines is probably the most cost-effective test. The sensitivity of different cell lines used for the diagnosis of HSV infection varies, the most sensitive

Fig. 7.2. HSV cytopathic effect in MRC-5 fibroblast cell lines. The herpes simplex viruses grow readily in many cell lines, including fibroblast cell lines. Infected cells begin to round up, becoming refractile and granular within 1–5 days; they are distributed throughout the cell sheet, not necessarily clustering or forming plaques. Infection spreads rapidly so that the entire sheet is involved within 1–2 days, often with sloughing of the monolayer.

being MRC-5, primary rabbit kidney, and mink lung fibroblasts. Once infected with HSV, the fibroblast cells round up, become refractile and demonstrate the classic cytopathic effect associated with this virus (Fig. 7.2).

Immunostaining is required to differentiate HSV-1 from HSV-2. While approximately 60% of the tube cultures are positive within 24 hours, optimal sensitivity for culture requires a further 4–7 days of culture. If more rapid test results are required, a spin-amplified culture method using shell vials can be applied. In the shell vial assay, patient specimens are inoculated onto cell monolayers growing on glass coverslips inside small sample vials. These cultures are centrifuged slowly to enhance viral infection into the cells prior to incubation. After 1–3 days of incubation, the inoculated cells may then be stained directly on the coverslip using fluorescently labelled monoclonal antibodies specific to either HSV-1 or HSV-2 (Fig. 7.3).

A genetically engineered system, ELVIS (enzyme-linked viral inducible) HSV detection culture (BioWhittaker), is commercially available. HSV is detected in shell vial cultures as peroxidase-staining plaques of infected cells. Recent changes in this

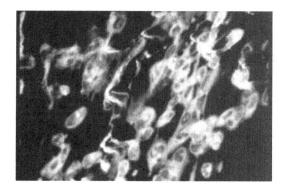

Fig. 7.3. Fluorescently stained HSV-2 infected MRC-5 cells in a shell vial culture. Infections with HSV-1 and -2 can be directly identified by staining infected cells on the cover slip with monoclonal fluorescently labelled antibodies. Individual cells thoughout this monolayer show fluorescent staining. Rounding and separation of the infected cells from the rest of the confluent monolayer is further evidence of the viral cytopathic effect.

system allow immediate review of positive cultures by fluorescence microscopy for speciation of HSV-2 infected cells.

In cases of suspected HSV-related encephalitis, culture of cerebrospinal fluid (CSF) is an insensitive method of diagnosis. In such cases, molecular detection is the preferred test. If HSV is isolated in culture, in vitro susceptibility testing is possible, but these techniques are not yet widely available for routine use.

Molecular diagnostic assays

Molecular diagnostic assays that detect viral DNA from a variety of samples are now available. Compared to culture, PCR offers higher sensitivity in diagnosis of acute genital or oral lesions. PCR is also more sensitive than culture for detecting HSV encephalitis and in detecting asymptomatic viral shedding from oral and genital sites. Two molecular assays are commercially available: Light cycler PCR (Roche Molecular Biochemicals, Indianapolis, IN) and the Hybrid Capture II Signal Amplification Probe test for HSV (Digene Corporation). These assays have shown excellent sensitivity and specificity for

detecting and differentiating the Herpes simplex viruses in ulcerative lesions and may be useful in detecting asymptomatic shedding in patients. They may be used in the future for detecting and speciating HSV in Thin-Prep PAP samples after cytological HSV identification. Currently, however, there are no FDA approved methods for diagnosing HSV infections by any amplified molecular technique, and results obtained using these techniques must be defined as 'for research purposes only'.

Serology

Serology may be helpful in detecting symptomatic shedding, or for identifying undiagnosed primary infections more than 4 months after initial presentation. Antibodies develop after 2–3 months in 70% of patients, but more than 6 months may be required before a measurable antibody response can be detected in 30% of patients. A negative HSV-2 antibody level should therefore be interpreted with caution in an individual who has been symptomatic for less than 4 months. Recent advances in technology have substantially improved our ability to detect and differentiate HSV specific antibodies, with several assays commercially available. Sensitivity and specificity of these assays in detection of HSV-1 antibodies are in the >90% range while the sensitivity of the HSV-2 assays varies from about 80–95%, depending on the manufacturer. FDA approved commercial kits are also available for recombinant immunoblot assays that reliably determine serostatus. These type-specific IgG assays are useful in monitoring serostatus and evaluating potentially transmitting partners.

Treatment

No currently available treatment is capable of eradicating a herpes simplex infection. Once a person has herpes, he or she will always have herpes and therefore prevention is the only effective manner of disease control. Although a barrier method of birth control such as the male and female condoms (but not the diaphragm) provides the best prevention of viral spread, these methods are not 100% effective. Failure of these condoms in preventing disease spread is probably not so much due to virus penetrating the latex barrier, but to incorrect or inconsistent use of condoms. In a study of mismatched couples (one partner with known herpes and one without), only 61% of couples reported ever using condoms and only 13% used condoms for each sexual encounter despite the known health risks.

Treatments are instead aimed towards shortening the length of active disease and viral shedding, or at decreasing the incidence of active recurrence, particularly during the first year of infection. Herpesviruses are one of the few viruses that code for their own DNA polymerase, and this is the target for antiviral therapy. Acyclovir (Zovirax) is an acyclic purine nucleoside analogue that cannot be metabolized by cells until phosphorylated by an HSV-specified thymidine kinase to acyclovir monophosphate. A host enzyme then converts this to acyclovir triphosphate, which acts as a competitive inhibitor for dGTP in DNA synthesis. Its incorporation into an elongating DNA chain interrupts elongation as it does not have an −OH group in the 3' position. Several commercial products are currently available for treatment, including topical over-the-counter medications, topical prescription medications or oral prescription medications. Guidelines for treatment with DNA polymerase inhibitors were recommended by the CDC in 2002. Dosage and dosing frequency are determined by the absorption and bioavailabiliy characteristics of each drug and the use of the drug as a suppressive or episodic treatment for symptomatic disease. Table 7.2 lists some of the treatment options.

Pencyclovir is marketed in a topical formulation for the symptomatic treatment of oral herpes labialis, requiring q8 or q12 hour applications of 5 mg/kg of drug. Cidofovir is an experimental drug currently being tested as a topical preparation in FDA Phase II trials for refractory and ophthalmic HSV infections.

Although these drugs are safe and effective, they must be administered early in infection for maximal antiviral activity, and drug-resistant viruses have been detected for most of the available agents.

Table 7.2. CDC Recommended treatment regimes for HSV

Recommended daily suppressive therapy:	
Acyclovir	400 mg p.o. ii qd
Famcyclovir	250 mg p.o. ii qd
Valacyclovir	500 mg p.o. qd
Valacyclovir	1.0 g p.o. i qd

Recommended therapy for episodic recurrent infections:	
Acyclovir	400 mg p.o. iii qd × 5 days
Acyclovir	200 mg p.o. v qd × 5 days
Acyclovir	800 mg p.o. ii qd × 5 days
Famcyclovir	125 mg p.o. ii qd × 5 days
Valacyclovir	500 mg p.o. ii qd × 3–5 days
Valacyclovir	1.0 g p.o. i qd × 5 days

Resistant forms arise from mutations in genes coding for thymidine kinase or DNA polymerase. Although the level of drug resistance is low in the immunocompetent patient population, it is increasing in the immunocompromised patient population: ACV-resistant HSV has been isolated from patients on prolonged therapy (e.g. AIDS patients). Newer drugs such as cidofovir will probably be used as an alternative therapy when acyclovir and the other nucleoside analogues fail due to the development of resistance, particularly in immunocompromised hosts. A new class of drugs that disrupt HSV replication through a different mechanism of action is now under development (Crute et al., 2002; Kleyman et al., 2002). These new drugs contain amino-thiazolylphenyl compounds and thiazole urea derivatives, and act by inhibiting the HSV helicase–primase complex that normally unwinds the double-stranded viral DNA and generates primers for viral DNA synthesis. On the basis of promising results in rodent models, these new drugs may soon be tested in clinical trials.

Vaccine availability

Immune response to infection with the herpes simplex viruses relies on the development of CD4 memory cells to produce IFN-gamma, CD8 T cells to proliferate and secrete cytokines, and production of neutralizing antibodies that are important for mediating antibody-dependent cell-mediated toxicity through the neutrophils, monocytes and NK-like cells. Although there is no consistent correlation between CD4 responses and disease severity, a brisk secretion of IFN-gamma by these cells generally produces a longer period of latency to the next symptomatic recurrence of HSV-1 disease compared to individuals in whom IFN-gamma secretion is poor. HSV-specific CD8 cells are low in number, but appear to be functionally very important. Local infiltration of infected tissues with the CD8 cells correlates with the rapid clearance of infective viral particles. Neutralizing antibody production has provided one of the important end points for vaccine evaluation and studies of seroprevalence or seroconversion.

HSV trial vaccines have included peptide and protein preparations, viral subunit mixtures, killed whole virus vaccines, live attenuated vaccine and genetically engineered live, non-replicative vaccines. Of the peptide vaccines, phase I human trials are ongoing for an HSV common type gB2 (272) and gD2 proteins administered in a heat shock protein adjuvant. Two subunit vaccines have completed phase II clinical trials. Vaccination with the Chiron subunit vaccine containing gB2 has partial and transient protective effects against HSV-2 seroconversion. This protective effect has been seen only in women, and only in those who were previously HSV-1 seronegative. The GSK vaccine was 75% effective in preventing clinically apparent genital lesions, although again, only women who were previously HSV-seronegative were protected. Subunit vaccines using truncated HSV-2 glycoprotein have demonstrated no correlation between antibody response and vaccine efficacy in preventing infection or disease manifestation. Killed virus vaccines have likewise failed to provide long-term benefit to vaccinated individuals, as have fractionated-viral particle vaccines. Replication-deficient gH-deleted HSV-2 vaccine has been demonstrated to be safe and immunogenic in clinical trials. When used in an immunotherapeutic trial, however, no clinical improvement in preventing symptomatic reactivation disease was seen for individuals receiving the vaccine. Finally, live viral vaccines with replication-competent HSV strains have been somewhat problematic in their development. HSV is neurotrophic, and even the vaccine strain may lead to neurologic complications. In addition, the live and replicating virus may develop latent and reactivation diseases. The most extensively studied attenuated viral strain, R7020, has been shown to trigger a dose-dependent antibody response in HSV seronegative patients, but trials were stopped due to the poor overall immunogenicity of the vaccine strain. Therefore, despite significant advances in vaccine development, we are left with no currently available options.

Syphilis

Treponema pallidum

Treponema pallidum is a spirochete – a long, slender, spiral, helically shaped unicellular bacterium, with several turns in the helix. It has a flexible cell wall with fibrils that are responsible for its motility. The organisms associate with animal and human hosts, are microaerophilic and die rapidly on drying. They reproduce by binary fission with a long (30-hour) generation time. Syphilis has been recognized as a significant sexually transmitted disease since the late 1400s. It has been suggested that Columbus's ships may have brought the disease back from the New World, but it may be that the disease was already present in Europe prior to its evolution into an epidemic spread. Following the French invasion of Italy to free Naples from Spanish control, troops began to fall ill with what was viewed as a new plague. The French army with its hired mercenaries from Britain and several European nations is credited with spreading the new scourge throughout Europe and into Britain during its retreat from battle. The disease was originally known as the 'Disease of Naples', after its presumed source of origin. This name was soon replaced with 'the French Disease' or the 'French Pox' after these troops spread it throughout Europe. The disease continued to spread as an epidemic between 1493 and the early eighteenth century; the virulence of the illness eventually decreased and then evolved into the sexually transmitted disease we recognize today. Whatever its origin, syphilis now has a worldwide distribution, and is the *second most common cause of genital ulcers* in the US and in the majority of the developed world. The overall number of new cases of syphilis has diminished greatly over the past half-decade. Males are affected more commonly than females, and the primary age group infected is 20–29 years. In the US the majority of cases occur in the black, non-Hispanic population.

Life cycle

Untreated syphilis has a very complicated life cycle, with primary, secondary and tertiary disease manifestations. Primary disease occurs at the initial site of inoculation, with the spirochete multiplying in the primary chancre. Following this initial infection, organisms are disseminated via the blood to every organ in the body. The spirochete undergoes extensive binary division locally within the primary lesion and, to a limited extent, in the disseminated sites. The patient becomes temporarily asymptomatic when the primary lesions heal and resolve, but the organisms continue to divide in disseminated sites. A secondary phase of cutaneous lesions (rash) follows, and the spirochetes multiply to yield huge numbers of organisms in the lesions. The organisms become confined in tissue sites all over the body and stimulate a gummatous granulomatous inflammatory response. There is little or no organism growth during this final phase of infection, and tissue damage and disease manifestations result instead from the extensive and characteristic inflammatory response.

Transmission

Syphilis is transmitted sexually in about 90% of cases. Sexual spread includes not only genital–genital contact, but also related acts where mucocutaneous sites from one individual are in direct contact with the infected lesions of another person. During the rash stage of secondary syphilis, infected lesions have a very high spirochetal load and direct casual contact with these lesions may lead to spread from one individual to another. Patients are highly infective

during the first year of disease, with no further sexual transmission seen after the fourth year. Vertical transmission is more common during the mother's first several years of infection and may be associated with repeated spontaneous abortions, as well as third trimester fetal death *in utero* and congenital syphilis in the newborn. During the early years of transfusion medicine when whole blood was transfused immediately after collection, syphilis was transmitted as a post-transfusion infection, but this risk was essentially eliminated by refrigeration of blood prior to transfusion. Although there is still a risk of infection from transfused platelets, routine testing of all donors for serologic evidence of syphilis has now all but eliminated the risk of transfusion-transmitted syphilis in most parts of the world.

Clinical presentation

The clinical presentation for syphilis depends upon the stage of infection at the time of diagnosis. Primary syphilis occurs between 3 to 90 days (mean 21 days) following infection and is characterized by the formation of a single, painless ulcer (chancre) at the point of inoculation. Although the primary chancre is most often located on the genitalia, it may also occur on the lips, oral mucosa, tongue or other sites that have been exposed to direct contact with lesions containing the infective spirochetes. Lymphadenopathy, if present, is hard and non-tender. The patient is infectious while the primary chancre is present and this primary chancre resolves spontaneously in about 3 weeks.

If left untreated, secondary disease generally develops around 3 weeks after the resolution of the primary lesion. Patients are systemically ill during this phase of disease, with generalized symptoms of fever, headache, weight loss, sore throat, nasal discharge, and arthralgias. The majority of patients develop generalized non-tender lymphadenopathy. The onset of secondary syphilis is characterized by a widespread cutaneous macular rash, starting on the lateral trunk region and extending to the upper arms. This evolves into a maculopapular rash, often involving the palms and soles, the middle of the face, back and trunk and the oral cavity. Syphilitic lesions may also progress to other morphologies. Pronounced, indurated dark red papular lesions follow the maculopapular rash, and **condyloma lata**, a form of papular lesion, occur in moist regions of the body. Condyloma lata are flat topped, variably pigmented, moist and may appear around the hairline ('Crown of Venus'), surround the neck ('Collar of Venus') or appear on the genitalia or oral mucosa. Pustular lesions or 'Great Pox' are loaded with spirochetes and are the most infectious lesions. Annular lesions are the final cutaneous manifestation.

Secondary syphilis with its various cutaneous manifestations typically lasts for several weeks, after which the lesions heal completely without scarring. In some patients, a second wave of symptomatic disease may occur weeks to months following the onset of secondary disease. While mucocutaneous manifestations are present, the patient is infectious to sexual and casual contacts that touch these lesions, and the female patient can transmit the disease to her fetus.

Following the resolution of secondary symptoms, the untreated patient goes into a latent phase of infection. Although there is serologic evidence of infection, he or she is no longer symptomatic. Disease can still be transmitted both vertically to the fetus and through sexual contact, but at a much lower rate than during the earlier disease phases. This phase of illness may persist for many years, but no further transmission of disease is generally seen after four years of infection.

Tertiary syphilis is a very late manifestation of *Treponema pallidum* infection, characterized by the formation of gummas in any organ. The gumma is a specialized form of granuloma that is specific to syphilis, with certain sites as characteristic targets. Cardiovascular gummas are very common, particularly involving the ascending aorta, and patients may present with aortic aneurysms as the late stage manifestation of disease. Neuronal involvement is also very common and may include gummatous inflammation in the brain, eye, auditory or other cranial nerves as well as spinal cord involvement. The posterior columns of the spinal cord are preferentially involved, leading to *Tabes dorsalis*, characterized by a slapping foot gait and subsequent knee joint abnor-

malities due to sensory nerve loss. Psychiatric disorders and dementia are common manifestations of neural syphilis.

An infected woman is capable of transmitting her infection transplacentally to the fetus throughout the course of pregnancy, with early first trimester abortions or late third trimester stillbirths. The majority of these aborted fetuses represent vertical transmission early in the pregnancy, and thus have evidence of extensive tissue damage from the infection, often with characteristic bone and central nervous system abnormalities. Those that survive to birth may also show evidence of congenital syphilitic syndromes. The diagnosis relies on the identification of radiographic bone abnormalities, demonstration of hepato-splenomegaly, cutaneous lesions and upper respiratory congestion. Abnormal tooth development is also frequently seen. Depending upon the degree of central nervous system involvement, these infants may demonstrate varying degrees of retardation, deafness and blindness. Microcephaly is also seen with some frequency. In countries where there is a recommended universal testing of pregnant women, the number of cases of congenital syphilis has steadily decreased over the past several decades.

Clinical diagnosis

Syphilis has been called 'The Great Imitator' because of the wide variety of symptoms that may be interpreted as being due to other diseases. The clinical diagnosis is complicated by having three distinct phases of presentation, with long intervening periods without signs or symptoms of infection. The terminal disease is far removed from the initial infection and may have an impact on every major organ system, making the diagnosis of disease decidedly difficult. Diagnosis is rarely made on the basis of clinical presentation alone.

Laboratory diagnosis

Diagnostic testing for syphilis relies on direct detection of infection, serology and (recently) PCR detection. There is no effective in vitro culture system

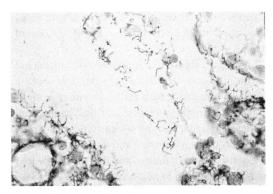

Fig. 7.4. Syphilis spirochetes in a tissue section stained with the Steiner stain. *Treponema pallidum* is a very thin spiral organism that does not stain well by conventional methods due to its very small diameter, and a special silver stain (Steiner stain) is used to detect the spirochetes in a tissue section. Organisms in this preparation are long (about 14 μm in length) and thin, the spirals are seen as multiple undulations.

for *T. pallidum. Direct examination* may be the only test that is positive during primary syphilis. The spirochete is very narrow, (1.0–1.5 μm), and therefore these bacteria cannot be detected by routine staining for light microscopy. They are visualized instead by illumination of the motile organisms using indirect light, appearing as bright bacteria in a dark background in the dark-field microscope. *T. pallidum* can be seen as tightly coiled spirals, measuring about twice the length of a red blood cell (10–20 μm). Other stains such as the Steiner silver stain may be used to detect the spirochetes in fixed tissue sections (Fig. 7.4). Direct fluorescent antibody stains are available in some laboratories, although the commercial availability of these stains is limited.

Serology is the gold standard for diagnosis of secondary, latent and tertiary syphilis; serology investigations are divided into treponemal and non-treponemal tests. *Non-treponemal* tests use an alcoholic solution of cardiolipin, cholesterol and lecithin that clumps in the presence of antibodies produced during a syphilis infection; four non-treponemal tests are used in screening for syphilis:
- Venereal Diseases Reference Laboratory test (VDRL) slide assay
- Untreated Serum Reagin test (USR) assay

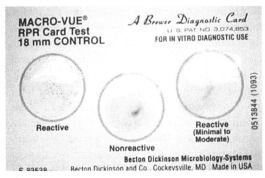

Fig. 7.5. Non-treponemal rapid plasma reagin (RPR) assay to screen for syphilis. The RPR is a standardized flocculation and co-agglutination assay used for serologic detection of *T. pallidum* infection. Patient's serum is mixed with a charcoal suspension containing cardiolipin antigen. The cardiolipin antigen reacts with 'reagin', an antibody-like substance present in the serum of syphilis patients, to produce a flocculation reaction and co-agglutinate the carbon particles in the assay. This Figure demonstrates typical reactive, minimally reactive (both considered as positive) and non-reactive (negative) results. This non-treponemal test is used to screen for syphilis, but must be confirmed using a treponemal assay (see Fig. 7.6).

- Rapid Plasma Reagin test (RPR) 18 mm circle card
- Toluidine Red Unheated Serum Test (TRUST) assay. VDRL and USR are flocculation assays and require a microscope to visualize reagent clumping. The RPR and TRUST assays cause agglutination that can be observed macroscopically, differing by their agglutination indicator: charcoal for the RPR (Fig. 7.5) and paint pigment for the TRUST assay. Patient serum and agglutination reagent are mixed on a card and rotated, and the agglutination agent is trapped in the antigen/antibody matrix that forms in reactive specimens. Although all four of these tests use serum as the antibody source, the VDRL is the only assay that may be used to detect antibody response in CSF samples in cases of neurosyphilis. Since the antigens used in these non-treponemal assays are not specific to *T. pallidum,* positive test results may be seen in other disease processes. All positive results therefore require confirmation using a treponemal test. The non-treponemal tests are useful for monitoring response to therapy, since they should become

non-reactive after successful treatment. Therapy can be monitored by following a decline in antibody titre as detected in these assays. Other assays such as the VISUWELL Reagin test, an indirect ELISA assay, are also available as screening tests for syphilis. This assay is useful for screening large numbers of patients, as in blood donor screening.

Treponemal tests confirm the presence of the spirochete
- Fluorescent treponemal antibody absorption test (FTA-ABS)
- FTA-ABS double staining
- Microagglutination test: either the microhemagglutination–*Treponema pallidum* (MHA–TP), or a *Treponema pallidum* particle agglutination (TPPA) assay.

These assays are based on the use of *Treponema*-derived antigens for the detection of antibodies produced during a syphilis infection. In the FTA-ABS and in the FTA-ABS double staining assays, patient-derived antibodies bound to the Nichols strain of *T. pallidum* are detected by fluorescent antibody staining. In the agglutination assays, passive agglutination of sensitized particles (red cells or gelatin particles) results in cells settling in clumps distributed over the entire bottom of the well in a microtitre well plate assay (Fig. 7.6). In the absence of treponemal antibodies, the cells pellet into a central tight button at the bottom of the well. These tests will remain positive for years or for life, even with appropriate therapy. Measuring antibody titre with these assays has no prognostic value and is not carried out. The treponemal tests remain the gold standard for diagnosis of syphilis.

PCR assays have been developed and are currently available for research purposes. These assays require extensive validation for use in the clinical lab, but may be useful for the detection of spirochetes in CSF or amniotic fluid. A multiplex PCR assay for the detection of the common causes of genital ulcer disease (HSV-1, HSV-2, syphilis, and chancroid) is under development. No PCR assays have been approved for patient testing by the FDA, which limits their usefulness in the United States.

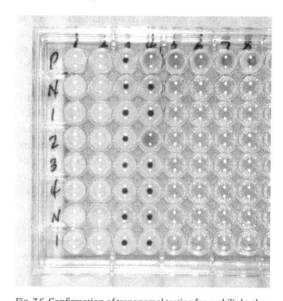

Fig. 7.6. Confirmation of treponemal testing for syphilis by the TPPA (*T. pallidum* particle agglutination) assay. All positive non-treponemal tests are confirmed by a treponemal assay such as the TPPA. Particle agglutination is similar to the red cell agglutination assay (MHA–TP), with sensitized gelatin particles used to mediate the agglutination reaction. In a microtitre well plate, a 1:10 dilution is prepared in the first column to the left and dilutions of 1:20, 1:40 and 1:80 are placed in the second, third and fourth columns, respectively. Serial dilutions are prepared in rows from 1:10 to 1:1280 for the positive control. Unsensitized gelatin particles are inoculated into the wells in column 3 as a reagent negative control (Column 3 from the left), and gelatin particles that have been sensitized with *T. pallidum* antigens from the Nichols' strain of the spirochete are added to the wells in columns 4–8 for the positive control. Patient and control wells with negative results demonstrate a solid small button of pelleted gelatin. In samples with sensitized gelatin and antibodies to *T. pallidum*, the gelatin does not pellet at the bottom of the well, but instead forms a thin matt over the bottom of the tube: the antibodies form cross-links with the sensitized gelatin particles to create a lattice that prevents pelleting (row 1 columns 4–8 for the positive control and row 4 from the top column 4 for a patient specimen).

Treatment

The Center for Disease Control (CDC) in the USA released recommendations for the management of patients with syphilis in 2002. Parenteral penicillin

G is the antibiotic of choice to treat all forms of syphilis, with dose and duration according to the stage being treated. Early disease in adults may be managed with a single intramuscular dose of 2.4 million units of benzathine penicillin G, while tertiary syphilis may require three injections, administered once per week over a period of 3 weeks. More aggressive management of neuro and ocular syphilis is recommended: penicillin every 4 hours for 2 weeks is required for cure. Management of sexual contacts is extremely important in limiting the spread of syphilis. All sexual contacts exposed within 90 days of primary lesions should be treated regardless of serologic status. Long-term partners of patients with latent or tertiary syphilis should be treated only if serology is positive, since the likelihood of transmission diminishes after a few years of infection.

Vaccine availability

There is no vaccine currently available to prevent syphilis.

Chancroid

Haemophilus ducreyi

Chancroid is caused by a fastidious gram-negative rod, *Haemophilus ducreyi*, transmitted almost exclusively during sexual contact – the human host is its only known reservoir. The disease is relatively uncommon in the USA and Europe (third most common cause of genital ulcers), but it is the most common cause of genital ulcer disease in tropical regions and developing nations. Regional outbreaks may be seen in non-endemic areas of the world, generally related to introduction of infection via the sex industry. Co-infection of *H. ducreyi* with other STDs is quite common. In Africa and other regions of the world where HIV is prevalent, chancroid is one of the most significant cofactors in acquisition of HIV infection: the presence of chancroid genital ulcers has been cited as one of the major factors

behind the ready transmission of HIV from women to men. Overall, chancroid is a disease of lower socio-economic classes; men are infected more often than females and non-whites more often than whites.

Life cycle

H. ducreyi is an extracellular gram-negative bacterium. It reproduces by binary fission, and produces no spore forms.

Transmission

Chancroid is almost exclusively a sexually transmitted disease, with *H. ducreyi* infection acquired by direct person-to-person contact with infected lesions.

Clinical presentation

Chancroid presents as one or more exquisitely painful soft genital ulcers. After an incubation period of about 3 to 4 days, papules appear that rapidly ulcerate. In comparison to the herpes simplex viruses that also produce painful ulcers, *H. ducreyi* never produces vesicular lesions. Primary lesions of chancroid often progress to form satellite lesions that may coalesce to become large, irregular shaped ulcers. The edges of the lesion are slightly indurated and excavate under the lesions' edge to produce a flask-shaped ulcer with a soft base. As in HSV disease, chancroid is often associated with tender inguinal lymphadenopathy but, unlike HSV disease, these may ulcerate to the overlying skin, becoming fluctuant and suppurative. Lymphatic involvement may impair flow of lymphatic fluid, leading to genital and lower extremity edema. If untreated, the infection will persist for several months before resolving.

Clinical diagnosis

Diagnostic laboratory tests for infection with *H. ducreyi* are very insensitive and therefore diagnoses are commonly made by exclusion: exquisitely painful genital ulcers with negative testing for

HSV and syphilis. Fluctuant and suppurative lymphadenopathy in the presence of painful non-vesicular genital lesions is almost pathognomonic for chancroid.

Laboratory diagnosis

Gram's stain of ulcer swab or scraping specimens is the direct examination of choice. On Gram's stain, the organisms will appear as gram-negative rods in chains ('railroad tracks') or aligned in the same direction in a cluster ('school of fish'). Tissue biopsies show three layers of inflammatory involvement: (i) acute inflammation and tissue necrosis characterized by fibrin and red blood cells at the surface of the ulcer, (ii) granulation tissue with extensive vascularization next, and (iii) a chronic inflammatory layer with plasma cells and lymphocytes at the lowest layer of tissue involvement.

Although culture is required for definitive diagnosis, *H. ducreyi* is extremely fastidious and may not grow even under optimal conditions in a support medium of enhanced chocolate agar with vancomycin (ECA-V, Nairobi Agar). Cultures must be grown under moist conditions at 33–37 °C in a candle jar, and held for 7–10 days. The bacteria grow very slowly to form small, tenacious tan colonies (Fig. 7.7).

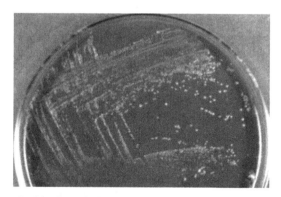

Fig. 7.7. Culture of *Hemophilus ducreyi*. *H. ducreyi* is a very fastidious organism that grows best on enhanced chocolate agar with vancomycin (Nairobi Agar). Colonies grow slowly and require high humidity in a candle jar atmosphere. Typical colonies seen in this figure are tan, moist and tenacious.

Positive culture under these optimal conditions may pick up 80% of cases. Biochemically, *H. ducreyi* is fairly inert. It requires X factor (heme) but not V Factor (nicotinamide adenine dinucleotide, NAD), and is δ-aminolevulinic acid (ALA)-porphyrin negative. The organism is catalase negative and oxidase positive. It is indole, urease and ornithine decarboxylase negative. *H. ducreyi* fails to produce acid from sucrose, lactose, fructose, ribose, xylose and mannose. It is the only *Haemophilus* species that fails to produce acids from glucose.

The difficulties in detecting *H. ducreyi* in culture have led to the development of non-culture techniques, including an enzyme immunoassay (EIA) to determine seroprevalence of *H. ducreyi* infection in patient populations. This assay has been useful for seroprevalence studies, but should not be used as the sole diagnostic test to detect chancroid. PCR amplification of *H. ducreyi* DNA has greater potential as a definitive diagnostic test and primers have been developed that are capable of detecting bacteria directly without culture amplification. When it becomes commercially available, this assay may be the test of choice in making a definitive diagnosis for this fastidious organism.

Treatment

Improved hygiene and male circumcision have decreased the spread of chancroid, even prior to the availability of antibiotics. Several antibiotics are now available, some of which may be administered in a single dose as directly observed therapy; this disease has now been marked for possible eradication. The CDC recommend several therapies for the treatment of chancroid, summarized in Table 7.3. Azithromycin and ceftriaxone are available as single dose treatments, to assure patient compliance. Multiple-dose regimens with ciprofloxacin and erythromycin are also recommended, the latter for use during pregnancy, lactation and for children under 18 years of age. However, intermediate drug resistance to both ciprofloxacin and erythromycin has been seen worldwide.

Table 7.3. Recommended alternative medical treatments for Chancroid

Azithromycin	1 g p.o. single dose
Ceftriaxone	250 mg im single dose
Ciprofloxacin	500 mg p.o. ii qd × 3 days
Erythromycin	500 mg p.o. iii qd × 7 days
(in pregnancy, lactation and <18 years)	

Antibiotic treatment is less effective in uncircumcised males and in HIV positive patients. Ulcers should show signs of symptomatic improvement after 3–7 days, and all patients should be re-examined after this period. Circumcision may be necessary for individuals with repeated infections or inadequate personal hygiene, and surgical intervention such as incision and drainage of inguinal buboes might also be required to expedite cure. All partners who have had sexual contact with an index case within 10 days of symptoms should be treated, regardless of symptoms.

Vaccine availability

There is no vaccine currently available to prevent infections with *Haemophilus ducreyi*.

Lymphogranuloma venereum (LGV)

Chlamydia trachomatis

Invasive serovars L1, L2, and L3 of *Chlamydia trachomatis*.

Epidemiology

Lymphogranuloma venereum is caused by the invasive serovars L1, L2, and L3 of *Chlamydia trachomatis*. Whereas the serovars that produce cervicitis and urethritis are widespread throughout the world, the LGV disease is rare in the US and the majority of industrialized countries. Pockets of endemic disease are seen in Southeast Asia, Africa, South America and Southeastern USA. A diagnosis of LGV should be considered when there is an appropriate travel history, or a history of intercourse with a person from an endemic area.

Life cycle

Like the non-invasive serovars of *C. trachomatis*, the invasive serovars are obligate intracellular parasites. They require the host cell as a source of ATP for replication and the life cycle also features the infectious, extracellular elementary body that is internalized and transformed into the replicative reticulate body. The organisms replicate for 1–3 days before causing host cell death, releasing elementary bodies that may initiate infection of additional epithelial cells (see Chapter 10 for further details).

Transmission

Lymphogranuloma venereum is transmitted as a typical STD. Receptive anogenital intercourse is commonly implicated in men and women presenting with rectal and anal involvement.

Clinical presentation

LGV has three distinct phases of infection. The *first stage* of disease consists of a painless inconspicuous vesicle or papule at the site of primary inoculation, appearing about one week after initial exposure. This evolves into an ulcerative nodule. In men, the nodule usually appears on the penis and in women the lesions are found either on the labia or on the cervix. Lesions usually resolve within 5 days and this initial disease is asymptomatic in about half of all patients.

Secondary syndromes occur after the primary lesion has healed. The most common presentation for heterosexual males is the inguinal syndrome, characterized by acute inguinal or femoral lymphadenopathy (buboes). This lymphadenopathy is usually unilateral, hard and extremely tender. The skin covering the involved lymph nodes becomes discolored. Although most of these infections heal without complication, some infected nodes may become fluctuant and rupture to form draining sinus tracts. Constitutional symptoms such as fever, chills, headache and malaise may also be seen during this secondary phase.

The *anogenital syndrome*, characterized by an acute hemorrhagic proctitis, is the most common presenting syndrome in women and in males infected during receptive anal intercourse. Inflammation of the perianal and perirectal lymphoid tissues often leads to fistula, strictures, intestinal obstruction and abscess formation in the tertiary stage of illness. Systemic dissemination is relatively uncommon, but may be accompanied by constitutional symptoms such as fever, chill, headache and malaise. If left untreated, the tertiary phase of disease resolves spontaneously after 2–3 months. Damage to the lymphatic drainage system of the genitalia may lead to scrotal elephantiasis.

Clinical diagnosis

Diagnosis of LGV is usually made during the secondary or tertiary stages of illness. Patients presenting with exquisitely tender lymphadenopathy, without significant history of prior or current genital ulcers should be evaluated for LGV. Similarly, proctitis, draining sinuses and abscesses involving the rectum, anus or inguinal or femoral lymph nodes should raise a suspicion of LGV.

Laboratory diagnosis

Laboratory diagnosis of LGV is carried out either by serology or culture. Serologic diagnosis relies on the identification of antibodies specific for the invasive LGV serovars of *Chlamydia trachomatis* L1, L2, and L3. These must be specifically requested, differentiated from the non-invasive serovars for which antibody tests are also available. Culture from aspirated lymph node or abscess contents may be diagnostic in about half of all cases. Since *C. trachomatis* is an obligate intracellular pathogen, culture requires a host cell for growth and McCoy cells in a shell vial assay are commonly used as the culture system. The specimen is inoculated onto the cell monolayer grown in a serum-enriched medium, and slowly centrifuged onto the monolayer to enhance infectivity. After 2–3 days, infected cells will demonstrate large cytoplasmic vacuoles containing the organism and starch. *C. trachomatis* is the only chlamydial species

that produces starch in cytoplasmic granules. The cells are fixed and stained either with *C. trachomatis* specific fluorescent monoclonal antibodies, or with iodine to identify infected cells. Organisms may then be identified using direct examination to visualize vacuolization of infected cells, or using electron microscopy to demonstrate the elementary and reticulate bodies of the organisms in infected tissues or aspirates.

Molecular diagnostic tests that detect 16s ribosomal RNA have been developed experimentally and may be used for diagnosis. Chlamydial plasmid-related DNA targets are not reliably present in the invasive serovars L1, 2, and 3, so that PCR and other amplified assays using these targets may not be reliable in making the diagnosis of LGV.

Treatment

LGV may be treated with either doxycycline (100 mg P.O. ii qd × 21 days) or erythromycin (500 mg P.O. iiii qd × 21 days during pregnancy and lactation). Individuals presenting with buboes or abscesses should also be treated with incision and drainage of lesions to expedite healing. All sexual contacts having had intercourse with the patient within 30 days of the onset of symptoms need to be evaluated and treated, regardless of symptoms.

Vaccine availability

There is no vaccine available for the prevention of LGV.

Granuloma inguinale (Donovanosis)

Calymmatobacterium granulomatis

Granuloma inguinale or Donovanosis is caused by *Calymmatobacterium granulomatis*, a gram-negative intracellular bacterium. This organism is very rare worldwide, but is found as an endemic infection in New Guinea, India, Central Australia, Southern Africa, the Caribbean and other tropical and subtropical locations. Sexual contact with someone from an endemic area is important in establishing a diagnosis outside of these areas.

Transmission

Infection with *C. granulomatis* is transmitted sexually in the majority of cases. Auto-inoculation of lesions to establish additional sites of involvement may be seen in chronic infections. This may lead to contiguous extension of existing lesions or inoculation of organisms into new areas of disease involvement. The occurrence of disease in children and in non-genital sites suggests that non-venereal modes of transmission may also take place but the preponderance of lesions on the genitalia, the scarcity of disease in virgins and the occurrence of Donovanosis with other STDs such as syphilis, supports the theory that this disease is predominantly transmitted sexually.

Life cycle

C. granulomatis is a very slow growing obligate intracellular bacterium, requiring 8–80 days of incubation before manifesting symptoms. Infections are generally chronic. Humans are the only known reservoir for this organism.

Clinical presentation

Infections with *Calymmatobacterium granulomatis* present as chronic infections of more than 6 weeks' duration, generally involving the genitalia. Mucous membranes of the mouth may also be involved. Initially, patients develop an indurated granulomatous nodule at the site of infection, which then ulcerates to form a painless and locally progressive destructive ulcer that extends across tissue planes. Satellite lesions arise by auto-inoculation. These coalesce over time, leaving large deficits that may be mutilating. Ulcers are raised and indurated with rolled edges, generally described as 'beefy red' in color. They are highly vascularized and therefore bleed very easily. The ulcers of *C. granulomatis* are often purulent secondary to mixed bacterial infections

but Donovanosis is not usually associated with lymphadenopathy. Untreated disease may lead to lymphatic obstruction and genital or lower extremity elephantiasis.

Extra-genital disease occurs in about 6% of patients and may be seen as primary or secondary disease. Although much of this spread is a result of auto-inoculation from genital disease to new sites, hematogenous spread to organs other than the skin is also seen. These patients may present with bone and visceral lesions; involvement of the oral mucosa is the most common extra-genital manifestation.

Clinical diagnosis

Donovanosis is generally diagnosed on the basis of clinical presentation: beefy red, destructive and mutilating lesions on the genitalia, particularly in an individual with a history of travel to an endemic area should suggest the diagnosis.

Laboratory diagnosis

There is very little testing available for the diagnosis of Donovanosis. Culture is not readily available for this organism, although monocyte and Hep-2 cell coinfection cultures have been described experimentally. For the majority of patients, diagnosis must be made on the basis of clinical presentation and direct examination of clinical materials. Organisms may be demonstrated using hematoxylin and eosin, Wright's Geimsa, and Gram's staining of preparations and Donovan bodies are seen as gram-negative encapsulated bacteria with a bulge of chromatin at one end, giving the organism the look of a 'closed safety pin'. Diagnosis may also be made on the basis of experimental PCR assays.

Treatment

Treatment must be long term if cure is expected: relapses at 6–18 months are seen even after initially successful therapy. Trimethoprim sulfamethoxazole, doxycycline and erythromycin are recommended for treatment, with therapy for at least 3 weeks or until all ulcerative lesions have healed (Table 7.4). Scarring

Table 7.4. Recommended medical treatments for Donovanosis

Recommended regimes:

Trimethoprim-sulfamethoxazole double strength tablet po ii qd × at least 3 weeks

Doxycycline   100 mg p.o. ii qd × at least 3 weeks

Alternative regimes:

Erythromycin 500 mg p.o. iv qd × at least 3 weeks

Ciprofloxacin 750 mg p.o. ii.qd × at least 3 weeks

Azithromycin 1g p.o. ii q.d. × at least 3 weeks

If pregnant, treat with erythromycin and add gentamicin

Treat until all ulcers are healed

is inevitable after extensive disease, and this may be very mutilating.

As with all sexually transmitted diseases, treatment of sexual contacts is very important. All current sex partners and sex contacts for the past 6 months need to be treated regardless of symptoms. Sexual contacts from prior to 6 months before patient presentation need to be treated only if symptomatic.

Vaccine availability

There is no vaccine currently available for the prevention of Donovanosis.

REFERENCES

HERPES SIMPLEX

Crute, J. J., Grygon, C. A., Hargrave, K. D. *et al.* (2002). Herpes simplex virus helicase-primase inhibitors are active in animal models of human disease. *Nature Medicine*, **8**(4): 386–91.

Kleyman, G., Fischer, R., Betz, U. A. K. *et al.* (2002). New helicase-primase inhibitors as drug candidates for the treatment of herpes simplex disease. *Nature Medicine*, **8**, (4): 392–8.

FURTHER READING

HERPES SIMPLEX

Arvin, A. M. & Pober, G. C. (1999). Herpes simplex viruses. In *Manual of Clinical Microbiology*, ed. P. R. Murray, E. J. Barton, M. A. Pfaller, F. C. Tenover & R. H. Yolken, 7th edn, pp. 878–87. ASM Press, Washington, DC: ASM Press.

Ashley, R. L. & Wald, A. (1999). Genital herpes: review of the epidemic and potential use of type-specific serology. *Clinical Microbiology Reviews*, **12**: 1–8.

Ashley, R., Cent, A., Maggs, V., Nahmias, A. & Corey, L. (1991). Inability of enzyme immunoassays to discriminate between infections with herpes simplex virus types 1 and 2. *Annals of Internal Medicine*, **115**: 520–6.

Ashley, R. L., Wu, L., Pickering, J. W., Tu, M. C. & Schnorenberg, L. (1998). Premarket evaluation of a commercial glycoprotein G-Based enzyme immunoassay for herpes simplex virus type-specific antibodies. *Journal of Clinical Microbiology*, **36**: 294–5.

Bader, C., Crumpacker, C. S., Schnipper, L. E. *et al.* (1978). The natural history of recurrent facial-oral infection with Herpes Simplex virus. *Journal of Infectious Diseases*, **138**: 897–905.

Baringer, J. R. (1974). Recovery of herpes simplex virus from human sacral ganglions. *New England Journal of Medicine*, **291**: 828–30.

Baringer, J. R. & Swoveland, P. (1973). Recovery of herpes-simplex virus from human trigeminal ganglions. *New England Journal of Medicine*, **288**: 648–50.

Barton, I. G., Kinghorn, G. R., Najem, S., Al-Omar, L. S. & Potter, C. W. (1982). Incidence of herpes simplex virus types 1 and 2 isolated in patients with herpes genitalis in Sheffield. *British Journal of Venereal Disease*, **58**: 44–7.

Benedetti, J., Corey, L. & Ashley, R. (1994). Recurrence rates in genital herpes after symptomatic first-episode infection. *Annals of Internal Medicine*, **121**: 847–54.

Benedetti, J. K., Zeh, J. & Corey, L. (1999). Clinical reactivation of genital herpes simplex virus infection decreases in frequency over time. *Annals of Internal Medicine*, **131**: 14–20.

CDC (2002). Guidelines for treatment of sexually transmitted diseases. *Morbidity and Mortality Weekly*, **47**(RR-1): 1–116.

Christenson, B., Bottiger, M., Svensson, A. & Jeansson, S. (1992). A 15-year surveillance study of antibodies to herpes simplex virus types 1 and 2 in a cohort of young girls. *Journal of Infectious Diseases*, **25**: 147–54.

Cone, R. W., Swenson, P. D., Hobson, A. C., Remington, M. & Corey, L. (1993). Herpes simplex virus detection from genital lesions: a comparative study using antigen detection (HerpChek) and culture. *Journal of Clinical Microbiology*, **31**: 1774–6.

Cotarelo, M., Catalan, P., Sanchez-Carrillo, C. *et al.* (1999). Cytopathic effect inhibition assay for determining the in-vitro susceptibility of herpes simplex virus to antiviral agents. *Journal of Antimicrobial Chemotherapy*, **44**: 705–8.

Crane, L. R. & Lerner, A. M. (1978). Herpetic whitlow: a manifestation of primary infection with herpes simplex virus 1 or type 2. *Journal of Infectious Diseases*, **137**: 855–6.

Cullen, A. P., Long, C. D. & Lorincz, A. T. (1997). Rapid detection and typing of herpes simplex virus DNA in clinical specimens by the hybrid capture II signal amplification probe test. *Journal of Clinical Microbiology*, **35**: 2275–8.

Embil, J. A., Stephens, R. G. & Manuel, F. R. (1975). Prevalence of recurrent herpes labialis and aphthous ulcers among young adults on six continents. *Canadian Medical Association Journal*, **113**: 627–30.

Espy, M. J. & Smith, T. F. (1988). Detection of herpes simplex virus in conventional tube cell culture and in shell vials with a DNA probe kit and monoclonal antibodies. *Journal of Clinical Microbiology*, **26**: 22–4.

Espy, M. J., Uhl, J. R., Mitchell, P. S. *et al.* (2000). Diagnosis of herpes simplex virus infections in the laboratory by LightCycler PCR. *Journal of Clinical Microbiology*, **38**: 795–9.

Fayram, S. L., Aarnaes, S. L., Peterson, E. M. & de la Maza, L. M. (1986). Evaluation of five cell types for the isolation of herpes simplex virus. *Diagnostic Microbiology and Infectious Diseases*, **5**: 127–33.

Fleming, D. T., McQuillan, G. M., Johnson, R. E. *et al.* (1997). Herpes simplex virus type 2 in the United States, 1976 to 1994. *New England Journal of Medicine*, **337**: 1105–11.

Forsgren, M. (1990). Genital herpes simplex virus infection and incidence of neonatal disease in Sweden. *Scandinavian Journal of Infectious Diseases*, **69**: 37–41.

Gibson, J. J., Hornung, C. A., Alexander, G. R., Lee, A. F., Potts, W. A. & Nahmais, A. J. (1990). A cross-sectional study of herpes simplex virus types 1 and 2 in college students: occurrence and determinants of infection. *Journal of Infectious Diseases*, **162**: 306–312.

Gleaves, C. A., Wilson, D. J., Wold, A. D. & Smith, T. F. (1985). Detection and serotyping of herpes simplex virus in MRC-5 cells by use of centrifugation and monoclonal antibodies 16 hours postinoculation. *Journal of Clinical Microbiology*, **221**: 29–32.

Glezen, W. P., Fernald, G. W. & Lohr, J. A. (1975). Acute respiratory disease of university students with special reference to the etiologic role of *Herpesvirus hominis*. *American Journal of Epidemiology*, **191**: 111–21.

Glogau, R., Hanna, L. & Jawetz, E. (1977). Herpetic whitlow as part of genital virus infection. *Journal of Infectious Diseases*, **136**: 689–92.

Goink, B., Seibel, M., Berkowitz, A., Woodin, M. B. & Mills, K. (1991). Comparison of two enzyme-linked immunosorbent assays for detection of herpes simplex virus antigen. *Journal of Clinical Microbiology*, **29**: 436–8.

Hardy, D. H., Arvin, A. M., Yasukawa, L. L. *et al.* (1990). Use of polymerase chain reaction for successful identification of asymptomatic genital infection with herpes simplex virus in pregnant women at delivery. *Journal of Infectious Diseases*, **162**: 1031–5.

Johnson, R. E., Nahmias, A. J., Magder, L. S., Lee, F. K., Brooks, C. A. & Snowden, C. B. (1989). A seroepidemiologic survey of the prevalence of herpes simplex virus type 2 infection in the United States. *New England Journal of Medicine*, **321**: 7–12.

Koelle, D. M. & Lawrence, C. (2003). Recent progress in herpes simplex virus immunobiology and vaccine research. *Clinical Microbiology Reviews*, **16**: 96–113.

Koelle, D. M., Benedetti, J., Langenberg, A. & Corey, L. (1992). Asymptomatic reactivation of herpes simplex virus in women after the first episode of genital herpes. *Annals of Internal Medicine*, **116**: 433–7.

Koenig, M., Reynolds, K. S., Aldous, W. & Hickman, M. (2001). Comparison of Light-Cycler PCR, enzyme immunoassay, and tissue culture for detection of herpes simplex virus. *Diagnostic Microbiology and Infectious Diseases*, **40**: 107–10.

Lafferty, W. E., Coombs, R. W., Benedetti, J., Critchlow, C. & Corey, L. (1987). Recurrences after oral and genital herpes simplex virus infection: influence of site of infection and viral type. *New England Journal of Medicine*, **316**:1444–9.

LaRocco, M. T. (2000). Evaluation of an enzyme-linked viral inducible system for rapid detection of herpes simplex virus. *European Journal of Clinical Microbiology and Infectious Diseases*, **19**: 233–5.

Mertz, G. J., Coombs, R. W., Ashley, R. *et al.* (1988). Transmission of genital herpes in couples with one symptomatic and one asymptomatic partner: a prospective study. *Journal of Infectious Diseases*, **157**: 1169–77.

Moseley, R. L., Corey, L., Benjamin, D., Winter, C. & Remington, M. L. (1981). Comparison of viral isolation, direct immunofluorescence and indirect immunoperoxidase techniques for detection of genital herpes simplex virus infection. *Journal of Clinical Microbiology*, **13**: 913–18.

Nahmias, A. J., DelBuono, I., Schneweis, K. E., Gordon, D. S. & Thies, D. (1971). Type-specific surface antigens of cells infected with herpes simplex virus (1 and 2). *Proceedings of the Society for Experimental Biology and Medicine*, **138**: 21–7.

Nahmias, A. J., Lee, F. K. & Beckman-Nahmias, S. (1990). Seroepidemiological and – sociological patterns of herpes simplex virus infection in the world. *Scandinavian Journal of Infectious Diseases (suppl.)*, **69**: 19–36.

Reeves, W. C., Corey, L., Adams, H. G., Vontver, L. A. & Holmes, K. K. (1981). Risk of recurrence after first episodes of genital herpes: relation to HSV type and antibody production. *New England Journal of Medicine*, **305**: 315–19.

Ribes, J. A., Hayes, M., Smith, A., Winters, J. L. & Baker, D. J. (2001a). Comparative performance of herpes simplex virus type-2 specific serologic assays from Meridian Diagnostics and MRL Diagnostics. *Journal of Clinical Microbiology*, **39**: 3740–2.

Ribes, J. A., Steele, A. D., Seabolt, J. P. & Baker, D. J. (2001b). Six-year study of the incidence of herpes in genital and nongenital cultures in a central Kentucky medical center patient population. *Journal of Clinical Microbiology*, **39**: 3321–5.

Rowe, N. H., Heine, C. S. & Kowalski, C. J. (1982). Herpetic whitlow: an occupational disease of practicing dentists. *Journal of the American Dental Association*, **105**: 471–3.

Sauerbrei, A., Eichhorn, U., Hottenrott, G. & Wutzler, P. (2000). Virological diagnosis of herpes simplex encephalitis. *Journal of Clinical Virology*, **17**: 31–6.

Tayal, S. C. & Pattman, R. S. (1994). High prevalence of herpes simplex virus type 1 in female anogenital herpes simplex in Newcastle upon Tyne 1983–1992. *International Journal of STD and AIDS*, **5**: 359–61.

Villarreal, E. C. (2001). Current and potential therapies for the treatment of herpes-virus infections. In *Antiviral Agents– Advances and Problems*, ed. E. Jucker, pp. 185–228. Basel, Switzerland.

Wald, A., Corey, L., Cone, R., Hobson, A., Davis, G. & Zeh, J. (1997). Frequent genital herpes simplex virus 2 shedding in immunocompetent women: effect of acyclovir treatment. *Journal of Clinical Investigation*, **99**: 1092–7.

Whitley, R. J. (1989). Herpes simplex virus infection of the central nervous system. A review. *American Journal of Medicine*, **85** (2A): 61–7.

SYPHILIS

Beck, S. V. (1997). Syphilis: The Great Pox. In *Plague, Pox and Pestilence: Disease in History*, ed. K. F. Kiple, pp. 110–15. New York: Weidenfield and Nicolson.

Centers for Disease Control and Prevention (2002). Guidelines for treatment of sexually transmitted diseases 2002. *Morbidity and Mortality Weekly*, **51**(RR-6), 1–78.

Fiumara, N. J. (1987). Syphilis. In *Pictoral Guide to Sexually Transmitted Diseases*. pp. 42–6. Secaucus, NJ: Hospital Publications Inc.

Ito, F., Hunter, E. F., George, R. W., Swisher, B. L. & Larsen, S. A. (1991). Specific immunofluorescence staining of *Treponema pallidum* in smears and tissues. *Journal of Clinical Microbiology*, **29**: 444–8.

Ito, F., Hunter, E. F., George, R. W., Pope, V. & Larsen, S. A. (1992). Specific immunofluorescent staining of pathogenic treponemes with a monoclonal antibody. *Journal of Clinical Microbiology*, **30**: 831–8.

Kaminester, L. H. (1991). Syphilis. In *Sexually Transmitted Diseases: An Illustrated Guide to Differential Diagnosis*, pp. 10–11. Research Triangle Park, NC: Burroughs Wellcome Co. Monograph.

Konemann, E. W., Allen, S. D., Janda, W. M., Schreckenberger, P. C. & Winn, W. C. (1997). Spirochetal infections. In *Color Atlas and Textbook of Diagnostic Microbiology*, 5th edn, pp. 953–981. Philadelphia, PA: Lippincott.

Larson, S. A., Steiner, B. M. & Rudolph, A. H. (1995). Laboratory diagnosis and interpretation of tests for syphilis. *Clinical Microbiology Reviews*, **8**: 1–21.

Larsen, S. A., Norris, S. J. & Pope, V. (1999). Treponema and other host-associated spirochetes. In *Manual of Clinical Microbiology*, 7th edn, ed. P. R. Murray, E. J. Baron, M. A, Pfaller, F. C. Tenover & R. H. Yolken, pp. 759–75. Washington, DC: ASM Press.

CHANCROID

Albritton, W. L. (1989). Biology of *Haemophilus ducreyi*. *Microbiology Reviews*, **53**: 377–98.

CDC (1995). Chancroid detected by polymerase chain reaction-Jackson, Mississippi, 1994–1995. *Morbidity and Mortality Weekly*, **44**: 567–74.

Centers for Disease Control and Prevention (2002). 2002 Guidelines for treatment of sexually transmitted diseases. *Morbidity and Mortality Weekly*, **51**(RR-6), 1–78.

Elkins, C., Yi, K., Olsen, B., Thomas, C., Thomas, K. & Morse, S. (2000). Development of a serologic test for *Haemophilus ducreyi* for seroprevalence studies. *Journal of Clinical Microbiology*, **38**(4): 1520–6.

Fiumara, N. J. (1987). Chancroid. In *Pictoral Guide to Sexually Transmitted Diseases*. pp. 2–4. Secaucus, NJ: Hospital Publications Inc.

Goens, J. I., Schwartz, R. A. & deWolf, K. (1994). Mucocutaneous manifestations of chancroid, lymphogranuloma venereum and granuloma inguinale. *American Family Physician*, **49**: 415–22.

Kaminester, L. H. (1991). Chancroid. In *Sexually Transmitted Diseases: An Illustrated Guide to Differential Diagnosis*, p. 1. Research Triangle Park, NC: Burroughs Wellcome Co. Monograph.

Konemann, E. W., Allen, S. D., Janda, W. M., Schreckenberger, P. C. & Winn, W. C. (1997). *Haemophilus.* In *Color Atlas and Textbook of Diagnostic Microbiology,* 5th edn, pp. 363–93. Philadelphia, PA: Lippincott.

Ronald, A. R. & Albritton, W. (2002). Chancroid and *Haemophilus ducreyi.* In *Sexually Transmitted Diseases,* 3rd edn, ed. K. K. Holmes, P. F. Sparling, P. A. Mardh *et al.* New York: McGraw-Hill.

Steen, R. (2001). Eradicating Chancroid. *Bulletin of WHO,* **79**: 818–26.

Schmidt, G. P., Sanders L. L., Blout, J. H. & Alexander, R. (1987). Chancroid in the United States: reestablishment of an old disease. *Journal of the American Medical Association,* **258**: 3265–8.

Van Dyck, E. & Piot, P. (1992). Laboratory techniques in the investigation of chancroid, lymphogranuloma venereum and Donovanosis. *Genitourinary Medicine,* **68**: 130–3.

West, B., Wilson, S. M., Changalucha, J. *et al.* (1995). Simplified PCR for detection of *Haemophilus ducreyi* and the diagnosis of chancroid. *Journal of Clinical Microbiology,* **33**: 787–90.

LYMPHOGRANULOMA VENEREUM

CDC (2002). 2002 Guidelines for treatment of sexually transmitted diseases. *Morbidity and Mortality Weekly,* **51**(RR-6): 1–78.

Fiumara, N. J. (1987). Lymphomagranuloma venereum. In *Pictoral Guide to Sexually Transmitted Diseases,* pp. 25–27. Secaucus, NJ: Hospital Publications Inc.

Goens, J. I., Schwartz, R. A. & deWolf, K. (1994). Mucocutaneous manifestations of chancroid, lymphogranuloma venereum and granuloma inguinale. *American Family Physician,* **49**: 415–22.

Hadfield, T. L., Lamy, Y. & Wear, D. J. (1995). Demonstration of *Chlamydia trachomatis* in inguinal lymphadenitis of lymphogranuloma venereum: A light microscopy, electron microscopy and polymerase chain reaction study. *Modern Pathology,* **8**: 924–9.

Kaminester, L. H. (1991). Lymphomagranuloma venereum. In *Sexually Transmitted Diseases: An Illustrated Guide to Differential Diagnosis,* pp. 12. Research Triangle Park, NC: Burroughs Wellcome Co. Monograph.

Lynch, C. M., Felder, T. L., Schwandt, R. A. & Shashy, R. G. (1999). Lymphogranuloma venereum presenting as a rectovaginal fistula. *Infectious Diseases in Obstetrics and Gynecology,* **7**: 199–201.

Perine, P. L. & Stamm, W. E. (2002). Lymphogranuloma venereum. In *Sexually Transmitted Diseases,* 3rd edn, ed. K. K. Holmes *et al.,* pp. 423–32. New York: McGraw-Hill.

Van Dyck, E. & Piot, P. (1992). Laboratory techniques in the investigation of chancroid, lymphogranuloma venereum and Donovanosis. *Genitourinary Medicine,* **68**: 130–3.

DONOVANOSIS

Bassa, A. G., Hoosen, A. A., Moodley, J. & Bramdev, A. (1993). Granuloma Inguinale (Donovanosis) in women. An analysis of 61 cases from Durban, South Africa. *Sexually Transmitted Diseases,* **20**: 164–7.

Carter, J., Hutton S., Spiprakash, K. S. *et al.* (1997). Culture of the causative organism of Donovanosis (*Calymmatobacterium granulomatis*) in Hep-2 cells. *Journal of Clinical Microbiology,* **35**: 2915–17.

Carter, J., Bowden, F. J., Sriprakash, K. S., Bastian I. & Kemp, D. J. (1999). Diagnostic polymerase chain reaction for Donovanosis. *Clinical and Infectious Diseases,* **28**: 1168–9.

Carter, J. S. & Kemp, D. J. (2000). A colorimetric detection system for *Calymmatobacterium granulomatis. Sexually Transmitted Diseases,* **76**: 134–6.

Fiumara, N. J. (1987). Granuloma Inguinale (Donovanosis), pp. 21–22. In *Pictoral Guide to Sexually Transmitted Diseases.* Secaucus, NJ: Hospital Publications Inc.

Goens, J. I., Schwartz, R. A. & deWolf, K. (1994). Mucocutaneous manifestations of chancroid, lymphogranuloma venereum and granuloma inguinale. *American Family Physician,* **49**: 415–22.

Hart, G. (1997). Donovanosis. *Clinical Infectious Diseases,* **25**: 24–32.

Kaminester, L. H. (1991). Granuloma Inguinale. In *Sexually Transmitted Diseases: An Illustrated Guide to Differential Diagnosis,* p. 13. Research Triangle Park, NC: Burroughs Wellcome Co. Monograph.

Kharsany, A. B. M., Hoosen, A. A., Kiepiela, P., Naicker, T. & Sturm, A. W. (1997). Growth and culture characteristics of *Calymmatobacterium granulomatis* – the aetiologic agent of granuloma inguinale (Donovanosis). *Journal of Medical Microbiology,* **46**: 579–85.

O'Farrell, N. (2002). Donovanosis. In *Sexually Transmitted Diseases,* 3rd edition, ed. K. K. Holmes *et al.,* pp. 525–31. New York: McGraw-Hill.

Van Dyck, E. & Piot, P. (1992). Laboratory techniques in the investigation of chancroid, lymphogranuloma venereum, and Donovanosis. *Genitourinary Medicine,* **68**: 130–3.

8

Vaginitis syndromes

The female genital tract hosts a variety of microbial organisms: composition of the normal flora varies according to the woman's age, site in the genital tract and hormonal status (prepubertal, different phases of the menstrual cycle, pregnancy, oral contraceptive use, hormone replacement therapy and post-menopausal). Vaginal secretions are usually clear, scanty and have a pH below 4.5. Normal vaginal flora usually favours colonization by the hydrogen peroxide producing *Lactobacillus* spp.; these organisms use epithelial glycogen and produce lactic acid, leading to the resultant normally acid pH of vaginal secretions. Imbalance in the vaginal flora or infection with some sexually transmitted pathogens may lead to abnormal vaginal discharges associated with inflammation. Not all vaginal discharges are vaginal in origin – uterine infections or mucopurulent cervicitis will also result in a discharge from the vagina.

Vulvo-vaginitis can have several different etiologies; three types of vulvo-vaginitis syndromes will be reviewed here:

(i) trichomoniasis, caused by the protozoan *Trichomonas vaginalis*;

(ii) candidiasis ('thrush'), caused by the yeast *Candida albicans*;

(iii) bacterial vaginosis, due to overgrowth with the anaerobic bacteria, *Mycoplasma hominis* and *Gardnerella vaginalis* or other *Candida* spp.

The vaginitis syndromes are significant from several standpoints.

- Trichomoniasis, and rarely some candidal infections, are considered to be sexually transmitted. The mode of transmission for bacterial vaginosis is unknown. Although there is some evidence to suggest that bacterial vaginosis is sexually transmitted, this conclusion is not supported by the bulk of the evidence.

- The presence of a vaginal inflammatory process places the patient at increased risk for developing other sexually transmitted diseases, including HIV, chlamydial and gonococcal infections.

- Vaginitis during pregnancy may be associated with an increased risk of premature rupture of the membranes, preterm birth and the development of post-partum maternal and neonatal infections.

In children, vulvo-vaginitis is most commonly caused by *Streptococcus pyogenes* or other β-hemolytic streptococci, *Haemophilus influenza*, *Streptococcus pneumoniae* or *Staphylococcus aureus*. Candidiasis and bacterial vaginosis/vaginitis syndromes in children are considered to be primarily non-sexually transmitted diseases, representing instead an imbalance in vaginal flora with an abnormal overgrowth of one or more agents normally found in the vagina. In contrast trichomoniasis, caused by *Trichomonas vaginalis*, is always considered to be a sexually transmitted disease.

Women with vaginitis usually present for evaluation with symptoms of vaginal discharge with vulvar itching or irritation, and these symptoms collectively characterize the vaginitis syndromes. They often report staining of the underwear with secretions and the presence of an abnormal, often foul smell that may be accentuated with menses or following intercourse. Some women may have few or no symptoms, or symptoms may develop weeks into the infection.

Table 8.1. Differentiating features of vaginal secretions in vaginitis syndromes

Syndrome	Etiologic agent	pH	Appearance	Odour	Direct microscopy
Bacterial Vaginosis	G. vaginalis, M. hominis, and mixed anaerobes in large numbers	>4.5, often 5.5–6.0	Milky white and uniform	Fishy (+ Whiff test)	Clue cells on Gram's stain
Trichomoniasis	T. vaginalis	5–5.5, sometimes higher	Yellow-green and frothy	Foul, fishy but does not enhance on Whiff test	Tumbling flagellates on wet prep
Candidiasis	C. albicans, C. glabrata in 3–5% of cases	<4.5	Thick, white, and pasty	Fermentative	Yeast and pseudohyphae on KOH

Diagnosis can be made in the physician office, laboratory or clinic by analysis of the vaginal secretion pH, odour (Whiff test: accentuated amine odour seen on the addition of potassium hydroxide to a clinical specimen) and presence of amines. Amines can also be detected using the Litmus card system that also assesses pH. Microscopic examination of vaginal secretions is also important for complete evaluation. The three etiologies responsible for vulvo-vaginitis may be separated by these simple outpatient tests (Table 8.1).

Trichomonas vaginalis

Trichomonas vaginalis is a flagellated protozoan whose only natural host is humans. The organism has a worldwide distribution, causing infections in all races and in all socio-economic strata. The Centers of Disease Control and Prevention (CDC) estimates that there are over 170 million cases each year worldwide. Consistent with its role as a sexually transmitted disease, the incidence of the disease is highest in women visiting STD clinics. Trichomoniasis is often associated with other STDs, particularly HIV, chlamydia and gonorrhea, and its diagnosis should always be followed by further STD evaluation, diagnosis, and treatment. In common with other sexually transmitted diseases, increased risk for infection is associated with increased numbers of sex

partners, employment as a prostitute, reproductive age (20–45 years) and black race. Females are infected and are symptomatic more often than men. Sexual contacts of women diagnosed with this infection also need to be identified and treated. Infected males may have symptoms of urethritis, but males are often asymptomatic and can serve as chronic carriers for the disease.

Life cycle

Unlike other flagellates that infect humans, *T. vaginalis* has no cyst form and has only a trophozoite stage. The trophozoite is therefore both the infective and replicative form of the organism and it reproduces by binary fission. The organisms are relatively unstable in the environment, outside of the human host and transmission usually requires close contact with an infected individual.

Transmission

The trophozoite of *T. vaginalis* is generally transmitted person to person during intercourse. Males and females can be chronic carriers, with few signs or symptoms of infection, but continuing to transmit the infection. In situations where antisepsis is poor, fomites such as shared douche nozzles, unclean specula and toilet seats may also be involved in transmitting the disease, although this is rarely seen. Trophozoites can survive up to several hours in urine, semen and pool water, and contact with infected fluids may sometimes initiate infection. If a mother is actively infected at the time of giving birth, the organism can be transmitted to the neonate during parturition. Vertical transmission across the placenta has not been described, but infection with *T. vaginalis* has been associated with infection of the amniotic membrane and subsequent premature rupture of the membranes.

Clinical presentation

Acute symptomatic disease is the most common presentation in women, but trichomoniasis is a chronic infection that can last for months in many cases. Patients experience vulvitis and vaginitis with a frothy yellow mucopurulent, often foul-smelling discharge. Small hemorrhages within the inflamed mucosal membranes produce a 'strawberry' vulva, vagina and cervix in some patients. Acute symptoms usually occur after 4–28 days of primary infection, but prolonged asymptomatic or minimally symptomatic phases of infection may also be seen. Symptoms are generally worse during menstruation, when the organism is maximally stimulated to reproduce. About 25–50% of infected women are asymptomatic carriers. In the chronically infected woman, infection may be characterized by mild pruritus and dyspareunia. Nearly 30% of these women will, however, develop symptomatic disease within 6 months of infection.

Although vaginitis is the most common presentation in women with *T. vaginalis* infection, other syndromes may also be seen, such as adnexitis, endometritis, pyosalpinx, cervical erosion and infertility. Increased risk of transmission of HIV has also been associated with *T. vaginalis* infections in women. In contrast, the majority of infections in males are asymptomatic. If symptomatic, men will present with either an acute mucopurulent or mild chronic urethritis. Rare complications of male infections include epididymitis, prostatitis and infertility.

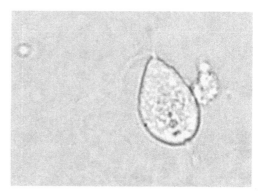

Fig. 8.1. Trichomonas vaginalis trophozoite from a male urine specimen (wet mount). *T. vaginalis* is seen in clinical specimens as a pyriform organism with tumbling motility; flagellar movement can be seen in fresh specimens. One of the organism's several flagella is just seen projecting from the posterior (pointed) aspect of the trophozoite.

Clinical diagnosis

The clinical diagnosis of trichomoniasis is suggested by the classic features of a yellow-green and foul-smelling frothy discharge, vulvar and perineal pruritus, dyspareunia and the presence of a 'strawberry' cervix on speculum exam. However, this classical presentation is seen in only 2% of patients and is not sufficient alone to make a definitive diagnosis.

Laboratory diagnosis

Several relatively easy out-patient tests may be used to make a definitive diagnosis of vulvo-vaginitis (Table 8.1). The majority of *Trichomonas vaginalis* cases will be diagnosed on direct exam. Trichomonads are flagellated organisms measuring 7–30 μm by 6–15 μm, pyriform in shape (Fig. 8.1) and the four flagella are sometimes detected even in unstained preparations.

Their random tumbling or jerking motility is readily detected in a saline wet mount of vaginal secretions or urine concentrates. Since motility requires the presence of live organisms, saline should be used as the dispersant for slide preparation, not

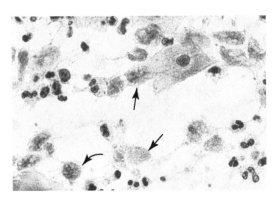

Fig. 8.2. Trichomonas vaginalis in a cervical PAP smear.
T. vaginalis trophozoites can be identified on a PAP smear as
poorly staining cells with little cellular detail (arrows). This
preparation also shows the acute inflammatory cell exudate
often seen with these infections.

10% potassium hydroxide. Infections are generally associated with a brisk acute inflammatory
process. Although this is the most common test used
to detect *T. vaginalis* infections, it is only about
60–70% sensitive. The organisms may be demonstrated on PAP stain, associated with an acute inflammatory response (Fig. 8.2). Vaginal pH in *T. vaginalis* infections is usually elevated, in the range of
5.0–5.5. Although the secretions are fishy or foul-
smelling, a positive Whiff test is not seen with this
infection.

Other tests are also available for the diagnosis of
trichomoniasis, but these tend to be more expensive and are not widely available. Culture is considered to be the most sensitive clinical assay currently
available commercially, but broth cultures require
a relatively large inoculum and 2–5 days growth
for optimal sensitivity. *T. vaginalis* liquid support
medium (Diamond's medium) is available in tube
form from some media suppliers. The InPouch is
another culture system (Fig. 8.3) that can detect low-
level infections. Genital swab specimens are inoculated directly into the media-containing pouch,
which is then sealed. The pouch is incubated at
33–35 °C to promote growth, and then examined
through the microscope to detect the tumbling parasites. The various culture methods are generally very
sensitive, 95% or higher.

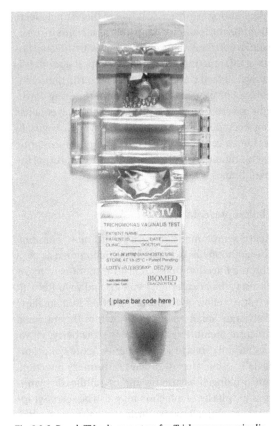

Fig. 8.3. InPouch TV culture system for *Trichomonas vaginalis.*
The InPouch system is a commercially available liquid culture
system for the detection of *T. vaginalis*, a modified Diamond's
medium prepackaged in a sterile clear plastic envelope. A
patient swab is introduced into the medium, the specimen
dispersed and the envelope is resealed with the plastic slide
holder clamped over a fluid-filled segment of the envelope.
The specimen is observed under the microscope for evidence
of tumbling motility.

Probe detection is also available: the Affirm probe
capture assay can detect the three major causes of
vaginitis syndrome in a single test. DNA is extracted
from vaginal or urethral samples and allowed to
hybridize to pathogen-specific DNA probes embedded on a plastic test card. Hybridized DNA is demonstrated with a synthetic oligonucleotide probe and
detected using horseradish peroxidase-mediated
colorimetric change. Dot blots have also been
developed to detect *T. vaginalis* DNA, but this assay
is not commercially available. Similarly, enzyme

immunoassays used to detect *T. vaginalis* antigens have been produced using monoclonal antibodies, but these assays are also not widely used or widely available. PCR assays have been developed for experimental purposes, but none are FDA approved for clinical use in the United States. An enzyme-linked immunoassay for the detection of *T. vaginalis* is not widely used due to its low sensitivity and specificity.

Treatment

The nitroimidazoles are the only drugs that are useful in treating infections with the trichomonads. Topical preparations are almost 50% less effective than oral treatment regimens. Non-nitroimidazole topical therapies may be attempted in the metronidazole-allergic patient, but these treatments also have a less than 50% cure rate. Neonatal infections are generally not treated since infections are dependent upon maternal estrogens and will resolve on their own without treatment. The CDC has updated its recommended treatment for trichomoniasis: metronidazole 2 grams given orally in a single dose may be given as directly observed therapy, and this is the preferred treatment during pregnancy. Metronidazole 500 mg taken twice each day for 7 days is an alternative therapy. All recent sexual contacts should be treated regardless of symptomatology. Patients should refrain from unprotected intercourse until both members have been successfully treated, measured either by completion of medical treatment or by microbiology testing to ensure that the organism has been eradicated.

Vaccine availability

There is no vaccine currently available for *Trichomonas vaginalis.*

Yeast vaginitis

Candida spp.

Genital tract yeast infections are extremely common among sexually active females. It is estimated that 75% of women will experience at least one episode of vulvo-vaginal yeast infection during their lifetime, with 45% having more than one episode. The vast majority of infections are caused by members of the *Candida* spp. Although *C. albicans* is the major pathogen accounting for over 90% of infections, other candidal species are also implicated. *C. glabrata* is the second most common isolate overall and comprises over 3–5% of all infections, seen with increasing frequency particularly in immuno-compromised patients and in patients receiving azole therapy. Studies of fungal genitourinary tract infections show that *C. albicans, C. glabrata, C. tropicalis,* and *C. krusei* are the isolates most frequently observed. Genital infections in the male (balantaniasis) are relatively uncommon, and are caused predominantly by *C. albicans.*

Life cycle

Candida spp. are eukaryotic fungal organisms that multiply in the human host asexually by budding or blastoconidia formation. They often form complex tertiary structures called pseudohyphae in vivo and in vitro, which may serve as a marker for locally invasive disease (as opposed to colonization).

Transmission

About 10% of women carry *C. albicans* as part of their normal vaginal and bowel flora, and this is the major source of infections. The vast majority of cases occur in otherwise healthy women during their reproductive years. Yeast infections are often linked to disruption in the normal balance of the microbial flora of the vagina, often associated with antibiotic use. Other influences associated with the development of vulvo-vaginal yeast infections include conditions where levels of progesterone and estrogen are elevated, particularly during the second and third trimesters of pregnancy, during oral contraceptive use and during the luteal phase of the menstrual cycle just prior to menstruation. Some vaginal yeast infections may be considered opportunistic, in patients with severe immune compromise. Patients on systemic steroids, those with significant neutropenia and individuals with diabetes mellitus are all at increased risk for

(a)
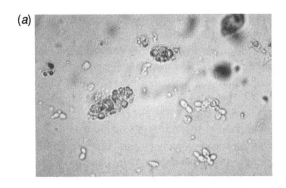

(b)
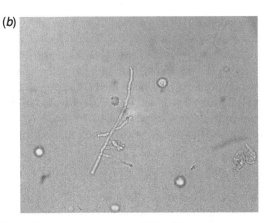

Fig. 8.4. (*a*) and (*b*) Morphologic characteristics of *Candida* spp. in direct KOH wet mount specimens. All *Candida* spp. except
C. glabrata demonstrate two forms in clinical specimens, budding yeast forms (or blastoconidia, frame (*a*)) and pseudohyphae
(frame (*b*)). The presence of pseudohyphae suggests invasive disease and the presence of yeast alone may reflect colonization only.
C. glabrata does not produce pseudohyphae, so that it is impossible to distinguish between colonization and symptomatic disease
by direct examination.

developing vaginal candidiasis. While the majority
of cases of vulvo-vaginal candidiasis are not sexually transmitted, occasional sexual transmission is
suggested by concurrent balanitis in the male sex
partner.

Clinical presentation

Fungal vulvo-vaginitis is characterized by a non-
homogeneous vaginal discharge associated with vulvar itching and irritation. The discharge is usually
thick, white and sticky, forming adherent clumps
on the mucosal surfaces. The characteristic odour
is that of fermentation, resembling the yeasty smell
associated with rising bread. Vulva and perineum are
often very erythematous and painful. Fungal genital
infections in men are relatively uncommon. When
present, balanitis is characterized by itching or pain
of the glans penis. The skin may appear flaking or
scaly with very prominent erythema.

Clinical diagnosis

Although the clinical diagnosis of vulvo-vaginal candidiasis is suggested by the presence of the typical
clumping, non-homogeneous, opaque and fermentative discharge in a patient at risk for infection,

a definitive diagnosis requires either potassium
hydroxide (KOH) examination or culture.

Laboratory diagnosis

Potassium hydroxide (KOH) wet mount to demonstrate budding yeast and/or pseudohyphae is the
direct exam of choice to detect vaginal candidiasis
(Fig. 8.4(*a*), (*b*)). KOH is used to clear the cellular contents so that fungal elements can be visualized. As
with any direct examination, a relatively large number of organisms is required to detect the infection;
the sensitivity of the assay is only 40–60%.

Fungal culture may be helpful for patients not
diagnosed on the basis of the KOH exam. *Candida*
spp. are relatively slow growing, producing small
colonies of dull, opaque and pasty appearance after
1–2 days (Fig. 8.5(*a*), (*b*)).

Since *Candida albicans* is the most common
etiologic agent in humans, most laboratories will
perform a screen for its rapid and efficient identification. The classic germ tube test is an efficient assay
used to identify a yeast such as *C. albicans* or a yeast
that requires further work-up for identification. The
germ tube test is performed by incubating yeast cells
at 37 °C for 2 hours in rabbit serum, during which
C. albicans will produce long processes (germ tubes)

(a) 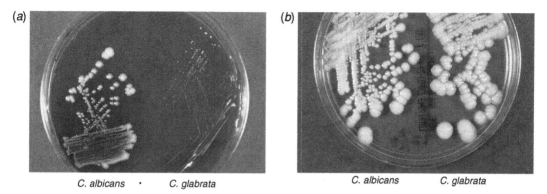 (b)

C. albicans · C. glabrata   C. albicans   C. glabrata

Fig. 8.5. (a) and (b) *Candida albicans* and *C. glabrata* colony morphology after 5 days' growth on a sheep blood agar plate (SBAP, frame (a)) and Sabaroud Dextrose Agar (SAB, frame (b)). *C. albicans* (on the left, frame (a)) demonstrates very slow growth on SBAP with small pinpoint colonies seen at 1–2 days and moderate-sized colonies seen after 5 days' incubation at 35 °C. *C. glabrata* has very small colonies even after 5 days' growth on SBAP (on the right, frame (a)). The colony morphology of these two yeasts is virtually indistinguishable on SAB agar (frame (b)). Growth of both *C. albicans* (left) and *C. glabrata* (right) is more luxurious on the SAB than on SBAP. The organisms both appear as dull opaque colonies with a 'rising bread' odour.

that grow out from the yeast cell; these processes are no more than half the width of the cell and at least 3–4 times the length of the cell (Fig. 8.6). The germ tube assay must be interpreted with care, as other candidal species may produce short, fat or pinched off germ tube-like processes. If the base of the tube is pinched off, if the tube is less than three times the length of the cell or if the width is greater than one half of the width of the cell, it is not considered to be a true germ tube.

Latex agglutination or biochemical assays are commercially available for the presumptive diagnosis of *C. albicans*. These either identify *C. albicans* specific antigens or combinations of enzymes produced by the species, providing rapid identification.

Further fungal culture is required if the yeast is not identified by one of these simple presumptive assays. This can be accomplished with sugar assimilation cultures such as the analytic profile index (API, BioMerieux) and by characteristics of morphology on Cornmeal agar growth. The sugar assimilation assay involves inoculating a suspension of yeast into cupules containing a single sugar. Growth in the presence of this sugar produces a turbid suspension within 2 days of culture (Fig. 8.7), and the sugar assimilation pattern is compared to a database for species identification.

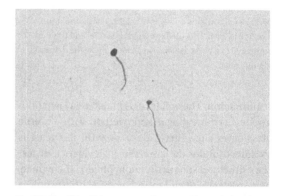

Fig. 8.6. Candida albicans germ tube assay. The majority of yeasts isolated from clinical specimens are identified as *C. albicans*, and a rapid screening test for its definitive identification is used in most laboratories. The germ tube assay is the standard test used to confirm diagnosis. A yeast colony is inoculated into rabbit serum and incubated at 37°C for no longer than 2 hours. At the end of the incubation period, the yeast suspension is examined under the microscope for evidence of germ tubes, tubular growths produced by the yeast cell that are no wider than half the cell diameter, longer than three times the cell length, and non-constricted at their origin from the yeast cell. This image demonstrates two good examples of *C. albicans* germ tubes.

Although the API database is extensive for the *Candida* spp., definitive diagnosis requires morphologic

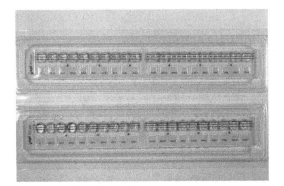

Fig. 8.7. Sugar assimilation assay for *C. albicans* (top) and *C. glabrata* (bottom). The sugar assimilation assay identifies yeasts based on their ability to utilize sugars as the sole source of nutrition. The yeast is inoculated into an agar medium to form a suspension, which is then used to inoculate cupules that each contain a single sugar. The strip is evaluated visually after 2 days' incubation: if growth has occurred, the cupule will show an increase in turbidity. The positive control contains glucose (second cupule from the left) and a negative control well contains no sugars (far left). The assimilation reaction as a whole is used to generate a code, and this is compared to a yeast database in order to make the definitive identification.

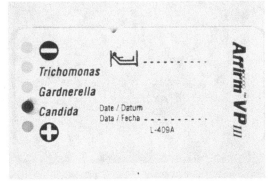

Fig. 8.8. Affirm VP III probe assay for the diagnosis of vaginitis syndromes. The Affirm VP system consists of a card that has been impregnated with probes to *T. vaginalis*, *G. vaginalis*, and *C. albicans*. DNA is extracted from vaginal swab specimens and the DNA solution is incubated with the card to allow specific probe-DNA binding. Unbound DNA is removed by washing and a secondary labelled probe is added. Specific pathogens are identified by peroxidase colour development. This card demonstrates a very strong reaction for *C. albicans* and negative reactions for the other two pathogens.

confirmation. The organism is plated as a lawn onto Tween-Corn meal agar and overlaid with a sterile glass cover slip. After 2 days' growth, the yeast is examined under the coverslip for evidence of tertiary structures such as pseudohyphae, giant hyphae, and arrangement and morphology of blastoconidia produced by the yeast strain. *C. albicans* is characterized morphologically by the formation of pseudohyphae with clusters of small round blastoconidia and the production of large refractile terminal chlamydospores. *Candida (Torulopsis) glabrata* on this same medium produces only small yeast cells and the API sugar assimilation is positive for the assimilation of glucose and trehalose only. Rapid trehalose assays are now commercially available to rapidly identify small yeasts as such *C. glabrata*.

Molecular testing for the fungal vaginitis syndromes is unnecessary, since the diagnosis can be efficiently reached with less expensive tests. The probe assay (Affirm VP system) has no significant advantage over direct detection with KOH, but if the technology is available, it does provide a single test for the three major etiologies of vaginitis (Fig. 8.8).

Treatment

A variety of short course therapies are available to treat fungal vulvo-vaginitis. Single dose and 1–3 day courses of azole-containing topical preparations are effective in 80–90% of patients. A number of acceptable antifungal regimens for symptomatic vaginitis use suppository cream preparations, vaginal tablets or oral agents. Butoconazole, clotrimazole, miconazole and tinoconazole cream suppositories are available over the counter, and require 1–14 days of treatment. Prescription strength preparations of these same agents in vaginal tablet or cream suppository form have the advantage of shorter treatment duration (single dose or several days). Nystatin preparations are overall less effective and are therefore not recommended. Oral fluconazole (150 mg p.o. in a single dose) is the only recommended oral preparation. If a non-albicans yeast is identified, then a longer course of therapy with a non-fluconazole-containing treatment is advised. Infections with *C. glabrata* have been treated successfully using topical boric acid when other antifungal therapies have failed. Sexual partners of women with yeast infections usually do not require treatment. Exceptions include male partners who develop symptomatic balanitis, and women who experience recurrent vaginitis. In both of those situations, treatment of the male partner is advisable.

Vaccine availability

No vaccine is available for the prevention of genital yeast infections.

Bacterial vaginosis

Bacterial vaginosis (BV) is the most common cause of vaginitis. This disease results from a shift in vaginal flora leading to an increase in vaginal pH, increased numbers of vaginal bacteria and a change in the types of bacteria present in the vagina. Hydrogen peroxide producing *Lactobacillus* spp. generally make up 95% of the normal flora in the healthy vagina. These lactobacilli utilize the glycogen produced by the vaginal epithelium, producing lactic acid that leads to the characteristic pH of below 4.5 found in normal women. In BV, the vaginal flora is altered, with *Gardnerella vaginalis*, anaerobes (*Bacteroide* spp., *Prevotella* spp., *Mobiluncus* spp.), and *Mycoplasma* spp. emerging as the predominant organisms. *Lactobacillus* spp. are notably diminished in number, and the overall bacterial load in the vagina is increased 20–1000-fold above normal levels.

Transmission

The mode of transmission for BV is unclear, complicated by the fact that the organisms associated with BV may be part of the normal flora of the vagina. Pathology is due to an imbalance in numbers of organisms and the relative proportions of each species present. Some studies suggest that transmission is linked to sexual activity and the disease is therefore an STD. BV is seen almost exclusively in sexually active women and is rarely seen in virgins. Onset of symptomatic disease in women is often associated with a change in sex partner and is also associated with increased numbers of sex partners, again suggesting sexual transmission. There is a relatively strong concurrence of BV with *T. vaginalis* infection, also pointing to a link with STD. However, unlike classic STDs, treatment of male partners to eradicate *G. vaginalis*, *M. hominis* and anaerobic colonization or carriage has little or no effect on recurrence of disease in female partners. The mode of transmission, therefore, remains obscure.

Clinical presentation

One-half of patients are asymptomatic for BV, but classic clinical features include:
- production of copious milky white vaginal discharge (stains the underwear),
- presence of a foul or fishy odour, particularly after intercourse.

Symptoms may be acute or chronic, sometimes lasting months or years. There is growing evidence of associated pathogenesis, such as increased rates of late miscarriage, premature rupture of the membranes, endometritis and preterm labour and delivery. *Gardnerella vaginalis* has been associated with irregular uterine bleeding and histologic endometritis. Liversedge *et al.* (1999) investigated the influence of bacterial vaginosis on the outcome of assisted conception treatment and made the observation that the prevalence of bacterial vaginosis in their group of 302 infertile patients was twice that found in patients attending obstetric and gynaecology clinics in the UK: 25.6% vs. 12 and 11%, respectively. Patients with tubal damage had a higher incidence of BV (31.5%) than did those with non-tubal infertility (19.7%), leading them to suggest that women with tubal factor infertility may have a predisposition to abnormal genital tract bacterial flora associated with BV.

Patients with non-tubal infertility also had an incidence of BV higher than that of the reference population. This study did not detect any adverse effect of BV on fertilization in vitro or on embryo implantation rates, but the authors suggest that treatment of BV could reduce later complications in pregnancy, and therefore patients with tubal infertility who achieve an IVF pregnancy should be a target group for antenatal screening for BV.

Clinical diagnosis

The clinical diagnosis is suggested by the presence of a homogeneous milky white discharge that is fishy in smell, even in vivo at the time of physical examination. There is no erythema or edema of the vaginal wall and there is generally a lack of inflammatory cells in the exudate. The diagnosis can be confirmed by inexpensive out-patient testing.

Laboratory diagnosis

The diagnosis of bacterial vaginosis is often made in the out-patient or physician office. Vaginal secretions are sampled during speculum exam by swabbing or scraping the vaginal wall at the superior aspect (high vaginal wall sampling). An altered pH of vaginal secretions, positive amine Whiff test and the presence of clue cells on direct examination provides a presumptive diagnosis. A pH greater than 4.5 (usually 5.0–6.0) is more than 80% sensitive in detecting infection when used as the sole diagnostic test. The anaerobes seen in this disease process produce amines, and their detection by the Whiff test is also helpful in making the diagnosis. The classic amine Whiff test is carried out by mixing a drop of vaginal secretions with a drop of 10% KOH: in the presence of alkali, amines produced as a result of anaerobic metabolism produce an enhanced fishy odour. Trimethylamine can also be specifically detected using the FemExam test card (Cooper Surgical, Shelton, CT, Fig. 8.9), and proline-aminopeptidase can be directly assayed using the Pip Activity TestCard (Litmus Concepts, Inc. Santa Clara, CA); both of these tests detect abnormal amine production in the secretions.

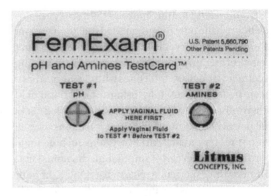

Fig. 8.9. FemExam card to detect abnormal pH and amine composition in vaginal discharges as an out-patient test. A vaginal discharge is directly inoculated onto two test areas. Test area 1 assesses pH elevation, and the other test area detects the presence of amines. Each test area has a built in positive control (the horizontal line), and pathology is detected by the presence of a vertical line. In this card, the pH is abnormally elevated but no amines have been detected.

BV can also be diagnosed by examining a wet prep or Gram's stain of vaginal discharge for the presence of 'clue cells', squamous epithelial cells that are covered with gram variable rods, i.e. a weak gram-positive reaction. These bacteria-covered cells have a very fuzzy or shaggy appearance that is typical of the disease process (Fig. 8.10).

Although BV is a polymicrobial process, the majority of the tests are focused on detection of *Gardnerella vaginalis*. *G. vaginalis* is part of the normal flora of the vagina, and although it can be cultured, this is no longer recommended as a diagnostic test. Culture requires special support medium (human blood agar or V agar) and incubation at 35 °C in 5% CO_2 for two days to demonstrate the typical soft beta hemolysis produced by the organisms in the presence of human blood (Fig. 8.11). Colonies are catalase-negative, oxidase-negative and positive for hippurate hydrolysis. *G. vaginalis* will also grow on other media such as Columbia–Colistin–Nalidixic acid (CNA), but will not give the characteristic hemolysis for colony selection. Culture for anaerobes in vaginal secretions is likewise not recommended and will not be performed by most microbiology laboratories.

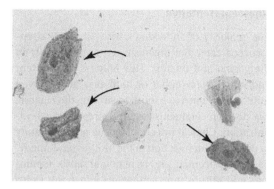

Fig. 8.10. Gram-stain preparation of clue cells in a vaginal discharge. Specimens collected from the wall of the vagina normally contain pale staining squamous epithelial cells (middle of the Figure). In bacterial vaginosis, these cells become covered in a shaggy layer of gram-variable bacilli (arrows); together with an elevated vaginal pH, these confirm the diagnosis of BV.

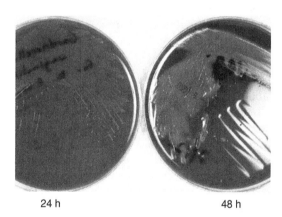

| 24 h | 48 h |

Fig. 8.11. Culture of *Gardnerella vaginalis* on human blood agar medium at 24 and 48 hours. *G. vaginalis* from vaginal exudates is softly beta hemolytic after growth on human blood agar, and non-hemolytic after growth on sheep blood agars. Hemolysis is barely evident at 24 hours (left plate), whereas a zone of complete hemolysis is readily seen after 48 hours (right plate).

Affirm VP System may be used for the molecular detection of *G. vaginalis* using a synthetic oligonucleotide probe. However, since it is part of the normal flora, the sensitivity of the assay may exceed its actual benefit, and it may be difficult to judge whether treatment is warranted if a weak positive result is obtained.

Table 8.2. Recommended medical treatments for BV

Metronidazole	500 mg p.o. ii qd × 7 days
Clindamycin cream 2%,	one full applicator (5 g) intravaginally at bedtime × 7 days
Metronidazole gel 0.75%,	one full applicator (5 g) intravaginally ii qd × 5 days
In pregnancy: Metronidazole	250 mg p.o. iii qd × 7 days to minimize fetal exposure

Treatment

All women with symptomatic BV require treatment, particularly during pregnancy. Patients who undergo therapeutic abortions or gynecologic surgery who have a diagnostic test positive for BV should also be treated. As there is no impact on subsequent chance of relapse when the partner has been treated, treatment of sexual partners is not recommended. The current CDC recommendations for treatment are listed in Table 8.2. The metronidazole therapies overall are more effective than topical or oral clindamycin preparations. Single dose metronidazole is also less effective than the recommended 5–7 day regimes.

Vaccine availability

There is no vaccine available to prevent bacterial vaginosis.

Vaginal colonization with Group B Streptococcus (GBS)

Streptococcus agalactiae

Streptococcus agalactiae is a gram-positive coccus (Group B streptococcus) that is found as normal flora of the human gut and vagina. Vaginal colonization has been associated with post-partum and neonatal sepsis, and therefore studies of *S. agalactiae* colonization have focused on women during pregnancy. Between 10% and 30% of pregnant women carry the organism in the vagina and/or rectum and this carriage may occur intermittently throughout pregnancy: first trimester colonization does not reflect what the status may be later in the pregnancy. The risk of maternal to neonate transmission increases with the presence of rectal/vaginal colonization at or near birth, and therefore diagnostic testing should be carried out near term, preferably at 35–37 weeks gestation, to determine whether prophylactic antibiotic treatment is required. Despite active surveillance to detect at risk pregnancies, *S. agalactiae* is still responsible for 1.8 neonatal infections per 1000 live births per year in the United States; neonatal colonization (without signs of infection) occurs in about 11% of babies. Fifty per cent of mothers with Group B streptococcal colonization who do not receive antibiotic treatment will transmit the infection to the neonates, putting the babies at risk of developing invasive disease.

Life cycle

Streptococcus agalactiae is a softly beta-hemolytic organism, classified as Lancefield's Group B. The bacterium reproduces by binary fission, grows in chains and does not produce spores.

Transmission

S. agalactiae is part of the normal flora of the gut, and this region probably serves as its principal reservoir. Colonization may occur in either the gut or the vagina, and vaginal carriage is probably maintained by seeding from the anorectal area. Intermittent colonization in pregnant women may reflect auto-inoculation from one site to the other, rather than occurring as a result of *de novo* infection from an external source. Neonatal infection can be caused either by vertical transmission across the placenta or from organisms present in the maternal vagina or intestine during birth. Young women of non-white race and low multiparity seem to be at greater risk for colonization; the major risk factor for neonatal disease is maternal colonization at the time of birth.

Clinical presentation

The majority of individuals with Group B streptococcus carry the organism asymptomatically in the vagina and rectum. This may be intermittent and may involve either or both sites at any given time. A baby born to a mother carrying the bacteria can develop cutaneous Group B streptococcus colonization. Clinical infections occur predominantly as post-partum infection in the mother (endometritis and septicemia), and as neonatal sepsis, meningitis and skin or mucocutaneous infections. Complications can be fatal in 5–20% of neonatal cases and in 15–32% of adults. An estimated 15–30% of babies who survive an episode of neonatal meningitis develop long-term neurological sequelae.

In the non-pregnant patient, Group B strep can sometimes cause urinary tract infections, bacteremia and soft tissue infections. Patients with diabetes mellitus, malignancies and cirrhosis of the liver are more susceptible to these GBS infections.

Laboratory diagnosis

Group B streptococcal colonization can be detected by routine culture of the organism from recto-vaginal swabs in women at 35–37 weeks gestation. The degree of colonization (i.e. the number of organisms detected) is irrelevant, as the presence of any *S. agalactiae* in the culture requires maternal prophylactic treatment. Direct cultures and direct detection assays for *S. agalactiae* from clinical specimens have low sensitivity and do not adequately detect colonization. Current guidelines recommend overnight enrichment culture in selective broth (Lim or Todd-Hewitt Broths) followed by culture, serologic or molecular techniques to identify the Group B strep. An inoculum from an overnight broth culture is plated onto blood agar plates, and checked for β-hemolytic colonies following overnight incubation. β-hemolytic colonies are then confirmed as Group B streptococci using serological methods, usually latex agglutination. Molecular probes that specifically identify GBS from the overnight broth culture have recently become available (AccuProbe

Table 8.3. CDC recommended intrapartum prophylaxis to prevent Group B streptococcal colonization

Recommended	Penicillin G	5 mU IV stat followed by	2.5 mU IV 4 hourly until delivery
Alternative,	Ampicillin	2 g IV stat followed by	1 g IV 4 hourly until delivery
if Penicillin	Clindamycin or	900 mg IV	8 hourly until delivery
allergic	Erythromycin	500 mg IV	6 hourly until delivery

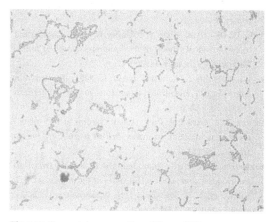

Fig. 8.12. Gram-stain preparation of Group B Streptococcus from a recto-vaginal culture. This slide demonstrates the characteristic Gram-stain morphology of Group B Streptococcus, gram-positive cocci in chains.

S. agalactiae ribosomal RNA probes assay, Gen-Probe, San Diego, CA). This technique is extremely sensitive and specific and expedites the diagnosis by eliminating the second day of culture.

Neonatal infections usually present with sepsis or meningitis. Cerebrospinal fluid (CSF) specimens have an elevated white cell count and elevated protein levels, low glucose levels and gram-positive chains of cocci are detected on Gram's stain. Direct antigen detection in the CSF is no more sensitive than Gram stain, and is of no benefit towards confirming a diagnosis. CSF and blood culture is the diagnostic test of choice for neonatal meningitis and sepsis. The organisms grow relatively rapidly and growth may be seen in broth blood culture systems within 12 hours. Blood agar plates show small colonies with a soft beta hemolysis, best visualized using indirect light. Gram stain of the cultured organism demonstrates gram-positive cocci in chains (Fig. 8.12).

In biochemical testing, the organism is catalase negative, hydrolyses arginine and hippurate but not esculin or PYR, and is Voges–Proskauer positive, reliably producing acids from ribose and trehalose. Appropriate minimal inhibitory concentration (MIC) testing is required to determine susceptibility in cases of invasive disease. The US National Committee for Clinical Laboratory Standards (NCCLS) for Group B streptococcal susceptibility testing approve both the commercially available frozen or lyophilized susceptibility test from Microscan (MicroSTREP panels, Dade Behring, West Sacramento, CA) and E-test susceptibility testing using Blood–Muller–Hinton medium. GBS are considered to be universally susceptible to penicillin; resistance to erythromycin and clindamycin has been seen.

Treatment

CDC guidelines recommend prophylactic treatment for all women confirmed with group B streptococcal colonization. Treatment immediately following the rupture of the membranes and prior to the delivery of the fetus provides adequate cover for both the mother and the neonate. Intrapartum penicillin G IV is the antibiotic treatment of choice, as Group B streptococci are still universally susceptible to penicillin (Table 8.3). The neonate requires no additional treatment if the antibiotics are administered prior to birth. If maternal *S. agalactiae* carriage status is not known, Pen G should be administered during labor in cases where delivery occurs before 37 weeks of gestation, membranes are ruptured for over 18 hours prior to delivery, or the mother has a temperature above 38 °C. If invasive disease is seen in either the mother or neonate, antibiotic susceptibility must be confirmed to ensure appropriate management, as resistance to clindamycin and erythromycin have been reported.

Vaccine availability

Although several vaccines are under development, none is currently available for the prevention of Group B streptococcal infections or colonization.

FURTHER READING

TRICHOMONAS VAGINALIS

Bickly, L. S., Krisher, K. K., Punsulang, A. *et al.* (1989). Comparison of direct fluorescent antibody, acridine orange, wet mount and culture for detection of *Trichomonas vaginalis* in women attending a sexually transmitted disease clinic. *Sexually Transmitted Diseases*, **16**: 127–31.

Borchardt, K. A. & Smith, R. F. (1991). An evaluation of an InPouch TV culture method for diagnosing *Trichomonas vaginalis* infection. *Genitourinary Medicine*, **67**:149–52.

Briselden, A. M. & Hillier, S. L. (1994). Evaluation of Affirm VP microbial identification test for *Gardnerella vaginalis* and *Trichomonas vaginalis*. *Journal of Clinical Microbiology*, **32**: 148–52.

Brown, H. L., Fuller, D. D., Davis, T. E., Schwebke, J. R. & Hillier, S. L. (2001). Evaluation of the Affirm ambient temperature transport system for the detection and identification of *Trichomonas vaginalis*, *Gardnerella vaginalis* and *Candida* species from vaginal fluid specimens. *Journal of Clinical Microbiology*, **39**: 3197–9.

Centers for Disease Control and Prevention (2002). Sexually transmitted diseases treatment guidelines 2002. *Morbidity and Mortality Weekly*, **51**(No. RR-6):1–76.

Draper, D., Parker, E., Patterson, W. *et al.* (1993). Detection of *Trichomonas vaginalis* in pregnant women with the InPouch TV culture system. *Journal of Clinical Microbiology*, **10**: 106–8.

Ferris, D. G., Hendrich, J., Payne, P. M. *et al.* (1995). Office laboratory diagnosis of vaginitis: Clinician-performed tests compared with a rapid nucleic acid hybridization test. *Journal of Family Practice*, **41**: 575–81.

Gardner, W. A., Culberson, D. E. & Bennett, B. D. (1986). *Trichomonas vaginalis* in the prostate gland. *Archives of Pathology and Laboratory Medicine*, **110**: 430–2.

Krieger, J. N. & Alderete, J. F. (1999). *Trichomonas vaginalis* and Trichomoniasis. In *Sexually Transmitted Diseases*, 3rd edn,

ed. K. K. Holmes, P. F. Sparling *et al.*, pp. 587–604. New York: McGraw-Hill.

Madico, G., Quinn, T. C., Rompalo, A., McKee, K. T. & Gaydos, C. A. (1998). Diagnosis of *Trichomonas vaginalis* infection by PCR using vaginal swab samples. *Journal of Clinical Microbiology*, **36**: 3205–10.

Patel, S. R., Wiese, W., Patel, S. C., Ohl, C., Byrd, J. C. & Estrada, C. A. (2000). Systemic review of diagnostic tests for vaginal trichomoniasis. *Infectious Diseases in Obstetrics and Gynecology*, **8**: 248–57.

Petrin, D., Delgaty, K., Bhatt, R. & Garber, G. (1998). Clinical and microbiological aspects of *Trichomonas vaginalis*. *Clinical Microbiology Reviews*, **11**: 300–17.

Sorvillo, F., Smith, L., Kerndt, P. & Ash, L. (2001). *Trichomonas vaginalis*, HIV, and African–Americans. *Emerging Infectious Disease*, **7**: 927–32.

Wetson, T. E. & Nichol, C. S. (1963). Natural history of trichomonas infection in males. *British Journal of Venerea Disease*, **35**: 251–4.

Wolner-Hassen, P. (1999). Trichomoniasis. In *Sexually Transmitted Diseases and Adverse Outcomes of Pregnancy*, ed. P. J. Hitchcock, H. T. MacKay & J. N. Wasserheit, pp. 209–24. Washington, DC: ASM Press.

YEAST VAGINITIS

Brown, H. L., Fuller, D. D., Davis, T. E., Schwebke, J. R. & Hillier, S. L. (2001). Evaluation of the Affirm ambient temperature transport system for the detection and identification of *Trichomonas vaginalis*, *Gardnerella vaginalis* and *Candida* Species from vaginal fluid species. *Journal of Clinical Microbiology*, **39**: 3197–9.

Centers for Disease Control and Prevention (2002). Sexually transmitted diseases treatment guidelines 2002. *Morbidity and Mortality Weekly*, **51**(No. RR-6): 1–76.

Denning, D. W. (1995). Fortnightly review: management of genital candidiasis. *British Medical Journal*, **310**: 1241–4.

Dun, E. (1999). Antifungal resistance in yeast vaginitis. *Yale Journal of Biological Medicine*, **72**: 281–5.

Ferris, D. G., Hendrich, J., Payne, P. M. *et al.* (1995). Office laboratory diagnosis of vaginitis: Clinician-performed tests compared with a rapid nucleic acid hybridization test. *Journal of Family Practice*, **41**: 575–81.

Fidel, P. L. (1998). Vaginal candidiasis: review and role of local immunity. *AIDS Patient Care STD*, **12**: 359–66.

Fidel, P. L., Vasquez, J. A. & Sobel, J. D. (1999). *Candida glabrata*: review of epidemiology, pathogenesis, and clinical disease with comparison to *C. albicans*. *Clinical Microbiology Reviews*, **12**: 80–96.

Fidel, P. L., Cutright, J. & Steele, C. (2000). Effects of reproductive hormones on experimental vaginal candidiasis. *Infection and Immunity*, **68**: 651–7.

Koneman, E. W., Allen, S. D., Janda, W. M., Schreckenberger, P. C. & Winn, W. C. (1997). Mycology. In *Color Atlas and Textbook of Diagnostic Microbiology*, 5th edn, pp. 983–1069. Philadelphia, PA: Lippincott.

Lanchares, J. L. & Hernandez, M. L. (2000). Recurrent vaginal candidiasis changes in etiolpathogenical patterns. *International Journal of Gynecology and Obstetrics*, **71**: S29–35.

Rex, J. H., Walsh, T. J., Sobel, J. D. *et al.* (2000). Practice guidelines for the treatment of candidiasis. *Clinical Infectious Diseases*, **30**: 662–78.

Sobel, J. D. (2002). Fungal infections of the genitourinary tract. In *Clinical Mycology*, ed. E. J. Anaisie, M. R. McGinnis & M. A. Pfaller, pp. 496–508. Philadelphia, PA: Churchill Livingstone, Elsevier Science.

Vasquez, J. A., Sobel, J. D., Peng, G. *et al.* (1999). Evolution of vaginal *Candida* species recovered from human immunodeficiency virus-infected women receiving fluconazole prophylaxis: the emergence of *Candida glabrata*? *Clinical Infectious Diseases*, **28**: 1025–31.

BACTERIAL VAGINOSIS

Briselden, A. M. & Hillier, S. L. (1994). Evaluation of Affirm VP microbial identification test for *Gardnerella vaginalis* and *Trichomonas vaginalis*. *Journal of Clinical Microbiology*, **32**: 148–52.

Brown, H. L., Fuller, D. D., Davis, T. E., Schwebke, J. R. & Hillier, S. L. (2001). Evaluation of the Affirm ambient temperature transport system for the detection and identification of *Trichomonas vaginalis*, *Gardnerella vaginalis* and *Candida* species from vaginal fluid specimens. *Journal of Clinical Microbiology*, **39**: 3197–9.

Centers for Disease Control and Prevention. (2002). Sexually transmitted diseases treatment guidelines 2002. *Morbidity and Mortality Weekly*, **51**(No. RR-6): 1–76.

Eschenbach, D. A. (1993). Bacterial vaginosis and anaerobes in obstetric-gynecologic infection. *Clinical Infectious Diseases*, **16**(suppl 4): S282–7.

Fanchin, R., Harmas, A., Benaoudia, F., Lundkvist, U., Olivennes, F. & Frydman, R. (1998). Microbial flora of the cervix assessed at the time of embryo transfer adversely affects in vitro fertilization outcome *Fertility and Sterility*, **70**(5): 866–70.

Ferris, D. G., Hendrich, J., Payne, P. M. *et al.* (1995). Office laboratory diagnosis of vaginitis: Clinician-performed tests compared with a rapid nucleic acid hybridization test. *Journal of Family Practice*, **41**: 575–81.

Gjerdingen, D., Fontaine, P., Bixby, M., Santilli, J. & Welsh, J. (2000). The impact of regular vaginal pH screening on the diagnosis of bacterial vaginosis in pregnancy. *Journal of Family Practice*, **49**:39–43.

Hillier, S. L., Nugent, R. P., Eschenbach, D. A. *et al.* (1995). Association between bacterial vaginosis and preterm delivery of a low-birth-weight infant. *New England Journal of Medicine*, **333**: 1737–42.

Hillier, S. L. (1998). Q & A identifying clue cells. *Laboratory Medicine*, **29**: 408.

Kristiansen, P. V., Oster, S. & Frost, L. (1987). Isolation of *Gardnerella vaginalis* in pure culture from the uterine cavity of patients with irregular bleeding. *British Journal of Obstetrics and Gynaecology*, **94**: 979–84.

Liversedge, N. H., Turner, A., Horner, P. J., Keay, S. D., Jenkins, J. M. & Hull, M. G. R. (1999). The influence of bacterial vaginosis on in-vitro fertilization and embryo implantation during assisted reproduction treatment. *Human Reproduction*, **14**(9): 2411–15.

Macsween, K. F. & Ridgway, G. L. (1998). The laboratory investigation of vaginal discharge. *Journal of Clinical Pathology*, **51**: 564–7.

Moller, B. R., Kristiansen, P. V. & Thorsen, P. (1995). Sterility of the uterine cavity. *Acta Obstetrica Gynaecologica Scandinavica*, **74**: 216–19.

Potter, J. (1999). Should sexual partners of women with bacterial vaginosis receive treatment? *British Journal of General Practice*, **49**: 913–18.

Sherrard, J. (2001). European guidelines for the management of vaginal discharge. *European Journal of STD and AIDS*, **12**: 73–7.

Spiegel, C. A. (1999). Bacterial vaginosis: changes in laboratory practice. *Clinical and Microbiological Newsletter*, **25**: 33–7.

Spiegel, C. A., Amsel, R., Eschenbach, D., Schoenknecht, F. & Holmes, K. K. (1980). Anaerobic bacteria in nonspecific vaginitis. *New England Journal of Medicine*, **303**: 601–6.

VAGINAL COLONIZATION WITH GROUP B STREPTOCOCCUS (GBS)

Badri, M., Zawaneh, S., Cruz, A. C. *et al.* (1977). Rectal colonization with group B streptococcus: relation to vaginal colonization of pregnant women. *Journal of Infectious Diseases*, **135**: 308–12.

Baker, C. J. (1996). Inadequacy of rapid immunoassays for intrapartum detection of group B streptococcal carriers. *Obstetrics and Gynecology*, **88**: 51–5.

Baker, C. J., Clark, D. J. & Barrett, F. F. (1973). Selective broth medium for isolation of group B streptococci. *Applied Microbiology*, **26**: 884–5.

Baker, C. J., Goroll, D. K., Alpert, S. *et al.* (1977). Vaginal colonization with group B streptococcus: a study in college women. *Journal of Infectious Diseases*, **135**: 392–7.

Bourbeau, P. P., Heiter, B. J. & Figdore, M. (1997). Use of Gen-Probe AccuProbe group B streptococcus test to detect group B streptococci in broth cultures of vaginal–anorectal specimens from pregnant women: comparison with traditional culture methods. *Journal of Clinical Microbiology*, **35**: 144–7.

Boyer, K. M., Gadsala, C. A., Kelly, P. D., Burd, L. I. & Gotoff, S. P. (1983). Selective intrapartum chemoprophylaxis of neonatal group B streptococcal early-onset disease. II. Predictive value of prenatal cultures. *Journal of Infectious Diseases*, **148**: 802–9.

Centers for Disease Control and Prevention (2002). Prevention of perinatal group B Streptococcal disease: revised guidelines from CDC. *Morbidity and Mortality Weekly*, **51** (RR-11): 1–22.

De Cueto, M., Sanchez, M. J., Sampedro, A., Miranda, J. A., Herruzo, A. J. & Rosa-Fraile, M. (1998). Timing of intrapartum ampicillin and prevention of vertical transmission of group B streptococcus. *Obstetrics and Gynecology*, **91**: 112–14.

Dillon, H. C., Gray, E., Pass, M. A. & Gray, B. M. (1982). Anorectal and vaginal carriage of group B streptococci during pregnancy. *Journal of Infectious Diseases*, **145**: 794–9.

Kircher, S. M., Meyer, M. P. & Jordan, J. A. (1996). Comparison, of a modified DNA hybridization assay with standard culture enrichment for detecting group B streptococci in obstetric patients. *Journal of Clinical Microbiology*, **34**: 342–4.

Koneman, E. W., Allen, S. D., Janda, W. M., Schreckenberger, P. C. & Winn, W. C. (1997). The Gram-positive cocci: Part II: Streptococci, Enterococci, and the 'Streptococcus-like' bacteria. In *Color Atlas and Textbook of Diagnostic Microbiology*, 5th edn, pp. 577–650. Philadelphia, PA: Lippincott.

Liu, J. W., Wu, J. J., Ko, W. C. & Chuang, Y. C. (1997). Clinical characteristics and antimicrobial susceptibility of invasive group B streptococcal infections in nonpregnant adults in Taiwan. *Journal of the Formosa Medical Association*, **96**: 628–33.

Morales, W. J., Dickey, S. S., Bornick, P. & Lim, D. V. (2002). Change in antibiotic resistance of group B streptococcus: impact on intrapartum management. *American Journal of Obstetrics and Gynecology*, **181**: 310–14.

Overman, S. B., Eley, D. D., Jacobs, B. E. & Ribes, J. A. (2002). Evaluation of methods to increase the sensitivity and timeliness of detection of *Streptococcus agalactiae* in pregnant women. *Journal of Clinical Microbiology*, **40**: 4329–31.

Philipson, E. H., Palerimino, D. A. & Robinson, A. (1995) Enhanced antenatal detection of group B streptococcus colonization. *Obstetrics and Gynecology*, **85**: 437–9.

Platt, M. W., McLaughlin, J. C., Gilson, G. J., Wellhoner, M. F. & Nims, L. J. (1995). Increased recovery of group B streptococcus by the inclusion of rectal culturing and enrichment. *Diagnosis Microbiology and Infectious Disease*, **21**: 65–8.

Rouse, D. J., Andrews, W. W., Lin, F. Y. C., Mott, C. W., Ware, J. C. & Philips, J. B. (1998). Antibiotic susceptibility profile of group B streptococcus acquired vertically. *Obstetrics and Gynecology*, **92**: 931–4.

Schrag, S. J., Zywicki, S., Farley, M. M. *et al.* (2000). Group B streptococcal disease in the era of intrapartum antibiotic prophylaxis. *New England Journal of Medicine*, **342**: 15–20.

Schrag, S. J., Zell, E. R., Lynfield, R. *et al.* (2002). A population-based comparison of strategies to prevent early-onset Group B streptococcal disease in neonates. *New England Journal of Medicine*, **347**: 233–9.

Williams-Bouyer, N., Reisner, B. S. & Woods, G. L. (2000). Comparison of Gen-Probe AccuProbe group B streptococcus culture identification test with conventional culture for the detection of group B streptococci in broth cultures of vaginal–anorectal specimens from pregnant women. *Diagnostic Microbiology and Infectious Disease*, **36**: 159–62.

9

Genital human papillomavirus infections (HPV)

The Family Papovaviridae has two genera:
 (i) papillomaviruses that produce warts in muco-cutaneous sites;
 (ii) polyomaviruses, the first class of DNA virus that was recognized to cause tumours in animals, including JC virus, BK virus and SV-40.

Papilloma viruses are non-enveloped DNA viruses with icosahedral symmetry, measuring 45–55 nm in diameter. The human papilloma viruses (HPV) represent a group of over 80 viruses that infect epithelial cells to produce warts in a number of sites: more than 30 types infect the genitalia. Over 90% of all HPV infections are caused by two low-risk (non-tumorogenic) strains of HPV, serotypes 6 and 11. These are usually associated with the visible genital lesions and may also be associated with laryngeal and upper respiratory tract condylomata. Other low-risk HPV serovars include 40, 42, 43, 44, 54, 61, 70, 72 and 81. High-risk serovars include HPV 16, 18, 31, 33, 35, 39, 45, 51, 52, 56, 58, 59, 68, 73 and 82. Overall, HPV 16, 18, and to a lesser extent 31, 33, 35, 45, 53 and 58 are the most common high-risk papilloma viruses causing infections in humans. HPV 16 infection represents about 50% of those infections associated with progression to carcinoma.

Genital warts and cervical cancer

Genital human popillomavirus infections (HPV)

Since genital HPV infections are not reportable to the CDC, the real prevalence and numbers of new infections is not really known. Recent estimates suggest that over 5 million new cases occur annually in the US, making this the most common STD – even more common than *Chlamydia trachomatis*. HPV infects all races and both sexes equally, and has been found more frequently in pregnant than in non-pregnant women. New infections are acquired most often in the 15–40 year age group, and are often seen in association with other STDs. Patients may be infected with multiple HPV serotypes at the same time.

Life cycle

As a virus, HPV is an obligate intracellular parasite. Its genome codes for several proteins required for viral DNA replication and for proteins required for malignant transformation. The E6 and E7 open reading frames produce proteins that lead to the evolution of malignancy. These proteins complex with tumor suppressors and lead to carcinogenesis. Viral DNA is integrated into the host cell genome in the oncogenic species of HPV, but remains episomal in the non-oncogenic strains.

The replicative cycle appears to be stimulated by increased levels of progesterone and other steroid hormones. Although HPV initially infects undifferentiated squamous epithelial cells, replication is linked to their differentiation, with viral capsid assembly occurring in the fully differentiated squamous epithelial cells. Following infection, there is an incubation period of about 4 months (range 1–20 months) before the development of detectable lesions; about 90% of individuals will remain totally asymptomatic. The majority of infections resolve spontaneously without intervention. Occasional infections will persist and may produce more or larger visible wart lesions. Infection with high-risk HPV serovars (HPV 16 and 18 particularly) may lead to malignant transformation with the development of squamous cell carcinoma. High-grade lesions arise most often in the cervix of younger women and in the vagina, vulva, penis or rectal/anal tissues of older patient populations.

Transmission

Transmission of the human papilloma viruses occurs by direct contact and via fomites. The genital HPV serovars are considered STDs, transmitted following direct contact with genital lesions. They are most commonly transmitted from genital sites to genital site, although inoculation into the oral mucosa or onto cutaneous sites, particularly on the peri-anal folds, thighs, abdomen and fingers may also occur. Use of male and female condoms has been shown to decrease, but not eliminate, the transmission of HPV between sexual contacts. Autoinfection of genital HPV to sites on the fingers and hands, as well as inoculation of common warts from fingers onto genital locations has also been described. HPV may be transmitted vertically to the neonate at the time of birth when the infant comes in direct contact with lesions in the birth canal. Iatrogenic fomite-mediated transmission has been described with reusable liquid nitrogen applicators used to treat genital HPV infections. Since HPV DNA has also been detected in the ejaculates of HPV-infected males, there is the potential for transmission during artificial insemination and assisted conception procedures, although no cases have yet been identified.

Clinical presentation

The clinical presentation for genital HPV infections differs according to the serovar of HPV causing infection: HPV serovars are divided into high and low risk for the development of carcinoma in the infected tissues. The vast majority of genital HPV infections are caused by low risk HPV strains, predominantly HPV 6 and 11. Over 90% of these cases are totally asymptomatic. When these strains produce symptomatic disease, exophytic fungating lesions in the external and internal genital epithelium are generally seen. In men, these low-risk genital warts most commonly occur on the penile frenulum, coronal sulcus or terminal urethra. Infection may also occur on the penile shaft, scrotum and in other cutaneous pubic and upper leg locations. In males practising unprotected anal and oral intercourse, lesions may also be seen in the rectal and peri-anal locations as well as in the oral mucosa. Individuals with demonstrated exophytic lesions often also have inconspicuous flat condylomata that can be detected by identification with aceto-whitening. Many individuals infected with HPV may have only these flat warts and will thus present with asymptomatic or subclinical infections. These subclinical HPV infections represent the majority of cases for both men and women.

Low-risk venereal warts in women occur most often on the vulva, perineum and anus; on the anus they appear as large fungating lesions. Visible external genital exophytic warts are caused predominantly by the low risk HPV 6 and HPV 11 serovars, although high-risk serovars 16, 18, 31, 33 and 35 may also be seen in these external locations. Co-infection with multiple serovars is common. Warts may also grow in the mucosa of the vaginal wall, cervix and recto-anal region. Intra-anal and rectal warts are usually seen in individuals practising receptive anal intercourse. Peri-anal lesions may occur in women, however, even in the absence of anal penetration. HPV 6 and 11 may also infect non-genital sites causing oral, nasal, conjunctival, laryngeal and cutaneous warts. In the neonate, vertically acquired HPV 6 and 11 may produce laryngeal papillomatosis in which bulky laryngeal lesions form and may produce symptomatic disease.

Although the high-risk HPV serovars may be associated with external exophytic genital lesions, the more important association of these high-risk serovars is with the development of squamous cell carcinoma and the precancerous genital lesions. These may present in a range from early asymptomatic or subclinical infection to low-grade to high-grade cervical intraepithelial neoplasia (CIN), usually seen on cervical Pap smear. Approximately 90% of patients spontaneously clear their infection without intervention, but cancerous lesions can develop in a minority of patients with high-risk HPV infections, most commonly in the cervix. Cervical cancer is seen primarily in young women, while vaginal, vulvar, anal and penile cancers are seen primarily in the older (over 50) patient populations. If left untreated, most cases of early infection and low-grade CIN will resolve; higher grade lesions should be removed to prevent metastatic disease.

Clinical diagnosis

Characteristic exophytic growths seen on the external genitalia may provide a clinical diagnosis of genital warts. Lesions may occur singly, or more commonly will occur as clusters of fungating structures: most patients will have less than ten lesions and 0.5–1 cm^2 of epithelial involvement. Immunocompromised hosts may have a larger overall disease burden. Lesions are seen commonly on the labia majora, perineum and anal opening, on the urethral opening, coronal sulcus or penile shaft, and in the peri-genital skin regions of the inner thighs, mons pubis and lower abdomen. Large and bulky external warts may become friable and bleed easily with minor trauma. Flat condylomata may not be easily recognized and may produce disease in the distal urethra, particularly in men, and in the mucosa of the vagina and cervix in women. Aceto-whitening with a 3–5% acetic acid solution is often used to aid detection of flat condylomata. Several minutes after painting the external and internal genitalia, epithelial lesions take up the weak acetic acid solution and appear white. In women with vaginal and cervical infections, colposcopy following aceto-whitening is often used to identify lesions for diagnostic biopsy or therapeutic removal.

Laboratory diagnosis

HPV infections at highest risk for malignant progression are generally identified via a PAP exam. Using the Bethesda System for classification delineated in the *Interim Guidelines for Management of Abnormal*

Cervical Cytology issued by the National Cancer Institute Consensus Panel, abnormal PAP smears may be divided into:

(i) low-grade squamous intraepithelial lesions (low-grade SIL);

(ii) high-grade SIL;

(iii) atypical squamous cells of undetermined significance (ASCUS).

Low-grade lesions include evidence of HPV cytological changes and mild dysplasia/cervical intraepithelial neoplasia (CIN1). Appropriate follow-up routinely includes repeat PAP evaluations every 4–6 months until three consecutive smears are negative. Patients with three negative repeat PAP smears may then be followed routinely every 1–2 years thereafter. Those with repeat abnormal PAP smears or detection of high-grade lesions should be referred for colposcopy and biopsy to rule out CIN.

High-grade SIL includes moderate dysplasia/CIN2, severe dysplasia/CIN3, and carcinoma *in situ*. Patients with high-grade SIL should undergo immediate colposcopy and biopsy to determine the degree of dysplasia, and high grade lesions confirmed by biopsy should be treated by cervical conization with cold-knife or laser excision, loop electrosurgical excision (LEEP) or loop electrosurgical conization. Since HPV is expected in any cases where cytology demonstrates either high- or low-grade SIL, molecular testing to detect high-risk serovars is not useful and is not recommended.

In patients with ASCUS detected on Pap stain, a protocol including reflexive testing for the detection of high-risk HPV DNA helps to identify those patients in need of closer follow-up. Since the majority of these patients are expected to spontaneously resolve their infections without surgical intervention (similar to low-grade SIL), colposcopy and biopsy are not initially recommended for patients with ASCUS. Patients with exophytic external genital warts that have no demonstrable cytological abnormality on PAP exam require no additional testing or evaluation beyond the yearly or every other year PAP exam used for other women with normal PAP cytologies.

Molecular diagnosis remains the most useful confirmatory test available for the differentiation of high and low risk HPV infections. The initial development of HPV diagnostic testing included a dot blot hybridization method for use with vaginal washings, first void male urine, or biopsy specimens. These assays were generally used to detect the high risk (16 and 18) and low risk (6 and 11) serotypes of HPV. They have largely been replaced with Hybrid probe capture assays now available in a semi-automated format that allows the detection of specific high or low risk HPV serovars. Probes used in these assays include a more extensive collection of sequences, detecting a greater number of the serovars that may cause genital infections. Specimens collected onto special collection swabs or fluid specimens submitted in the form of the Thin-prep PAP specimens may be used to detect either high- or low-risk HPV serovars. Although PCR assays have also been developed, none are FDA-approved for diagnostic testing. The American Society for Colposcopy and Cervical Pathology (ASCCP) consensus guidelines recommend that all first-time ASCUS specimens submitted in thin prep format should be tested for high-risk HPV serovars only, since low-risk serovars are not associated with genital tract cancer. *In situ* hybridization in tissue sections may also be used to identify serotypes, but this is expensive and therefore used relatively infrequently. Current CDC guidelines do not recommend routine screening of sexual contacts to detect subclinical infections.

HPV has not been successfully cultured in vitro due to the need for fully differentiated squamous epithelial cells that cannot be maintained in culture, and a culture test for HPV is not currently available.

Treatment

Treatment of patients with external exophytic warts should be dictated by the presence of symptomatic disease, essentially in order to alleviate symptoms. Since no treatment modality or combination of treatments is known to totally alleviate infections with HPV, routine removal of asymptomatic lesions is not generally required. For painful lesions, lesions that bleed and those that are debilitating for other reasons (bulky disease), removal of wart tissue may

be attempted using cryotherapy, laser therapy, surgical excision or caustic agents to destroy infected tissues. The most commonly used caustics include 10–25% podophyllin in tincture of benzoin, 80–90% trichloroacetic acid (TCA) or bichloroacetic acid (BCA), each agent applied topically weekly until the lesions are no longer evident. Patients can expect to see hypopigmented scar lesions post treatment.

Identification of SIL in HPV-infected tissues requires the removal of the tissues containing the neoplasia. Cervical conization or removal of the involved vaginal, anal or penile lesions is required to limit the potential metastatic spread of the squamous cell carcinoma. Further details on patient management is available in the 2001 consensus guidelines suggested by the ASCCP.

Vaccine availability

Monovalent and multivalent preventative vaccines, and vaccines to be used in treatment of invasive HPV-related carcinomas are under development. Preventative vaccines are in stages I–III of research trials, and there have been some preclinical studies to evaluate the long-term antibody response. The most promising vaccine under development so far utilizes a monovalent virus-like particle (VLP) containing the major capsid protein L1. Initial studies with this vaccine have shown a high antibody response that persists for over 2.5 years after vaccination. This vaccine appears to be well tolerated and safe in the volunteers tested thus far. A quadrivalent vaccine utilizing antigens from HPV 6, 11, 16 and 18 has demonstrated similar efficacy to the monovalent product. Therapeutic vaccines using E6 and E7 proteins from HPV 16 are currently being tested in human volunteers with high-grade SIL and these have shown some efficacy in decreasing the size of HPV-related tumours and in diminishing the size of non-neoplastic lesions. However, this has not been effective in all cases. Since HPV infections are often composed of multiple different serotypes, this type of vaccine would not be useful in treating disease in all patients with neoplastic lesions.

FURTHER READING

HPV

Burd, EM. (2003). Human papillomavirus and cervical cancer. *Clinical Microbiology Reviews*, **16**: 1–17.

Centers for Disease Control and Prevention (2002). Sexually transmitted disease treatment guidelines 2002. *Morbidity and Mortality Weekly Report*, **51**(No. RR-6): 1–76.

Eppel, W., Worda, C., Frigo, P., Ulm, M., Kucera, E. & Czerwenka, K. (2000). Human papillomavirus in the cervix and placenta. *Obstetrics and Gynecology*, **96**: 337–41.

Hildesheim, A., Han, C. L., Brinton, L. A., Kurman, R. J. & Schiller, J. T. (1997). Human papillomavirus type 16 and risk of preinvasive vulvar cancer: results from a seroepidemiological case-control study. *Obstetrics and Gynecology*, **90**: 748–54.

Jonsson, M., Karlsson, R., Evander, M., Gustavsson, A., Rylander, E. & Wadell, G. (1997). Acetowhitening of the cervix and vulva as a predictor of subclinical human papillomavirus infection: sensitivity and specificity in a population-based study. *Obstetrics and Gynecology*, **90**: 744–7.

Koutsky, L. A., Ault, K. A., Wheeler, C. M. *et al.* (2002). A controlled trial of human papillomavirus type 16 vaccine. *New England Journal of Medicine*, **347**: 1645–51.

Kulasingam, S. I., Hughes, J. P., Kiviat, N. B. *et al.* (2002). Evaluation of human papillomavirus testing in primary screening for cervical abnormalities. *Journal of the American Medical Association*, **288**: 1749–57.

Mork, J., Lie, A. K., Glattrem E. *et al.* (2001). Human papillomavirus infection as a risk factor for squamous-cell carcinoma of the head and neck. *New England Journal of Medicine*, **344**: 1125–31.

Muderspach, L., Wilcznski, S., Roman, L. *et al.* (2000). A phase I trial of a human papillomavirus (HPV) peptide vaccine for women with high-grade cervical and vulvar intraepithelial neoplasia who are HPV 16 positive. *Clinical Cancer Research*, **6**: 3406–16.

Muñoz, N., Bosch, F. X., de Sanjose, S. *et al.* (2003). Epidemiologic classification of human papillomavirus types associated with cervical cancer. *New England Journal of Medicine*, **348**: 518–27.

Olatunbosun, O., Deneer, H. & Pierson, R. (1995). Human papillomavirus DNA detection in sperm using polymerase chain reaction. *Obstetrics and Gynecology*, **97**: 357–60.

Sideri, M., Spinaci, L., Spolti, N. & Schettino, F. (1999). Evaluation of CO_2 laser excision or vaporization for the treatment of vulvar intraepithelial neoplasia. *Gynecologic Oncology*, **75**: 277–81.

Solomon, D., Davey, D., Kurman, R. *et al.* (2002). The 2001 Bethesda system terminology for reporting results of cervical cytology. *Journal of the American Medical Association*, **287**: 2114–19.

Touze, A., de Sanjose, S., Coursaget, P. *et al.* (2001). Prevalence of anti-human papillomavirus type 16, 18, 31, and 58 virus-like particles in women in the general population and in prostitutes. *Journal of Clinical Microbiology*, **39**: 4344–8.

Venturoli, S., Cricca, M., Bonvicini, F. *et al.* (2002). Human papillomavirus DNA testing by PCR-ELISA and hybrid capture II from a single cytological specimen: concordance and correlation with cytological results. *Journal of Clinical Virology*, **25**: 177–85.

Wright, T. C., Cox, J. T., Massas, L. S., Twiggs, L. B. & Wilkinson, E. J. (2002). 2001 Consensus guidelines for the management of women with cervical cytologic abnormalities. *Journal of the American Medical Association*, **287**: 2120–9.

10

Urethritis and cervicitis syndromes

Male urethritis

Inflammation of the male urethra can be either infectious, caused by sexually transmitted diseases, or due to trauma following urological procedures, intermittent catheterization, insertion of foreign bodies, anatomical abnormalities or following accidental injury. Traditionally, the infectious causes have been divided into gonococcal urethritis, caused by *N. gonorrheae*, or non-gonococcal (also known as 'non-specific' urethritis, NSU). *Chlamydia trachomatis* is the most common agent of NSU, but other agents include *Ureaplasma urealyticum, Mycoplasma hominis* and *Trichomonas vaginalis*. Mixed infections can occur in a minority of cases. Other rare causes include lymphogranuloma venereum, herpes genitalis, syphilis, mycobacterium and typical bacteria (usually gram-negative rods) that are associated with cystitis in the presence of a urethral stricture. In vitro experiments have demonstrated that some bacteria, in particular the urogenital pathogens, can adhere to spermatozoa; this property might be an important mechanism by which infections may be spread throughout the female reproductive tract, with sperm acting as vectors of disease (Hosseinzadeh *et al.*, 2000). Urethritis may also be seen in association with other infectious syndromes such as epididymitis, orchitis, prostatitis, proctitis, Reiter's syndrome, iritis, pneumonia, otitis media or urinary tract infection.

Signs and symptoms

Infections may be asymptomatic; patients sometimes present following partner screening. Symptoms may include urethral discharge, urethral itch, and dysuria. Urinary frequency and urgency are typically absent and, if present, should suggest prostatitis or cystitis. Systemic symptoms such as fever, chills, sweats, and nausea are also usually absent and their presence may suggest disseminated gonococcaemia, pyelonephritis, orchitis or other infection. Gonococcal, chlamydial and mycoplasmal infections may also have associated arthritis, conjunctivitis, proctitis, prostatitis, epididymo-orchitis, pneumonia, otitis media, low back pain, iritis and skin rash. The disease usually resolves without complication, even if untreated, but in rare cases can result in urethral stricture, stenosis or abscess formation.

Female urethritis/cervicitis

Urinary tract infections are more common in women because of the short urethra and the proximity to the anus, but the short length of the female urethra makes female urethritis less common. However, young women in their reproductive years are at risk from the same pathogens that affect the male, with a clinical presentation of dysuria, frequency and urgency. Risk factors include age < 20 years, multiple sexual partners and a prior history of STD.

Cervicitis, inflammation of the uterine cervix, can be regarded as the 'silent partner' of urethritis in males: although it occurs with similar frequency, it is more difficult to recognize. It is caused by the same sexually transmitted organisms, *C. trachomatis*, *N. gonorrhoeae*, *Trichomonal vaginalis* and Herpes simplex virus. Non-infectious causes include local trauma, malignancy and exposure to radiation. There is some overlap between the syndromes of vulvo-vaginitis and cervicitis, and an abnormal cervical discharge is usually interpreted by the patient as an abnormal vaginal discharge – cervicitis may accompany vaginitis due to *Candida albicans* or *Trichomonas vaginalis*, but cervicitis without vaginitis is caused primarily by *N. gonorrhoeae*, *C. trachomatis* or Herpes simplex virus. Gonorrhoeal, chlamydial and *T. vaginalis* cervical infections are often completely asymptomatic. When symptoms are present, they are often non-specific: increased vaginal discharge, dysuria, urinary frequency and intermenstrual or postcoital bleeding. Long-standing infections may present with lower abdominal or lower back pain. Complications from untreated infectious cervicitis depend on the pathogen, and include pelvic inflammatory disease, infertility, ectopic pregnancy, spontaneous abortion, cervical cancer, premature rupture of the membranes and preterm delivery. Perinatal and neonatal infections can cause mental retardation, blindness, low birth weight, stillbirth, meningitis and death.

Gonorrheal disease

Gonorrhea ('The Clap') is a disease that causes purulent inflammation of the mucous membranes that is sexually transmitted by the organism *Neisseria gonorrhoeae*. Virtually any mucous membrane can be infected. Gonococcal urethritis has been described in the earliest writings of recorded history: Hippocrates (460–377BC) is credited with the first scientific observations, describing dissected infected urethrae. Galen (AD 129–210) used the word *gonorrhoea*, which literally means 'a flow of semen'. It

is still a major cause of morbidity worldwide, with 200 million new cases per year reported internationally; many cases and contacts remain undiagnosed or under-reported and the prevalence is therefore thought to be greater. The disease occurs in all age groups, but most often in sexually active young adults. In the US, over 80% of reported cases occur in the 15–29-year age group, with significant clustering in the 20–24-year-old group. The level of risk increases with the number of sex partners and in the presence of other STDs. The risk of acquiring active disease after exposure is mediated by the individual's immune status, antigenic composition of the organism and the infectious dose of the particular strain. As with other lower genital tract infections, the affected individual is also at risk of acquiring other STDs, including HIV. Gonococcal infections are 1.5 times more common in men than in women, but serious sequelae are much more common in women, in particular pelvic inflammatory disease (PID), ectopic pregnancy and infertility. Disseminated infection is also more common in women.

Neisseria gonorrhea

Neisseria gonorrhoeae, or **gonococcus (GC)** belongs to the family *Neisseriaceae*. It is a gram-negative, non-spore forming, non-motile diplococcus that is flattened on one side, giving it the appearance of a 'kidney bean' or 'coffee bean'. The organisms can frequently be seen in pairs, with the flattened sides adjacent to each other. They have no capsule, but have hair-like filaments, **pili**, that are associated with the virulence of the genital strain. The presence of pili seems to influence the bacterium's ability to adhere to sperm, and this might facilitate the spread of disease through the male and female reproductive tracts (Hosseinzadeh *et al.*, 2000). Gonococci inhabit mucous membranes of the human urogenital, alimentary and respiratory tracts in humans, their only natural host. Some *Neisseriacea* can be found as normal flora in the naso- and oro-pharynx.

Life cycle

When the organisms come into contact with stratified columnar epithelium of the cervix, conjunctiva, pharyngeal surface, anorectal area or male urethra, adherence to the mucosal cells is mediated by an outer membrane protein (Protein II) and by the pili. An IgA1 protease also facilitates attachment. The bacteria penetrate columnar epithelium through the intercellular spaces and multiply in subepithelial connective tissue, releasing a lipooligosaccharide (LOS) that attracts polymorphonuclear leukocytes (PMNs). Together with host complement components, this induces a severe acute inflammatory response. Both pili and Protein II also mediate attachment to the PMNs and the organisms are eventually phagocytosed and killed. Clinically, this process is manifested by a 2 to 8-day incubation period followed by sudden onset of fever, abdominal pain, burning and frequency of urination and a purulent creamy-yellow discharge. The extent of the phagocytic process influences subsequent invasion or cure.

Expression of pili is turned on and off genetically, and the genes have variable domains. The antigenically variable domains of pili are coded by dominant genes and are not associated with attachment. Conserved recessive regions are critically involved in adherence. Intragenic recombination and gene conversion cause antigenic variation in pili, so that each gonococcal cell carries different DNA sequences representing portions of the pilus that vary among the different possible antigenic types. The high frequency of antigenic variation is responsible for antigenic heterogeneity and numerous types of pili among strains. This property gives the gonococcus a mechanism of evading host immune response, allowing it to cause repeated infection in the same host.

Transmission

Transmission of gonococcus is exclusively by exogenous routes, either by sexual contact (including oral, genital and anal) or from an infected pregnant mother to the newborn. Pharyngeal infections are generally seen following receptive oral intercourse. Anal infections are seen in both male and female patients following receptive anal intercourse, but females may have rectal involvement via autoinoculation from a primary genital infection in the absence of anal penetration. Conjunctivitis in adults can occur as a result of autoinoculation or transfer of infected genital secretions via fingers and hands. Neonatal infections are commonly ocular or genital, following direct contact with infected maternal cervical secretions during parturition. Transmission from fomites (such as toilet seats) does not occur, as gonococci are highly susceptible to chemical and physical agents and are rapidly destroyed in the environment.

Virulence factors

Outer membrane proteins (OMP)

Three **outer membrane proteins** (**OMP**) have been studied extensively:

Protein I

Protein I, the major OMP, varies antigenically between different strains, and functions as a porin in complex with Protein III. A porin is an OMP trimer that forms channels (pores) that allow small molecular weight solutes to diffuse across the outer membrane. They resist passage of large molecules, and may contribute to the organism's resistance to antimicrobial agents. Gonococci that contain high molecular weight Protein I molecules are associated with primary genital disease, and are serum sensitive. Serum-resistant organisms are more often associated with disseminated disease; these organisms contain low molecular weight Protein I.

Protein II

Protein II mediates attachment to host cells, along with pili, and has the capacity to undergo extensive antigenic variation; this contributes to evasion of immune response and the risk of recurrent infection. Protein II is present in opaque gonococcal colonies and is sometimes referred to as the 'opacity protein'.

Protein III

Protein III forms a porin complex with Protein I. It also seems to be the binding site for IgG blocking antibody: this feature prevents complement-mediated antibody function, thus contributing to disease dissemination. Protein III does not display antigenic diversity or variation.

Lipooligosaccharide (LOS)

Lipooligosaccharide (LOS) is a major gonococcal component, released during multiplication and autolysis. It attracts polymorphonuclear leukocytes to the primary site of infection, and has been implicated as a potential cause of fallopian tube damage. LOS may also contribute to other toxic manifestations of the disease such as joint inflammation in cases of gonococcal arthritis. The molecule has short, non-repeat O-antigenic side chains that differ antigenically in different gonococcal strains, and sialic acid on the LOS makes the microbes more resistant to the killing action of human serum. Experimentally, sialylation of LOS has been shown to occur on gonococci incubated with human PMNs and on gonococci present within PMNs from male urethral exudates. The sialylated LOS may be antigenically similar to antigens present on human erythrocytes, and this similarity to 'self' may interfere with an effective immune response to these LOS antigens.

Harvey *et al.* (2000) proposed that the asialoglycoprotein receptor (ASGP-R) on human sperm serves as a binding and attachment site for *N. gonorrhoeae*, with LOS as the complementary ligand on the bacterium.

IgA1 protease

IgA1 protease produced by the organism inactivates local secretory IgA, and thus may play a role in facilitating gonococcal adherence to mucosal surfaces.

Clinical presentation

Infection of the lower genital tract is the most common clinical presentation, acute urethritis in the male and endocervicitis in the female. Both present with purulent discharge, dysuria, bleeding and pain. Asymptomatic infection occurs in about 10% of males and 20–80% of females, and these asymptomatic individuals are communicable and capable of developing disseminated disease. Infection of the pharynx, rectum and female urethra also occur frequently, but these are less likely to be symptomatic. Vulvo-vaginitis occurs in children aged 2–8 following sexual abuse. The incubation period averages 2–5 days, but may be as long as 2–3 weeks. Those men who develop signs and symptoms after the incubation period have an abrupt onset of severe dysuria followed by thick purulent exudate at the urethral meatus; unfortunately, this presentation occurs in only approximately 40% of cases, and asymptomatic urethral carriage is an important mode of disease transmission. Symptomatic and asymptomatic disease may be associated with different strains of the organism. Ascending infection or systemic spread results in more serious clinical syndromes:

(i) In the female, infection spreads in 20% of cases from primary foci in the cervix or urethra to the fallopian tubes and pelvic peritoneum, causing pelvic inflammatory disease with salpingitis, endometritis and tubo-ovarian abscess. Further retrograde spread can lead to abdominal peritonitis and a perihepatitis known as Fitz-Hugh Curtis syndrome: the liver capsule becomes infected, with subsequent adhesions and pain.

(ii) In the male, the infection spreads from the anterior to the posterior urethra and Cowper's glands; subsequent fibrosis can lead to urethral strictures. Gonococcal urethritis can spread to the prostate and epididymis, causing prostatitis, epididymitis or epididymo-orchitis. Fibrotic obstruction following the infection can result in obstructive azoospermia.

(iii) Direct inoculation of organisms by perinatal transmission (*Ophthalmia Neonatorum*) or hand–eye contact in adults can cause conjunctivitis, and this can lead to blindness. Prophylaxis for neonatal eye infection is a routine in most parts of the developed world.

(iv) Disseminated gonococcal infection (DGI) occurs in approximately 1% of all patients, most frequently in those with asymptomatic genital infection. Three-fourths of the cases occur in women, who are more susceptible if the primary mucosal infection occurs during menstruation or pregnancy. Changes in the vaginal environment at these times may influence surface features and phenotype of the gonococcus, making it more resistant to host defences in the bloodstream and allowing dissemination. Strains of GC isolated from DGI, in contrast to those that produce only primary or invasive disease, have surface Protein III binding sites for IgG blocking antibody. This prevents complement-mediated bactericidal antibody function, making these strains resistant to killing by normal serum.

Gonococci usually invade the circulation from primary genital sites, but occasionally from secondary sites. A deficiency of complement factors C5–C8 predisposes to bacteremia and the resulting septicemia is exacerbated by toxic effects of LOS, causing chills, fever, malaise, arthralgia and a characteristic rash of petechial or papular skin lesions with central necrosis. The organism can invade joints to cause arthritis and tenosynovitis. *N. gonorrhoeae* bacteremia is the number one cause of monoarticular arthritis, usually affecting the knee joint, in teenagers and young adults. Females are more commonly affected and there is an association between the syndrome and HLA-B27 genotype. Rarely, dissemination from the circulation can also reach the heart valves and meninges to cause endocarditis and meningitis, which, if unrecognized and untreated are usually fatal.

The most common long-term sequelae of gonorrhea are: (i) chronic pelvic pain following PID, (ii) septic abortion and chorioamnionitis in pregnancy, (iii) infertility in both males and females and (iv) blindness after neonatal or adult conjunctivitis.

Laboratory diagnosis

Gonorrheal disease is caused by a variety of strains of the organism. These strains are antigenically distinct, have variable nutrition requirements and differ in their virulence and distribution within the population. The bacteria are strict aerobes and are oxidase-positive. Commensals do not require enriched media and grow at room temperature, whereas pathogens are very fastidious, require enriched media and grow at body temperature.

Specimen collection and transport

Pathogenic *Neisseria* are sensitive to drying and to extremes of temperature: specimens for lab diagnosis must therefore be fastidiously collected. The type of specimen depends upon the disease process: correct choice of specimen is critical to successful isolation and identification of the organism. Exudate samples may be taken from urethra, endocervix, rectum, pharynx and conjunctiva. In cases of DGI, samples should be cultured from blood, skin scrapings, joint fluid and cerebrospinal fluid. Specimens from potential sites of infection should be cultured for both gonorrhea and chlamydia and the possibility of other STDs should be considered.

N. gonorrhoeae is sensitive to SPS (sodium polyanetholsulfonate) found in blood culture bottles: these should contain no more than 0.025% SPS. The organism is sensitive to cold; body fluids should be left at room temperature or placed in a 37 °C incubator before plating.

Female patients in whom asymptomatic infection or primary or invasive genital disease is suspected should have specimens cultured from the cervix and from the rectum. Rectal and pharyngeal specimens must be obtained when a history of oral and/or anal sex is elicited.

- Swabs are acceptable if the specimen is plated within 6 hours. Cotton swabs contain fatty acids that are toxic to *N. gonorrhoeae*; if cotton swabs are used the transport medium should contain charcoal to inhibit the toxic fatty acids. Calcium alginate or rayon swabs are preferred.
- Ideally, specimens should be plated immediately, using a JEMBEC system. This consists of a tray

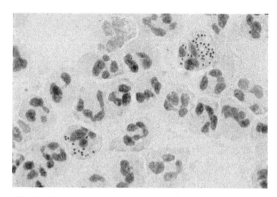

Fig. 10.1. Gram-stain preparation of *Neisseria gonorrhoeae* in a cervical specimen demonstrating gram-negative intracellular cocci with characteristic kidney bean shape. In male urethral exudates this provides a presumptive diagnosis for gonococcus infection, but in a woman this requires additional confirmation to rule out potential normal vaginal flora that may have a similar appearance on Gram-stain.

containing modified Thayer–Martin agar, a CO_2 generating system and zip-lock container for the medium. The JEMBEC system is transported to the laboratory at room temperature. In the laboratory, the plate should be streaked for isolation and incubated at 35 °C in 5% CO_2.

Direct detection: Gram stain

Gram-stained preparations containing *N. gonorrhea* demonstrate acute inflammatory cell exudates with intra- and extracellular gram-negative diplococci. The organisms are described as 'kidney bean shaped' with flattened adjacent sides (Fig. 10.1).

The direct detection of organisms in Gram-stained material is very insensitive, requiring a microbial concentration of about 1×10^6 per ml of sample for detection. Therefore, fluids that are normally sterile should first be concentrated by centrifugation in order to increase the level of sensitivity. Gram-stain smears can be equivocal and direct detection of characteristic gram-negative intracellular diplococci within PMNs can only be considered diagnostic in the appropriate clinical context, in urethral exudates of males with the characteristic clinical manifestations. Gram-stains of smears

from female urethral and cervical exudates, from rectal, pharyngeal and conjunctival exudates and from asymptomatic patients are unreliable, as other nonpathogenic organisms with similar morphology may be present. All such specimens must be cultured for identification of the isolated organism. In patients with DGI, gram-negative intracellular diplococci can be demonstrated in 30–50% of smears from skin scrapings, joint fluid and CSF. This must be differentiated from the meningococcal *Neisseria* by culture and biochemistry.

Antigen detection

An enzyme-linked immunosorbent assay (ELISA) is available to detect gonococcal antigen in urethral and endocervical discharge. Results from ELISA are available more rapidly than from culture but the result is only presumptive, as it may cross-react with saprophytic *Neisseria*.

Culture

Culture is about ten times more sensitive than direct examination in detecting infection. *N. gonorrhoea* requires enriched chocolate agar formulations for growth on primary culture, often supplemented with antibiotics to inhibit the growth of flora. Thayer–Martin medium is one selective agar that is used to inhibit normal flora in genital specimens. This medium contains:

colistin to inhibit gram-negative organisms,
anisomycin to inhibit yeasts,
vancomycin to inhibit gram-positive organisms,
trimethoprim to inhibit swarming *Proteus*.

Some *N. gonorrhoea* strains are inhibited by the concentration of vancomycin in selective media. New York City Medium (contains lysed horse blood, horse plasma, yeast dialysate and the same antibiotics as MTM) can also be used. NYC medium has the advantage of also supporting the growth of *Mycoplasma hominis* and *Ureaplasma urealyticum*. Samples are initially incubated on Thayer–Martin or other selective media (MTM, NYC medium, or Martin–Lewis agar) for 48 hours at 35–37 °C under

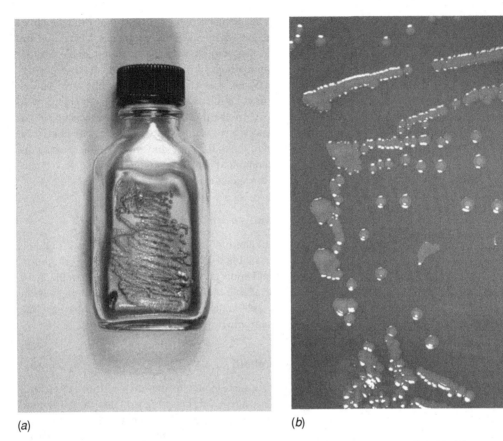

(a) (b)

Fig. 10.2. (a) *Neisseria gonorrhoeae* colony morphology in a Transgrow bottle (a) and (b) on Thayer–Martin Medium.
N. gonorrhoeae has very fastidious growth requirements, and The Transgrow bottle (a) is designed so that the sample can be plated directly onto agar at the patient's bedside. Antibiotics in the selective chocolate-based media inhibit the majority of normal flora in a genital specimen. Close inspection of colonies on Thayer–Martin medium (b) demonstrates moist grey colonies typical of gonococcus.

aerobic conditions in the presence of 3–10% carbon dioxide. Colonies on these selective chocolate agars are small, transparent or grey-white, convex, translucent and glistening with either smooth or irregular margins (Fig. 10.2(a), (b)); there may be up to five different colony types on a primary plate.

- Colony types 1 and 2 are small, raised, moist, have pili and are virulent.
- Types 3, 4, 5 are larger, lack pili and are non-virulent.

Some gonococci are arginine, hypoxanthine and uracil (AHU) deficient, and require these three fac-tors for growth. Suspicious colonies are selected for biochemical testing, including spot catalase and oxidase, both of which are positive for gono-cocci. The RapID NH system (Innovative Diagnos-tic Systems, Inc., Atlanta, GA) or other commer-cially available biochemical identification panels may be used to definitively differentiate *Neisse-ria*, *Haemophilus*, *Moraxella*, *Kingella* species and other related gram-negative bacteria. The RapID NH panel utilizes microbial reactivity to 12 different sub-strates or sugars to provide definitive identification. *N. gonorrhoeae* is very biochemically inert and in this system reliably produces positive reactions only for proline p-nitroanilide hydrolysis and glucose utilization. Many laboratories additionally confirm isolate identification using GC-specific RNA probe testing with an assay such as the Genprobe GC probe. This non-amplified molecular assay detects GC-specific nucleic acids directly from colonies chosen from selective media and provides a very specific identification required for medical legal cases such as child abuse and rape.

Molecular diagnostic testing

Because of the fastidious nature of *N. gonorrhoeae*, culture is no longer considered to be the most efficient or sensitive method to detect infections. Both amplified and non-amplified molecular assays are available that can identify GC directly from clinical specimens. The first molecular diagnostic test to be widely used was Gen-Probe PACE 2C (San Diego, CA), with a sensitivity of about 1×10^4 organisms per aliquot tested. This assay uses a ribosomal target and is therefore at least ten times more sensitive than other probe assays that use DNA targets. It is approved for testing urethral and cervical swabs, but not first void urines. The sensitivity of amplified molecular assays reaches one organism in the aliquot tested and these methods have largely replaced the non-amplified probe assays as the tests of choice. PCR (Amplicore PCR Assay, Roche Diagnostics, Indianapolis, IN), strand displacement amplification (BD ProbeTek ET, BD Biosciences, Sparks, MD) and transcription mediated amplification (Gen-Probe, San Diego, CA) are all commercially available for use on direct specimens. Some of these assays may also be used to detect GC in first void urine specimens, as well as in urethral and cervical swabs that are more invasive to obtain. However, first void urines may not be approved specimens for some assay systems if the patient is asymptomatic. This information is crucial if the test is used to screen semen donors for asymptomatic GC infections. Non-genital sources should be tested with caution, since they may cross-react with non-gonococcal *Neisseria* species. The ultimate choice of amplified assay should also take into consideration the required sensitivity, specificity and other issues specific to each laboratory, such as work-flow, logistics and technology.

Treatment

Antibiotic treatment should be initiated as soon as possible, if necessary even before the complete laboratory evaluation is available. The signs and symptoms of gonococcal urethritis/cervicitis overlap with those of chlamydial infection, and the latter is also found frequently in patients with gonorrhoea; therefore empiric antibiotic therapy should be aimed towards treating both infections. Until several years ago, gonorrhoea was treated with penicillin injections or oral therapy for up to 10 days. Antigenic shifts with redistribution of strain types has resulted in a progressive increase in antibiotic resistance, due to both genetic and plasmid-mediated mechanisms in response to antibiotic treatment. Plasmids that carry antibiotic-resistance genes have been well characterized. The exchange of surface protein genes means that infection prompts a polyantigenic host immune response, and this generally fails to provide long-term protection against genital reinfection. The exchange of antibiotic resistance genes has led to extremely high levels of resistance to beta-lactam (penicillin) antibiotics, with the emergence of penicillinase-producing *N. gonorrhoea* (PPNG) during the early 1980s. Fluoroquinolone resistance has also been documented more recently on multiple continents. Treatment regimes now recommended by the CDC in the US are based upon the rapid development of PPNG, as well as the high frequency of co-existing chlamydial infections.

Uncomplicated urethritis, cervicitis, or proctitis

250 mg ceftriaxone IM in a single injection, plus 100 mg doxycycline p.o. ii qd $\times$ 7 days as first-line therapy.

Spectinomycin 2g IM in a single dose may be used for patients who do not tolerate ceftriaxone.

For pregnant women: 500 mg erythromycin p.o. iv qd × 7 days is recommended as a substitute for doxycycline.

Uncomplicated pharyngitis

The ceftriaxone régime is recommended for uncomplicated pharyngitis, but 500 mg ciprofloxacin as a single oral dose may be substituted.

Patients with DGI

Require admission to hospital and aggressive IM or IV therapy with either ceftriaxone, ceftizoxime, or cefotaxime. Spectinomycin may be used if the patient is allergic to the other antibiotics.

Infants and children

Ceftriaxone or cefotaxime is recommended, in doses depending on the disease process and the weight of the child.

Gonococcal ophthalmia neonatorum

Instillation of 0.5% erythromycin, 1% tetracycline, or 1% silver nitrate into the conjunctiva of newborns at birth is required by law in the USA as prophylactic treatment.

Information and patient counselling should emphasize the use of condoms to avoid future STDs and unwanted pregnancies and the patient should be encouraged to abstain from sexual activity until full treatment is completed. All sexual partners should be tested and treated. Patients with epididymitis, PID and DGI may also require medication for pain relief, as well as referral to appropriate specialists for follow-up. In cases of arthritis, aspiration of purulent joint effusions may speed recovery of affected joints. Every patient presenting with gonococcal conjunctivitis should be urgently referred to an ophthalmologist, as this disease can progress rapidly with permanent loss of vision.

Vaccine availability

The gonococcus is a complex organism that infects only humans. Development of an effective vaccine has been hampered by the lack of a suitable animal model for gonococcal disease. Although experimental vaccines are under development, vaccine trials to prevent gonorrhea have thus far met with little success. Strategies for producing a vaccine include using the bacterial surface proteins to elicit an IgA response in order to prevent adherence and colonization. However, the gonococcus has a remarkable ability to protect itself by changing or mutating: it varies its surface antigens, as well as turning them on/off, so that the original IgA response becomes obsolete. As a result, immunity is incomplete and an individual may experience repeated infections with GC.

Chlamydial disease

Chlamydial infection is the most common bacterial sexually transmitted disease in industrialized countries, occurring mostly in young men and women under the age of 25. In women, it is the most frequent cause of PID, and can also infect the cervix, urethra, Bartholin's gland ducts, fallopian tubes and rectum. Disease can also be transmitted to the newborn baby via an infected birth canal. In men, chlamydial infection is an important cause of non-specific/non-gonococcal urethritis (NSU/NGU), epididymitis and Reiter's syndrome (urethritis/arthritis/conjunctivitis).

Recurrent or persistent infection is common, with greater tissue damage and scarring than results from initial infection. In 1996, it was estimated that there are 50–70 million new cases of *C. trachomatis* infection worldwide annually (Paavonen & Lehtinen, 1996). Many men and women who are infected do not experience any symptoms, and there is therefore a large reservoir of unrecognized infected individuals capable of transmitting the infection to their sexual partners. Undiagnosed and untreated infections in women can have considerable consequences, increasing the risk for PID, tubal infertility, ectopic pregnancy and post-partum fever.

Chlamydia trachomatis

Chlamydia infections are caused by the bacterium *Chlamydia trachomatis*: the word *chlamys* is Greek for 'cloak draped around the shoulder', which describes the appearance of its intracytoplasmic inclusions 'draped' around the infected cell nucleus. The infections are often latent, persistent and inapparent; disease manifestation depends upon an interaction between host cell defence mechanisms and persistent low levels of chlamydial replication. *Chlamydiae* have the appearance of small gram-negative cocci, but they are obligate intracellular parasites and therefore were originally thought to be viruses. However, like true bacteria, they contain both RNA and DNA as well as 70S ribosomes, with a genome size of 500–1000 kilobases. They are primarily energy parasites, highly adapted to intracellular life; the organisms shut down host cell macromolecular synthesis and divert host substrates to the synthesis of chlamydial proteins and lipids. They have a unique cell wall containing cysteine-rich proteins instead of peptidoglycan, and an outer lipopolysaccharide membrane. This cell wall structure contributes to the organism's virulence by inhibiting phagolysosome fusion in lysosomes. Because of their unique developmental cycle, these microorganisms have been classified into a separate order, *Chlamydiales*, with one family, *Chlamydiaceaea*, containing one genus, *Chlamydia*. There are three species, differing in their tissue tropism and spectrum of diseases: *C. trachomatis, C. psittaci and C. pneumoniae*.

C. trachomatis, the organism responsible for disease of the reproductive tract, has at least 15 different serotypes that interact serologically: the host serological response is complex and the presence of antibodies does not appear to be protective. It is responsible for four major diseases in humans:

  (i) endemic trachoma that can lead to blindness: serotypes A, B, Ba and C;
  (ii) sexually transmitted disease: serotypes D through K;

  (iii) inclusion conjunctivitis associated with STD, that does not lead to blindness: serotypes D through K;
  (iv) lymphogranuloma venereum: serotypes L1, L2, and L3.

Life cycle

The organism initiates colonization by attaching to sialic acid receptors on the genitalia, throat or eye. It has a special preference for columnar epithelial cells, but can also survive and persist in macrophages and at body sites that are inaccessible to phagocytes, T-cells and B-cells. Its life cycle consists of two stages.

Elementary body (EB)

A small, infectious, metabolically inactive form with a rigid outer membrane adapted for surviving outside the cell. This is the dispersal form, approximately 0.3 μm in diameter, analogous to a spore. It is relatively impermeable and resistant to sonication or trypsin treatment as methods of disinfection. In vitro, EBs will adhere to human spermatozoa (Wølner-Hanssen & Mardh, 1984) and can penetrate the tail structure (Erbengi, 1993).

Reticulate body (RB)

A larger, metabolically active intracellular replicating form that is non-infectious and unstable outside of the cell. This structure divides actively by binary fission. Reticulate bodies are more permeable, and are sensitive to sonication and trypsin treatment (Fig. 10.3). Ultrastructural studies demonstrate that both elementary and reticulate bodies can be found in the sperm nucleus after in vitro co-incubation with *C. trachomatis* (Erbengi, 1993).

The elementary body (EB) is adapted for extracellular survival and for establishing infection, but does not produce ATP as source of energy: therefore it cannot reproduce outside a cell. During the infectious phase, the EB adheres to mucosal epithelium,

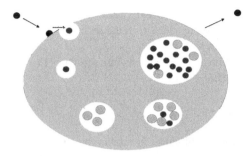

● Elementary body (infective phase)
● Reticulate body (replicative phase)

Fig. 10.3. Cartoon demonstrating the *Chlamydia* life cycle. The infective elementary body binds to the cell surface and is internalized in a phagocytic vacuole. Inside the vacuole, the elementary body converts into the replicative reticulate body, which reproduces by binary fission. Reticulate bodies are converted to elementary bodies, and new infective particles are released when the cell lyses 2–3 days later.

attaching to sialic acid receptors. This induces endocytosis in its target cells, where it is uncoated and loses its infectivity. EBs direct the fusion of lysosomes, so that they lie in a host-derived vacuole, protected from the action of lysozyme. Endocytosis and growth within the vacuole do not incite phagolysosomal fusion, which normally forms the basis for the subsequent killing of any foreign agent directed against the cell's integrity. Therefore, *Chlamydiae* escape the normal cellular defence mechanisms and are able to survive intracellularly. Once inside the cell, the EB enlarges over a period of approximately 12 hours and uses EB polymerase to produce mRNA and form the metabolically active Reticulate Body. The phagosome moves centripetally towards the host cell nucleus, where the RB undergoes binary fission to form other RBs during the next 2–3 hours. After division, the RBs condense to form EBs + intermediate stages and these EBs are further replaced by RBs. The mature intracellular inclusions release infectious EBs within 36–48 hours after the initial infection, with sequential damage to the host cell membrane, until the cell ruptures. One phagolysosome usually produces 100–1000 elementary bodies (Fig. 10.3).

Transmission

C. trachomatis infects mainly mucosal membranes of the urethra, cervix, rectum, throat and conjunctiva. The organism is transmitted via transfer of infected secretions and although transmission is most often seen as an STD, it can also occur through direct non-sexual contact. Transmission is most efficient via heterosexual or male homosexual contact; it is not easily spread among women. Transmission from an infected mother to the neonate may occur during parturition: *C. trachomatis* may be directly inoculated into the mucosa of the eyes, oropharynx, genital tract, urethra and rectum.

Clinical presentation

Symptoms are very variable and infection is frequently asymptomatic: 70–80% of women and 25–50% of men with chlamydia show no symptoms at all. In women, infection usually begins at the cervix and symptoms include vaginal discharge, dysuria, vulval irritation, bleeding after sexual intercourse, lower abdominal pain and abnormal vaginal bleeding. Women with endocervical infections have a high risk of developing ascending infections during uterine instrumentation such as hysterosalpingography (HSG), hydrotubation and hysteroscopy (Land *et al.*, 2002; Thomas & Simms, 2002), and these interventions can also reactivate a latent infection from past disease. Statistics indicate that one chlamydial infection can lead to a 12% risk of infertility, two infections can lead to 40% risk, and three infections increases the risk of infertility to 80%.

Symptoms in men can resemble those of gonococcal urethritis, including mild dysuria that sometimes resolves without treatment, clear, white or yellow urethral discharge, tingling or itching sensations, hemospermia or proctitis. Chronic infection may remain after the symptoms resolve and untreated infection can lead to fever, testicular pain and swelling and epididymitis. Subsequent scarring can lead to infertility.

Infection in men and women can also spread to the eyes to cause conjunctivitis and transmission from mother to infant during labour can cause trachoma in the infant; scarring from this disease can ultimately lead to blindness.

Laboratory diagnosis

Chlamydiae are extremely temperature sensitive: specimens for diagnosis must be kept at 4 °C as soon as the sample is obtained.

Staining

Chlamydia's cell wall lacks the peptidoglycan that reacts with Gram-stain; they stain very poorly and therefore this is not the diagnostic stain of choice for these organisms. A Gram-stain of genital secretions from women with chlamydial infections will demonstrate an acute inflammatory exudate, which is a non-specific finding. A neutrophilic inflammatory cell exudate seen in a PAP stain of cervical specimens may serve as an initial indication of *C. trachomatis* infection. Infected epithelial cells with the characteristic intracellular cytoplasmic vacuole harboring the replicating bacteria may be detected in the PAP smear (Fig. 10.4). A systematic study of these inclusions as indicators for chlamydial infection showed that their detection was only 8.3% sensitive, and the majority of culture positive cases were missed (Arroyo *et al.*, 1989). Inter-observer variation in interpretation is a problem; many cytologists are reluctant to interpret these inclusions as chlamydia-specific and report non-specific inflammatory changes without comment as to the etiology.

Direct fluorescence antibody (DFA) staining of cervical specimens with antibodies specific to either major outer membrane protein (MOMP) or lipopolysaccharide (LPS) provides a more specific and sensitive method for chlamydial detection. A fixed direct specimen slide stained with the fluorescently labelled monoclonal antibody is examined under fluorescence microscopy. MOMP antibodies are used to detect the *C. trachomatis*-specific elementary bodies and LPS reagent detects chlamydial species. These assays require interpretation by a skilled and experienced microscopist for optimal

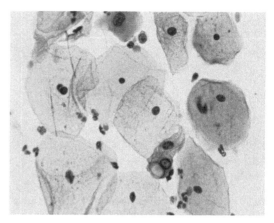

Fig. 10.4. Intracytoplasmic inclusions of *Chlamydia trachomatis* in a PAP smear. Chlamydia-infected cells in a PAP smear contain one or more prominent intracytoplasmic vacuoles, which are the replicative vacuoles that shelter the organism prior to cell lysis. This finding may be non-specific, and culture is required for a definitive diagnosis.

sensitivity and specificity, and have been largely replaced by molecular diagnostic assays.

Enzyme Immunoassays (EIA)

Several LPS-based enzyme immunoassays to detect chlamydial infections have been developed. These assays are generally based on anti-LPS antibody-coated microwell plates. Urine sediments or swab eluates are incubated in the microwell to allow for protein binding and LPS is demonstrated by indirect immunoperoxidase staining using a second anti-LPS antibody. The sensitivity of most EIAs is in the range of 10^5 to 10^7 organisms/ml, at least ten-fold less sensitive than the probe assays targeted at non-amplified ribosomal RNA. Positive results using this assay may be confirmed by DFA in order to improve the specificity of the assay.

Culture

Chlamydia trachomatis is cultured by using the shell vial assay or a 96-well McCoy cell culture plate. Specimens are slowly centrifuged over the cell monolayer at the start of the culture and the cells are fixed and

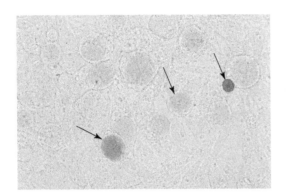

Fig. 10.5. Culture of *C. trachomatis* in a McCoy's shell vial assay. Chlamydiae are obligate intracellular parasites that require a host cell to provide energy, and culture can be accomplished in a cell culture system similar to that used for growing viruses. McCoy's cells are used for *C. trachomatis* culture. Intracytoplasmic inclusions (arrows) may be demonstrated after about 48 hours; starch produced by the organism is stained with iodine in this slide. A lytic phase will be seen every 72 hours, so timing of the review is important in order to visualize the infected cells before they lyse.

stained after 48–72 hours of incubation at 35–37 °C. A direct fluorescent antibody against MOMP specifically identifies *Chlamydia trachomatis* cytoplasmic inclusions; anti-LPS antibodies can be used for a more sensitive stain. Other non-specific stains such as Giemsa or iodine that stain the starch also present in these vacuoles (Fig. 10.5) have a much lower sensitivity and are no longer recommended for routine use. A lytic phase in *C. trachomatis* growth occurs between 72 and 96 hours and therefore the timing of the culture is important. Cell lysis destroys the cells; staining the monolayer after lysis will give a false negative result. The sensitivity of the culture technique can be improved by blind passaging primary cultures onto new monolayers, essentially increasing the number of infected cells following a first lytic amplification of the organism.

Serology

Serology is of little value in making a diagnosis of acute chlamydial infections and should not be used in screening for the disease. Serology may, however be used to determine past exposure in individuals undergoing evaluation of infertility. Chlamydial antibodies have a long half-life, but different types of serological assays may demonstrate cross-reactivity between the different chlamydial species that can cause disease in man. It is estimated that antibodies to *C. psittacci* and *C. pneumoniae* account for up to half of the chlamydia-specific antibodies detected in the indirect fluorescent antibody (IFA) and EIA assays currently available commercially.

Molecular diagnostics

Molecular detection of infection may be accomplished either by non-amplified or by amplified molecular techniques. The sensitivity of detection varies greatly, depending upon the type of test used. A non-amplified probe using ribosomal RNA targets (Gen-Probe PACE 2 Assay) was the first molecular assay to be used extensively in the detection of chlamydial disease. The sensitivity of this assay is in the rage of about 10^4 organisms/mL, much more sensitive than any of the direct exams or EIAs currently available. This assay is of approximately the same sensitivity as culture, but the Gen-Probe PACE 2 assay has the advantage of very good specimen stability characteristics. Culture requires fastidious attention to specimen transport and storage conditions to ensure a reliable diagnosis. Digene Hybrid Capture II assay uses a genomic DNA or plasmid DNA target, and likewise has the advantage that specimens remain stable for up to 7 days before testing is compromised.

Amplified molecular diagnostic assays (also called nucleic acid amplification tests or NAATs) are generally considered the most sensitive assays currently available for detecting infections with *C. trachomatis*. Theoretically, a single target RNA or DNA sequence can be detected in the specimen aliquot tested. There are three types of NAAT assays commercially available for the detection of *C. trachomatis* in cervical or urethral swabs and from first void urine sediments: polymerase chain reaction (PCR), strand displacement amplification and transcription-mediated amplification (TMA). The reported sensitivities for these assays exceed that of culture and the non-amplified probe assays all have a sensitivity greater than 90%. Disease can be detected equally from first void urine and from swab specimens. Although the amplification reaction may sometimes be inhibited in urine specimens, inhibited reactions are identified by internal positive controls in many of these assays. The assays also have high specificity, generally over 95%.

Screening

Screening for chlamydia is still a subject of debate, particularly in patients attending fertility clinics. Acute infection occurs mainly in women < 25 years of age, and subfertile women tend to be in an older age group. However, the vast majority of subfertile women will undergo invasive procedures either diagnostically or therapeutically, with risk of introducing ascending infection into the upper genital tract. Studies indicate that *C. trachomatis* may persist in a viable state in fallopian tubes for a long period, even several years after antibiotic treatment, and reactivation can therefore occur, possibly during uterine instrumentation (Patton *et al.*, 1994; Land *et al.*, 2002). The use of azithromycin in a single oral 1 g dose, 12 hours before the planned procedure, has therefore been encouraged as prophylaxis in subfertility patients who might be at risk of chlamydial reactivation. The risk of post-procedure PID in these women has been quoted in a range from 0.3–4% (Macmillan, 2002), and the risk is higher in the presence of tubal pathology. It has been suggested that prophylactic antibiotic cover is more effective than screen-and-treat in the population of patients undergoing induced abortion, but this strategy is not necessarily applicable to subfertility patients who are likely to undergo several diagnostic and therapeutic procedures. Furthermore, the issue of antibiotic resistance cannot be ignored: if the overall prevalence of genital tract chlamydial infection is low, blanket prophylaxis in cases of no relevant past history or tubal pathology may increase the problem of resistance and maintain the bacterial load of CT in the community. Screening of the lower genital tract by a sensitive test is recommended for:

- gamete donors,
- women <25 years of age,
- women >25 years with risk factors such as concurrent sexual partners or partners working in an STD endemic region,
- women with a current or past history of STD, PID, ectopic pregnancy or tubal factor infertility,
- men with risk factors.

In 1996, the Royal College of Obstetricians and Gynaecologists recommended that all women undergoing uterine instrumentation should be screened for chlamydial infection or be treated prophylactically with antibiotics. More recently, these guidelines have been updated to recommend screening for chlamydia prior to uterine instrumentation only in patients at risk, i.e. women < 25 years of age, but protection against upper genital tract infection should be considered in all women presenting for infertility investigations (Royal College of Obstetrics and Gynaecology, 2000). Controversy remains between screen-and-treat vs. prophylactic antibiotics (for review see debate: Land *et al.*, 2002; Thomas & Simms, 2002).

Treatment

Patient treatment is important in preventing disease complications and to prevent potential transmission to future sex partners. Infected pregnant women must be treated to prevent transmission to the neonate during parturition. Sex partners must also be evaluated and treated to prevent reinfection of additional transmission. Doxycycline (100 mg bd for 7 days) is the antibiotic of choice for patients in whom compliance is anticipated. Azithromycin 1 g p.o. has recently been proven as an effective single-dose therapy and should be considered equivalent to doxycycline in eliminating disease. Although it is more expensive than the other antibiotics, it does improve patient compliance as it may be administered as a directly observed therapy (the CDC recommends that the first dose of antibiotics should be directly observed, even for mutiple dose regimens). Since GC and CT may present with overlapping symptoms, patients receiving treatment without confirmation from testing should be treated with antibiotics to cover both infections.

Alternative regimens are considered to be less effective or are more costly. Although erythromycin is less effective than azithromycin or doxycycline, it is the recommended treatment during pregnancy (500 mg erythromycin base iv qd × 7 days) and for neonatal infections (erythromycin base or ethylsuccinate 50 mg/kg/day orally, divided into 4 daily doses for 14 days). Neonatal eye infections (*Ophthalmia neonatorum*) should be managed with the same systemic protocol and not with topical treatment.

Chlamydia infection is a sexually transmitted disease that is preventable and could be eradicated by implementing appropriate activities such as behavioural changes and consistent access to good quality health care. Important preventative measures include the use of condoms, delaying the age of first intercourse and monogamy. Treatment of all sexual contacts for identified cases is also important for infection control.

Vaccine availability

Research at Johns Hopkins University is directed towards developing a vaccine targetted towards a chlamydial cell wall exolipid antigen that induces a weak immune response. A protein version of the antigen was experimentally produced by injecting *C. trachomatis* into mice, isolating and amplifying the antibodies produced, and then using these antibodies to create a protein resembling the exoglyco-lipid antigen (Coghlan, 1996). The next step will be to adapt the procedure to humans.

Genital mollicutes

Mycoplasma and *ureaplasma* spp.

Mollicutes, 'soft skin' bacteria, are the smallest free-living microbes known, similar in size to the Poxvirus ($0.3 \times 0.7\ \mu$m). The mollicutes are ancestors of gram-positive anaerobes, derived from *Clostridia* spp. by gene deletion. Although they have a cell membrane, they lack a cell wall and thus do not retain the Gram stain. Therefore, despite their gram-positive heritage, they are considered neither gram-positive nor gram-negative, but are referred to as gram-null. Together with their very small size, this makes them extremely difficult to identify microscopically and by other conventional laboratory methods. The mollicutes are also extremely fastidious, preferring to grow under nearly anaerobic conditions; they require cholesterol and nucleic acid precursors in growth medium in order to detect proliferation. In liquid culture, growth produces little or no turbidity in the culture medium, and on solid medium they produce small colonies, only the largest of which can be detected by the unaided eye.

Several mollicutes have been identified that colonize or produce infection in the human genital tract:

Ureaplasma urealyticum	*Mycoplasma hominis*
M. genitalium	*M. spermatophilum*
M. penetrans	*M. primatum*
M. fermentans (M. incognitus)	

U. urealyticum and *M. hominis* are the mollicutes most commonly isolated from the human genitourinary tract. Infection is associated with sexual promiscuity, detected more often in women than men, more often in black people than in white people. Vaginal colonization is more frequent in sexually active women. *M. genitalium* is seen only as a colonizer in women, but it has been detected in men with prostatitis. *M. genitalium*, *M. penetrans* and *M. fermentans* have been identified in association with HIV infection, and have a questionable association with a more rapid progression of HIV to AIDS. Co-incubation of sperm with *U. urealyticum* leads to a reduction in human sperm motility, possibly due to increased sperm death. Overnight incubation of sperm with *U. urealyticum* and *M. hominis* has also been shown to have an effect on sperm physiology, including expression of hyperactivated motility, the ability to undergo ionophore-induced acrosome reaction (Rose & Scott, 1994), and their ability to penetrate zona-free hamster oocytes. It has also been reported that *U. urealyticum* can cause premature chromatin decondensation and sperm DNA damage without an apparent loss of sperm viability, and that men with infection ejaculate greater numbers of sperm showing evidence of apoptotic damage (Shang *et al.*, 1999, Reichert *et al.*, 2000).

Life cycle

Similar to other bacteria, the genital mollicutes reproduce by binary fission. Unlike their clostridial ancestors, the mollicutes do not produce spores.

Transmission

U. urealyticum and *M. hominis* are commensal colonizers of the genitourinary tract. Studies in pregnant women estimate that 15–25% are colonized with *M. hominis*, and 57–80% with *U. urealyticum*. They are known to be transmitted vertically *in utero* to the fetus during pregnancy and by direct contact with contaminated vaginal fluids during parturition. When the mother is known to be colonized, vertical transmission rates of from 26% to 66% have been reported (Dinsmoor *et al.*, 1989; Cassell *et al.*, 1991), with infants found to have positive cultures from the eye, throat, vagina and rectum. Although the route of vaginal colonization in adults is not known, the close association with sexual activity, particularly with increased numbers of sex partners, suggests that they might be sexually transmitted.

The mode of *M. penetrans* and *M. fermentans* transmission is unknown, although their linkage with HIV infection and with sexual activity suggests that these are also sexually transmitted diseases. *M. genitalium* has been identified in oral and genital secretions, suggesting that oral–genital contact has a role in its spread. *M. genitalium* is also associated with HIV infection, again suggesting sexual transmission.

Clinical presentation

Clinical presentations differ for each of the genital mollicutes and also differ markedly depending upon age and gender.

U. urealyticum causes significant disease in both males and females and can also cause disease in the fetus and neonate. In males, *U. urealyticum* has been shown to produce non-gonococcal urethritis, epididymitis and orchitis, but not prostatitis. Infection has also been linked with decreased sperm motility and abnormal sperm morphology, suggesting a role in male subfertility, although the topic remains controversial. *Ureaplasma* has been seen in cases of renal calculus formation, probably linked to the fact that the organism produces ureases that may initiate the formation of struvite and calcium phosphate crystals. In women, *U. urealyticum* is a commensal colonizer of the vagina in a large proportion of sexually active women. This organism does not play a role in the pathogenesis of bacterial vaginosis, but may be involved in mixed infections of the fallopian tubes and pelvis. It may play a role in the female urethral syndrome and has been strongly associated with post-partum and post-abortion sepsis and PID. The role of *Ureaplasma* infections in female subfertility is again tenuous, the main effect on female reproductive health being linked to fetal wastage and disease in the fetus and neonate. *U. urealyticum* has been associated with spontaneous abortions, chorioamnionitis, central nervous system infections and congenital and neonatal pneumonia. Several investigators have cultured *U. urealyticum* from spontaneously aborted fetuses, cases of fetal death *in utero* and in placentas or amniotic membranes. Infection during pregnancy has been linked to premature labor and premature rupture of the membranes. Infants with neonatal *Ureaplasma* infections are generally severely premature, have low birth weights and have a variety of disease manifestations. The vast burden of disease consists of pulmonary infections with the development of broncho-pulmonary dysplasia, although sepsis and meningitis have also been described, usually in association with a pulmonary infection. The majority of infants in whom *Ureaplasma* has been isolated are asymptomatically colonized, acquired via contact with contaminated vaginal secretions. It is therefore seen in children born by vaginal delivery following extended rupture of the membranes.

M. hominis demonstrates a very different constellation of disease in humans. *M. hominis* is not considered to be a pathogen in males and the bulk of disease is seen in women. This organism is known to proliferate in bacterial vaginosis and may cause vaginitis in prepubescent girls. *M. hominis* has been cultured from about 10% of cases of PID in which it has been sought, and has been isolated in pure culture from about 10% of women with post-partum or post-abortion fever. In the neonate, it can produce respiratory disease, meningitis and sepsis similar to *U. urealyticum*, but with a much lower frequency.

M. genitalium is an organism with limited pathogenicity. It has been demonstrated as a cause of non-gonococcal urethritis in males, but has not been shown to cause epididymitis or prostatitis. In women, the significance of vaginal colonization is unknown, and probably reflects asymptomatic colonization only. Similar to *U. urealyticum*, this organism does not appear to play a role in the pathogenesis of bacterial vaginosis.

M. fermentans, *M. penetrans* and *M. genitalium* have all been associated with HIV infections and may have a role in accelerating the progression of HIV to AIDS. This association is widely disputed, with some studies finding no direct evidence for a meaningful role in causing disease progression. Most of the data relies on the molecular detection of these organisms in genital and blood specimens.

M. spermatophilum was identified in semen samples from males attending an infertility clinic and is suspected to affect sperm motility and morphology (Hill, 1991).

Clinical diagnosis

Clinically, if a patient presents with symptoms and routine investigations fail to reveal the etiologic agent, infections with the genital mollicutes may be suspected. Circumstances in which infection should be suspected include cases of bacterial vaginosis (where *M. hominis* is known to proliferate), culture negative prostatitis, post-partum sepsis, and in cases of neonatal pneumonia, sepsis or meningitis, particularly in the premature infant.

Laboratory diagnosis

Culture

U. urealyticum and *M. hominis* can be detected by culture, and this remains the primary mode of diagnostic testing for these two organisms. The remaining *Mycoplasma* species are not easily cultured using the currently available culture techniques; they require prolonged incubation times and specific nutrients for recovery. They are rarely identified without specific culture, due to their fastidious growth requirements and the fact that their colony size on solid medium is very small.

U. urealyticum and *M. hominis* culture is usually accomplished in two stages, a fluid phase and a solid culture phase. Specimens are first inoculated into a fluid medium containing specific nutrients and a pH indicator.

U. urealyticum culture

Specimens for *U. urealyticum* culture are inoculated into enriched selective SP-4 liquid medium supplemented with urea (U medium). Rapid growth (1–2 days) of *U. urealyticum* in the medium produces an increase in pH in colour from salmon uninoculated medium colour to red, with no increase in turbidity. Cultures demonstrating the typical colour change are then plated onto Shepard's A7 or A8 solid agar and incubated under anaerobic conditions. *U. urealyticum* produces small dark colonies that turn brown when exposed to an Mg^{2+} salt solution (Fig. 10.6(*a*)). The colonies are not visible to the naked eye and must be visualized with the use of a dissecting or inverted scope. Alternatively, U broth and U agar may be used to isolate the Ureaplasmas. Identification of this organism is definitive, with no further testing required for speciation.

M. hominis culture

M. hominis culture requires an enriched fluid medium supplemented with arginine. Specimens are inoculated into SP-4 liquid medium containing arginine (M medium) and incubated for 7 days;

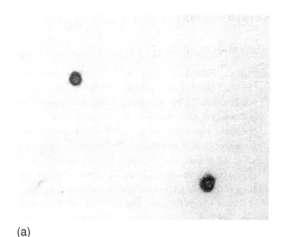

(a)

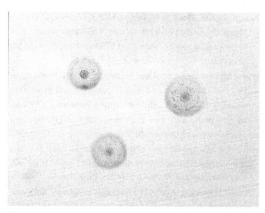

(b)

Fig. 10.6. (*a*) Colony morphology of *Ureaplasma urealyticum* and (*b*) *Mycoplasma hominis* in culture: growth in a fluid medium supplemented with urea (U medium) or arginine (M medium) is generally linked with subsequent culture on solid medium for these two organisms. *Ureaplasma* growth is identified in the U broth liquid medium by an alkaline change in pH, seen as a change in color from salmon to red. Cultures with this increased pH change are then plated onto solid medium, and characteristic colony morphology can be detected by microscopy. (*a*) *U. urealyticum* produces diagnostic small darkly staining colonies on solid U agar containing magnesium sulfate. (*b*) *M. hominis* requires arginine in the liquid medium, and increasing pH in the M medium changes the color from salmon to red-purple. (*b*) This culture plated onto solid medium produces large colonies with a characteristic 'fried egg' morphology.

growth produces an increase in pH, turning the medium from salmon to red-purple. Although the culture does not become frankly turbid, it may turn slightly cloudy. Using the change in pH as the screen for growth, specimens are then inoculated onto A7 or A8 solid agar and incubated under anaerobic conditions. An alternative culture system (H broth and H agar) may also be used. *M. hominis* produces larger (300 μm) colonies with a typical 'fried egg' morphology (Fig. 10.6(*b*)). In comparison with other bacteria, these are very small colonies, and cannot be detected without the use of a stereo-dissecting scope or other low magnification microscope. Identification of the typical colony morphology provides a presumptive diagnosis.

Commercially available culture systems such as Mycotrim GU broth and Mycotrim Triphasic flask systems can also be used to identify *M. hominis* and *U. urealyticum*. The broth culture requires subsequent plating onto A7 or A8 medium for colony morphology, and the triphasic system provides both the liquid and solid phase culture conditions. Identification is again based upon pH changes and colony morphology.

Mycoplasmas may occasionally be isolated from blood culture bottles that have been incubated under anaerobic conditions. Blood cultures require blind subculture and prolonged incubation to detect infection; the organisms fail to take up the Gram-stain and are identified from the blood culture with alternate stains such as acridine orange. Similarly, mycoplasmas may be isolated from routine culture medium in anaerobic cultures after extended culture. The plates must be viewed under magnification to detect the growth of small colonies.

Serology

Serology may be used to detect infections with the genital mollicutes, with varying degrees of success. Assays for the detection of anti-ureaplasmal antibodies are relatively specific and suggest recent or current infections. Reliable serologic assays for the detection of anti-*M. hominis* antibodies have also been developed, but are not widely available. The assays that have been developed to detect infections with *M. genitalium* are not widely used since there is a high degree of cross reactivity between *M. genitalium* and *M. pneumoniae*.

Molecular diagnosis

PCR assays have been developed for research purposes, and are not yet commercially available. PCR primer and probe sequences have been determined for *M. genitalium*, *M. fermentans* and *M. penetrans*, and molecular diagnosis of the non-culturable mollicutes provides the bulk of evidence that these organisms are responsible for causing human disease.

Treatment

Because they lack a cell wall, the mollicutes are intrinsically resistant to any of the beta-lactam antibiotics.

U. urealyticum: the majority of isolates are sensitive to tetracycline, erythromycin and clarithromycin, but up to 10% of isolates are resistant to tetracycline. *M. hominis* is not susceptible to erythromycin but is susceptible to clindamycin and lincomycin. *M. hominis* is also generally susceptible to tetracycline, ciprofloxacin and difloxacin, with about 10% of isolates reported as resistant to tetracycline. *M. genitalium* isolates are generally sensitive to tetracycline, erythromycin, clarithromycin, azithromycin, streptomycin and spectinomycin.

Vaccine availability

No vaccine is currently available to help prevent any infections with the genital mollicutes.

REFERENCES

GONORRHOEAL DISEASE

Harvey, H. A., Porat, N., Campbell, C. A. *et al.* (2000). Gonococcal lipooligosaccharide is a ligand for the asialoglycoprotein receptor on human sperm. *Molecular Microbiology*, **36**: 1059–70.

FURTHER READING

GONORRHOEAL DISEASE

Carroll, K. C., Aldeen, W. E., Morrison, M., Anderson, R., Lee, D. & Mottice, S. (1998). Evaluation of the Abbott LCx Ligase chain reaction assay for the detection of *Chlamydia trachomatis* and *Neisseria gonorrhoeae* in urine and genital swab specimens from a sexually transmitted disease clinic population. *Journal of Clinical Microbiology*, **36**: 1630–3.

Chan, E. L., Brandt, K., Olineus, K., Antonishyn, N. & Horsman, G. B. (2000). Performance characteristics of the Becton Dickinson ProbeTec system for direct detection of *Chlamydia trachomatis* and *Neisseria gonorrhoeae* in male and female urine specimens in comparison with the Roche Cobas system. *Archives of Pathology and Laboratory Medicine*, **124**: 1649–52.

Ching, S., Lee, H., Hook, E. W., Jacobs, M. R. & Zenilman, J. (1995). Ligase chain reaction for detection of *Neisseria gonorrhoeae* in urogenital swabs. *Journal of Clinical Microbiology*, **33**: 3111–14.

Centers for Disease Control and Prevention (1999). High prevalence of chlamydial and gonococcal infection in women entering jail and juvenile detention centers – Chicago, Birmingham, and San Francisco, 1998. *Morbidity and Mortality Weekly Report*, **48**: 793–6.

Centers for Disease Control and Prevention (2002a). Sexually transmitted disease treatment guidelines 2002. *Morbidity and Mortality Weekly Report*, **51**(No. RR-6): 48–53.

(2002b). Screening to detect *Chlamydia trachomatis* and *Neisseria gonorrhoeae* infections – 2002. *Morbidity and Mortality Weekly Report*, **51**(No. RR-15): 1–38.

Evangelista, A. T. & Beilstein, H. R. (1993). *Cumitech 4A – Laboratory Diagnosis of Gonorrhea*. Washington DC: ASM Press Cammarata.

Farrell, D. J. (1999). Evaluation of amplicor *Neisseria gonorrhoeae* PCR using cppB nested PCR abd 16s rRNA PCR. *Journal of Clinical Microbiology*, **37**: 386–90.

Fiumara, N. J. (1972). Short case report: transmission of gonorrhea by artificial insemination. *British Journal of Venereal Disease*, **48**: 308–9.

Gaydos, C. A., Quinn, T. C., Willis, D. *et al.* (2003). Performance of the APTIMA Combo 2 assay for detection of *Chlamydia trachomatis* and *Neisseria gonorrhoeae* in female urine and endocervical swab specimens. *Journal of Clinical Microbiology*, **41**: 304–9.

Hosseinzadeh, S., Brewis, I. A., Pacey, A. A., Moore, H. D. M. & Eley, A. (2000). Co-incubation of human spermatozoa with *Chlamydia trachomatis in vitro* causes increased tyrosine phosphorylation of sperm proteins. *Infection and Immunity*, **68**: 4872–4976.

Hosseinzadeh, S., Brewis, I. A., Eley, A. & Pacey, A. A. (2001). Co-incubation of human spermatozoa with *Chlamydis trachomatis* serovar E causes premature sperm death. *Human Reproduction*, **16**: 293–299.

Hosseinzadeh S., Eley, A., & Pacey, A. A., (2004). Semen quality of men with aymptomatic chlamydial infection. *Journal of Andrology*, **25**: 104–110.

Howard, T. L. (1971). Bacterial hitch-hikers. *Journal of Urology*, **106**: 94.

Jephcott, A. E. (1997). Microbiological diagnosis of gonorrhoea. *Genitourinary Medicine*, **73**: 245–52.

Knapp, J. S. & Koumans, E. H. (1999). Neisseria and Branhamella. In *Manual of Clinical Microbiology*, 7th edn, ed. P. R. Murray, E. J. Barton, M. A. Pfaller, F. C. Tenover & R. H. Yolken, pp. 586–603. Washington, DC: ASM Press.

Koneman, E. W., Allen, S. D., Janda, W. M., Schreckenberger, P. C. & Winn, W. C. (1997). *Neisseria* species and *Moraxella catarrhalis* In *Color Atlas and Textbook of Diagnostic Microbiology*, 5th edn, pp. 491–538, Philadelphia, PA: Lippincott.

Limberger, R. J., Biega, R., Evancoe, A., McCarthy, L., Slivienski, L. & Krikwood, M. (1992). Evaluation of culture and the Gen-Probe PACE 2 assay for detection of *Neisseria gonorrhoeae* and *Chlamydia trachomatis* in endocervical specimens transported to a state health laboratory. *Journal of Clinical Microbiology*, **30**: 1162–6.

Palmer, H. M., Mallinson, H., Wood, R. L. & Herring, A. J. (2003). Evaluation of the specificities of five DNA amplification methods for the detection of *Neisseria gonorrhoeae*. *Journal of Clinical Microbiology*, **41**: 835–7.

Van der Pol, B., Martin, D. H. & Schachter, J. (2001). Enhancing the specificity of the COBAS AMPLICOR CT/NG test for *Neisseria gonorrhoeae* by retesting specimens with equivocal results. *Journal of Clinical Microbiology*, **39**: 3092–8.

REFERENCES

CHLAMYDIAL DISEASE

Arroyo, G., Linnemann, C. & Wesseler, T. (1989). Role of the Papanicolaou smear in diagnosis of chlamydial infections *Sexually Transmitted Diseases*, **16**: 11–14.

Coghlan, A. (1996). Shapely vaccine targets Chlamydia. *New Scientist*, **152**: 18.

Erbengi, T. (1993). Ultrastructural observations on the entry of *Chlamydia trachomatis* into human spermatozoa. *Human Reproduction*, **3**: 416–21.

Land, J. A., Gijsen, A. P., Evers, K. I. H. & Bruggeman, C. A. (2002). *Chlamydia trachomatis* in subfertile women undergoing uterine instrumentation. *Human Reproduction*, **17**(6): 525–7.

Macmillan, S. (2002). Avoiding iatrogenic PID: the clinician's role. *Human Reproduction*, **17**(6): 1433–6.

Paavonen, J. & Lehtinen, M. (1996). Chlamydial pelvic inflammatory disease. *Human Reproduction Update*, **2**(6): 515.

Patton, D. L., Askienazy-Elbhar, M., Henry-Suchet, J. *et al.* (1994). Detection of *Chlamydia trachomatis* in fallopian tube tissue in women with postinfectious infertility. *American Journal of Obstetrics and Gynecology*, **171**: 95–101.

Royal College of Obstetricians and Gynaecologists (1996). *The Initial Investigation and Management of the Infertile Couple*. London, UK: RCOG Press.

Royal College of Obstetricians and Gynaecologists (2000). The management of infertility in tertiary care. www.rcog.org.uk/guidelines/tertiarycare.html

Thomas, K. & Simms, I. (2002). *Chlamydia trachomatis* in subfertile women undergoing uterine instrumentation. How can we help in the avoidance of iatrogenic pelvic inflammatory disease? *Human Reproduction*, **17**(6): 1431–2.

Wølner-Hanssen, P. & Mardh, P-A. (1984). In vitro tests of the adherence of *Chlamydia trachomatis* to human spermatozoa. *Fertility and Sterility*, **42**: 102–7.

FURTHER READING

CHLAMYDIAL DISEASE

Black, C. M. (1997). Current methods of laboratory diagnosis for *Chlamydia trachomatis* infections. *Clinical Microbiology Reviews*, **10**: 160–84.

Black, C. M., Marrazzo, J., Johnson, R. E. *et al.* (2002). Head-to head multicenter comparison of DNA probe and nucleic acid amplification tests for *Chlamydia trachomatis* infection in women performed with an improved reference standard. *Journal of Clinical Microbiology*, **40**: 3757–63.

Burstein, G. R., Gaydos, C. A., Diener-West, M., Howell, M. R., Zenilman, J. M. & Quinn, T. C. (1998). Incident *Chlamydia trachomatis* infection among inner-city adolescent females. *Journal of the American Medical Association*, **280**: 521–6.

Carroll, K. C., Aldeen, W. E., Morrison, M., Anderson, R., Lee, D. & Mottice, S. (1998). Evaluation of the Abbott LCx Ligase chain reaction assay for the detection of *Chlamydia trachomatis* and *Neisseria gonorrhoeae* in urine and genital swab specimens from a sexually transmitted disease clinic population. *Journal of Clinical Microbiology*, **136**: 1630–3.

Chan, E. L., Brandt, K., Olineus, K., Antonishyn, N. & Horsman, G. B. (2000a). Performance characteristics of the Becton Dickinson ProbeTec system for direct detection of *Chlamydia trachomatis* and *Neisseria gonorrhoeae* in male and female urine specimens in comparison with the Roche Cobas system. *Archives of Pathology and Laboratory Medicine*, **124**: 1649–52.

Chan, E. L., Brandt, K., Stoneham, H., Anonishyn, N. & Horsman, G. B. (2000b). Comparison of the effectiveness of polymerase chain reaction and enzyme immunoassay in detecting *Chlamydia trachomatis* in different female genitourinary specimens. *Archives of Pathology and Laboratory Medicine*, **124**: 840–934.

Centers for Disease Control and Prevention (1999). High prevalence of chlamydial and gonococcal infection in women entering jail and juvenile detention centers – Chicago, Birmingham, and San Francisco, 1998. *Morbidity and Mortality Weekly Report*, **48**: 793–6.

(2002a). Sexually transmitted disease treatment guidelines 2002. *Morbidity and Mortality Weekly Report*, **51**(No. RR-6): 48–53.

(2002b). Screening to detect *Chlamydia trachomatis* and *Neisseria gonorrhoeae* infections – 2002. *Morbidity and Mortality Weekly Report*, **51**(No. RR-15): 1–38.

Goessens, W. H. F., Mouton, J. W., van der Meijden, W. I. *et al.* (1997). Comparison of three commercially available amplification assays, AMP CT, LCx, and Cobas Amplicore, for detection of *Chlamydia trachomatis* in first void urine. *Journal of Clinical Microbiology*, **35**: 2628–33.

Gaydos, C. A., Howell, M. R., Pare, B. *et al.* (1998). *Chlamydia trachomatis* infections in female military recruits. *New England Journal of Medicine*, **339**: 739–44.

Gaydos, C. A., Quinn, T. C., Willis, D. *et al.* (2003). Performance of the APTIMA Combo 2 assay for detection of *Chlamydia trachomatis* and *Neisseria gonorrhoeae* in female urine and endocervical swab specimens. *Journal of Clinical Microbiology*, **41**: 304–9.

Hatch, T. P. (1996). Disulfide cross-linked envelope proteins: the functional equivalent of peptidoglycan in Chlamydia? *Journal of Bacteriology*, **178**: 1–5.

Kalman, S., Mitchell, M., Marathe, R. *et al.* (1999). Comparative genomes of *Chlamydia pneumoniae* and *C. trachomatis*. *Nature Genetics*, **21**(4): 385–9.

Kilstrom, E., Lindgren, R. & Ryden, G. (1990). Antibodies to *Chlamydia trachomatis* in women with infertility, pelvic inflammatory disease and ectopic pregnancy. *European Journal of Obstetrics and Reproductive Biology*, **35**: 119–204.

Koneman, E. W., Allen, S. D., Janda, W. M., Schreckenberger, P. C. & Winn, W. C. (1997) Diagnosis of infections caused by viruses, chlamydia, richettsia and related organisms. In *Color Atlas and Textbook of Diagnostic Microbiology*, 5th edn, pp. 1177–293. Philadelphia, PA: Lippincott.

Lauderdale, T. L., Landers, L., Thorneycroft, I. & Chapin, K. (1999). Comparison of the PACE 2 assay, two amplification assays, and clearview EIA for detection of *Chlamydia trachomatis* in female endocervical and urine specimens. *Journal of Clinical Microbiology*, **37**: 2223–9.

Limburger, R. J., Beige, R., Evince, A., McCarthy, L., Slivienski, L. & Krikwood, M. (1992) Evaluation of culture and the Gen-Probe PACE 2 assay for detection of *Neisseria gonorrhoeae* and *Chlamydia trachomatis* in endocervical specimens transported to a state health laboratory. *Journal of Clinical Microbiology*, **30**: 1162–6.

Moore, D. E., Spandoni, L. R., Foy, H. M. *et al.* (1982). Increased frequency of serum antibodies to *Chlamydia trachomatis* in infertility due to distal tubal disease. *Lancet*, **ii**: 574–7.

Nagel, T. C., Tagatz, G. E. & Campbell, B. F. (1986). Transmission of *Chlamydia trachomatis* by artificial insemination. *Fertility and Sterility*, **46**: 959–60.

Newhall, W. J., Johnson, R. E., DeLisle, S. *et al.* (1999). Head-to-head evaluation of five chlamydia tests relative to a quality-assured culture standard. *Journal of Clinical Microbiology*, **37**: 681–5.

Pannekoek, Y., Westenberg, S. M., De Vries, J. *et al.* (2000). PCR assessment of *Chlamydia trachomatis* infection of semen specimens processed for artificial insemination. *Journal of Clinical Microbiology*, **38**: 3763–7.

Quinn, T. C., Gaydos, C., Shepherd, M. *et al.* (1996). Epidemiologic and microbiologic correlates of *Chlamydia trachomatis* infection in sexual partnerships. *Journal of the American Medical Association*, **276**: 1737–42.

Radcliffe, K. W., Rowen, D., Mercey, D. E. *et al.* (1990). Is a test of cure necessary following treatment for cervical infection with *Chlamydia trachomatis*? *Genitourinary Medicine*, **66**: 444–66.

Rowland, G., Forsey, T., Moss, T. R., Steptoe, P. C., Hewitt, J. & Darougar, S. (1985). Failure of *in vitro* fertilization and embryo replacement following infection with *Chlamydia trachomatis*. *Journal for In-vitro Fertilization and Embryo Transfer*, **2**: 151–5.

Schachter, J. & Stamm, W. E. (1999). Chlamydia. In *Manual of Clinical Microbiology*, 7th edn, ed. P. R. Murray, E. J. Barton, M. A. Pfaller, F. C. Tenover & R. H. Yolken, pp. 795–806. Washington, DC: ASM Press.

Schachter, J., Stoner, E. & Moncada, J. (1983). Screening for Chlamydial infection in women attending family planning clinics. *Western Journal of Medicine*, **138**: 375–9.

Stamm, W. E. & Cole, B. (1986). Asymptomatic *Chlamydia trachomatis* urethritis in men. *Sexually Transmitted Diseases*, **13**: 163–5.

Stamm, W. E., Tam, M., Koester, M. & Cles, L. (1983). Detection of *Chlamydia trachomatis* inclusions in McCoy cell cultures with fluorescein-conjugated monoclonal antibodies. *Journal of Clinical Microbiology*, **17**: 666–8.

Stary, A., Tmazic-Allen, S., Choueiri, B., Burczak, G., Steyrer, K. & Lee, H. (1996). Comparison of DNA amplification methods for the detection of *Chlamydia trachomatis* in first-void urine from asymptomatic military recruits. *Sexually Transmitted Diseases*, **23**: 97–102.

Uyeda, C. T., Welborn, P., Ellison-Birang, N., Shunk, K. & Tsaouse, B. (1984). Rapid diagnosis of chlamydial infections with the MicroTrak direct test. *Journal of Clinical Microbiology*, **20**: 948–50.

Zellin, J. M., Robinson, A. J., Ridgway, G. L., Allason-Jones, E. & Williams, P. (1995). Chlamydial urethritis in heterosexual men attending a genito-urinary medicine clinic: prevalence, symptoms, condom usage and partner change. *International Journal for STD and AIDS*, **6**: 27–30.

REFERENCES

GENITAL MOLLICUTES

Cassell, G. H., Waites, K. B. & Crouse, D. T. (1991). Perinatal mycoplasmal infections. *Clinical Perinatology*, **18**: 241–64.

Dinsmoor, M. J., Ramamurthy, R. S. & Gibbs, R. S. (1989). Transmission of genital mycoplasma from mother to neonate in women with prolonged membrane rupture. *Pediatric Infectious Disease Journal*, **8**: 483–7.

Hill, A. C. (1991). *Mycoplasma spermatophilum*, a new species isolated from human spermatozoa and cervix. *International Journal of Systematic Bacteriology*, **41**(2): 229–33.

Reichart, M., Kahane, I. & Bartoov, B. (2000). *In vivo* and *in vitro* impairment of human and ram sperm nuclear chomatin integrity by sexually transmitted *Ureaplasma urealyticum* infection. *Biological Reproduction*, **63**: 1041–9.

Rose, B. I. & Scott, B. (1994). Sperm motility, morphology, hyperactivation, and ionophore-induced acrosome reactions after overnight incubation with mycoplasmas. *Fertility and Sterility*, **61**: 341–8.

Shang, X-J., Huang, T-F., Xiong, C-L., Xu, J-P., Yin, L. & Wan, C.-C. (1999). *Ureaplasma urealyticum* infection and apoptosis of spermatogenic cells. *Asian Journal of Andrology*, **1**: 127–9.

GENITAL MOLLICUTES

Busolo, F. & Zanchetta, R. (1985). The effect of *Mycoplasma hominis* and *Ureaplasma urealyticum* on hamster egg *in vitro* penetration by human spermatozoa. *Fertility and Sterility*, **43**: 110–14.

Cassell, G. H. (1999). Ureaplasma infection. In *Sexually Transmitted Diseases and Adverse Outcomes of Pregnancy*, ed. P. J. Hitchcock, H. T. MacKay, J. N. Wasserheit & R. Binder, pp. 175–93. Washington DC: ASM Press.

Cassell, G. H., Davis, R. O., Waites, K. B. *et al.* (1983). Isolation of *Mycoplasma hominis* and *Ureaplasma urealyticum* from amniotic fluid at 16–20 weeks gestation: potential effect on pregnancy outcome. *Sexually Transmitted Diseases*, **10**: 294–302.

Cassell, G. H., Crouse, D. T., Canupp, K. C., Waites, K. B., Rudd, P. T. & Stagno, S. (1988a). Association of *Ureaplasma urealyticum* infection of the lower respiratory tract with chronic lung disease and death in very low birth weight infants. *Lancet*, **ii**: 240–5.

Cassell, G. H., Crouse, D. T., Waites, K. B., Rudd, P. T. & Davis, J. K. (1988b). Does *Ureaplasma urealyticum* cause respiratory disease in newborns? *Pediatric Infectious Disease Journal*, **7**: 535–41.

Elshibly, S., Kallings, I., Hellberg, D. & Mardh, P. A. (1996). Sexual risk behaviour in women carriers of *Myocoplasma hominis*. *British Journal of Obstetrics and Gynaecology*, **103**: 1124–8.

Eschenbach, D. A. (1999). Bacterial vaginosis. In *Sexually Transmitted Diseases and Adverse Outcomes of Pregnancy*, ed. P. J. Hitchcock, H. T. MacKay, J. N. Wasserheit & R. Binder, pp. 103–23. Washington DC: ASM Press.

Fowlkes, D. M., Dooher, G. B. & O'Leary, W. M. (1975). Evidence by scanning electron microscopy for an association between spermatozoa and T-mycoplasmas in men of infertile marriages. *Fertility and Sterility*, **26**: 1203–5.

Friberg, J. (1980). Mycoplasmas and ureaplasmas in infertility and abortion. *Fertility and Sterility*, **33**: 351–9.

Garland, S. M. & Murton, L. J. (1987). Neonatal meningitis caused by *Ureaplasma urealyticum*. *Pediatric Infectious Disease Journal*, **6**: 868–70.

Gump, D. W., Gibson, M. & Ashikaga, T. (1984). Lack of association between genital mycoplasma and infertility. *New England Journal of Medicine*, **310**: 937–41.

Hentschel, J., Abele-Horn, M. & Peters, J. (1993). *Ureaplasma urealyticum* in the cerebrospinal fluid of a premature infant. *Acta Paediatrica*, **82**: 690–3.

Knox, C. L., Cave, D. G., Farrell, D. J., Eastment, H. T. & Timms, P. (1997). The role of *Ureaplasma urealyticum* in adverse pregnancy outcomes. *Australia and NZ Journal of Obstetrics and Gynecology*, **37**: 45–51.

Koneman, E. W., Allen, S. D., Janda, W. M., Schreckenberger, P. C. & Winn, W. C. (1997). Mycoplasmas and ureaplasmas. In *Color Atlas and Textbook of Diagnostic Microbiology*, 5th edn, pp. 857–92. Philadelphia, PA: Lippincott.

Lumpkin, M. M., Smith, T. S., Coulam, C. B. & O'Brien, P. C. (1987). *Ureaplasma urealyticum* in semen for artificial insemination: its effect on conception and semen analysis parameters. *International Journal of Fertility*, **32**: 122–30.

McCormack, W. M., Almeida, P. C., Bailey, P. E., Grady, E. M. & Lee, Y. H. (1972). Sexual activity and vaginal colonization with genital mycoplasmas. *Journal of the American Medical Association*, **221**: 1375–7.

Quinn, P. A., Gillain, J. E., Markstad, T., St. John, M. A., Daneman, A. & Lie, K. I. (1985) Intrauterine infection with *Ureaplasma urealyticum* as a cause of fatal neonatal pneumonia. *Pediatric Infectious Disease Journal*, **4**: 538–43.

Quinn, P. A., Butany, J., Chipman, M. *et al.* (1985). A prospective study of microbial infection in stillbirths and early neonatal death. *American Journal of Obstetrics and Gynecology*, **151**: 238–49.

Rudd, P. T. & Carrington, D. (1985). A prospective study of chlamydial, mycoplasmal and viral infections in a neonatal intensive care unit. *Archive of Diseases in Children*, **59**: 120–5.

Sanchez, P. J. & Regan, J. A. (1987). Vertical transmission of *Ureaplasma urealyticum* in full term infants. *Pediatric Infectious Disease Journal*, **6**: 825–8.

Shaw, N. J., Pratt, B. C. & Weindling, A. M. (1989). Ureaplasma and mycoplasma infections of the central nervous system in preterm infants. *Lancet*, **ii**: 1530–1.

Sompolinsky, D., Solomon, F., Elkina, L., Weinraub, Z., Bukovsky, I. & Caspi, E. (1975). Infections with mycoplasma and bacteria in induced midtrimester abortion and fetal loss. *American Journal of Obstetrics and Gynecology*, **121**: 611–6.

Stahelin-Massik, J., Levy, F., Friderich, P. & Schadd, U. B. (1994). Meningitis caused by *Ureaplasma urealyticum* in full term neonate. *Pediatric Infectious Disease Journal*, **13**: 419–20.

Taylor-Robinson, D., Csonka, G. W. & Prentice, M. J. (1977). Human intra-urethral inoculation of ureaplasmas. *Quarterly Journal of Medicine*, **XLVI**: 309–26.

Taylor-Robinson, D., Ainsworth, J. G. & McCormack, W. W. (1999). Genital mycoplasmas. In *Sexually Transmitted Diseases*, 3rd edn, ed. K. K. Holmes, P. F. Sparling, P. A. Mardh *et al.*, pp. 533–48. New York, NY: McGraw-Hill.

Waites, K. B. & Taylor-Robinson, D. (1999). Mycoplasma and Ureaplasma. In *Manual of Clinical Microbiology*, 7th edn, ed. P. R. Murray, E. J. Barton, M. A. Pfaller, F. C. Tenover & R. H. Yolken, pp. 782–94. Washington, DC: ASM Press.

Waites, K. B., Rudd, P. T., Crouse, D. T. *et al.* (1988). Chronic *Ureaplasma urealyticum* and *Mycoplasma hominis* infections of central nervous system in preterm infants. *Lancet*, **1**: 17–21.

Waites, K. B., Duffy, L. B. & Crouse, D. T. (1990). Mycoplasmal infections of cerebrospinal fluid in newborn infants from a community hospital population. *Pediatric Infectious Disease Journal*, **9**: 241–5.

Wang, E. E. L., Frayha, H., Watts, J. *et al.* (1988). Role of *Ureaplasma urealyticum* and other pathogens in the development of chronic lung disease of prematurity. *Pediatric Infectious Disease Journal*, **7**: 547–51.

11

Pathology of the upper genitourinary tract

Pathology in the male upper GU tract can be due to epididymitis, orchitis and prostatitis, i.e. inflammation of the epididymis, testis and prostate. In the female, salpingitis, oophoritis, endometritis and 'pelvic inflammatory disease' (PID) describe infection or inflammation of the fallopian tubes, ovaries, endometrium, and pelvis.

Male upper GU infections

Epididymitis

The epididymis, which lies on the posterior surface of the testicle, is responsible for transport, storage, and maturation of sperm. Epididymitis is the most common cause of intrascrotal inflammation, and is likely to be due to retrograde extension of organisms from the vas deferens. Hematogenous spread is very rare. It is primarily a disease of adults, most commonly in the age range of 19–40 years. The onset of pain and swelling is usually gradual, and there may be initial abdominal or flank pain because the inflammation typically begins in the vas deferens. Younger patients may have symptoms of urethritis, and there may be a urethral discharge. A recent history of instrumentation or urinary tract infection is more common in the older patient. The disease is usually unilateral; bilateral involvement is seen in only 10% of cases. Peritubular fibrosis can lead to occlusion of the ductules and obstructive azoospermia. Progression of the infection can lead to an epididymal abscess, epididymo-orchitis, or testicular abscess.

The causative agent can be identified in 80% of cases, varying with the age of the patient. *E.coli* is the most common cause in prepubertal males, and at least 50% of these cases are associated with a genitourinary anomaly. Sexually transmitted pathogens are usually responsible for epididymitis in males younger than 35 years of age, with *C. trachomatis* being the most common organism (50–60% of cases), followed by *N. gonorrheae*. In older males, coliform bacteria are more common because of underlying obstructive urinary disease. Rarely, chemical epididymitis can result from reflux of sterile urine. Males with AIDS may have candidal epididymitis.

Diagnosis

Other causes of scrotal pain and swelling must be excluded, especially testicular torsion – the most common misdiagnosis for testicular torsion is epididymitis. Urine culture should be performed, especially for prepubertal and older patients. Gram stain can be performed on urethral discharge, if this is present. Patients in whom sexually transmitted etiology is probable or suspected should be tested with urethral swab culture, as well as serology for syphilis and HIV.

Treatment

Antibiotic treatment is recommended in all cases of epididymitis, regardless of negative urinalysis or urethral Gram stain result. Males younger than 35 years of age need empiric treatment for *C. trachomatis* and

N. gonorrheae, and partners should also be investigated and treated. Prepubertal and older age patients should have empiric treatment for coliforms. Occasionally, a testicular tumour is the true cause of the symptoms, and therefore a patient who presents with possible epididymitis should be referred for urological evaluation within 3–7 days.

Orchitis

Viral or bacterial infection that reaches the testis causes an acute inflammatory reaction, orchitis. Isolated orchitis is normally due to a viral infection.

Epididymo-orchitis

Epididymo-orchitis is more common, and usually has a bacterial cause. Orchitis presents with acute scrotal pain and swelling, varying from mild discomfort to severe pain. There may be associated systemic symptoms of fatigue, malaise, myalgias, fever, chills, nausea and headache. The majority of cases are associated with the mumps virus; other rare viral etiologies include Coxsackie virus, infectious mononucleosis, varicella, and echovirus. Approximately 20% of young boys with mumps develop orchitis 4 to 7 days following the parotitis, and therefore cases of mumps orchitis often occur in prepubertal males (<10 years of age); 70% of cases present unilaterally, and in 30% the contralateral testis is involved from 1 to 9 days later. The majority of cases resolve spontaneously in 3–10 days.

Bacterial orchitis

Bacterial orchitis rarely occurs without an associated epididymitis, and is usually due to infection spreading from the epididymis in sexually active males, or in men >50 years of age with benign prostatic hypertrophy (BPH). This orchitis presents with a gradual onset of pain and swelling, and unilateral testicular edema is seen in 90% of cases. The etiologic agents include *Neisseria gonorrhoeae*, *C. trachomatis*, *Escherischia coli*, *Klebsiella pneumoniae* and other coliforms, *Pseudomonas aeruginosa*, *Haemophilus influenzae* and staphylococcus and streptococcus species. In immunocompromised patients, cases of

orchitis have been reported due to *Mycobacterium tuberculosis*, *Mycobacterium avium intracellulare* complex, *Cryptococcus neoformans*, *Toxoplasma gondii*, *Haemophilus parainfluenzae*, and *Candida albicans*.

Diagnosis

Since orchitis often presents with acute swelling and pain, as in the case of epididymitis, testicular torsion must first be excluded. The differential diagnosis must also include hernia, testicular tumour, reactive hydrocoele, scrotal pyocoele and torsion of the testicular appendage. Ultrasound is the investigation of choice, with colour doppler ultrasound the most helpful imaging test. Diagnosis of mumps orchitis can be made on the basis of history and examination, and can be confirmed with serum immunofluorescent antibody testing.

Treatment

No medication other than analgesia or anti-emetics is indicated for treatment of viral orchitis. If there is a question of epididymo-orchitis, urinalysis and urethral cultures should be assessed and appropriate antibiotic treatment for the suspected infectious agents arranged. In sexually active patients, antibiotic cover should include STDs and the partner must also be treated. Older patients with possible BPH require additional cover for other gram-negative bacteria. Some degree of testicular atrophy occurs in 60% of patients with orchitis, and impaired fertility is reported at a rate of 7–13%. Unilateral orchitis is rarely associated with infertility.

Prostatitis

Inflammation of the prostate is notoriously difficult to diagnose and to treat effectively. It has been estimated that up to half of all men suffer from symptoms of prostatitis at some time in their life, and a wide range of putative etiologies have been described, including infection, immune disorder, neuromuscular tension, stones, stricture, tumour – it has even been associated with food allergies. Four different prostatitis syndromes can be identified.

Acute bacterial prostatitis

Acute bacterial prostatitis is the least common of the four types but also the easiest to diagnose and treat effectively. It can occur as a result of ascending urethral infection, or by reflux of infected urine into prostatic ducts. Other possible routes of infection include invasion of rectal bacteria through direct extension or via the lymphatics or bloodstream. Symptoms include sudden onset of chills, fever, pain in the lower back and genital area, urinary frequency and urgency (often at night), burning or painful urination, body aches, and infection of the urinary tract. White blood cells and bacteria can often be demonstrated in the urine. In order to obtain a sample that will localize the infection to the prostate gland, urine samples are collected before and after prostatic massage. Urethral swabbing must not be performed prior to obtaining the sample; prostatic secretions are obtained by systematic massage of each lobe of the prostate gland. Positive cultures can be obtained from expressed prostatic secretions and from post-massage voided urine, which also show high numbers of polymorphonuclear leukocytes and macrophages. This type of prostatitis can be treated with appropriate antibiotic therapy.

Chronic bacterial prostatitis

Chronic bacterial prostatitis is also relatively uncommon, and is characterized by relapsing recurrent urinary tract infection (UTI) and persistence of bacteria in prostatic secretions despite multiple courses of antibiotic therapy. It is usually associated with an underlying defect in the prostate that acts as a focal point for bacterial persistence in the urinary tract, and effective treatment may require identification and removal of the defect. The organism most commonly identified in bacterial prostatitis is *Escherichia coli*, as well as other *Enterobacteriacea* (e.g. *Klebsiella, Proteus, Serratia)*, pseudomonads and other less common gram-negative bacteria. Obligate anaerobes are rarely implicated. Gram-positive cocci remain controversial as an infective cause; coagulase-negative staphylococci and coryneform bacteria have also been found in prostatic

secretions. *Enterococcus faecalis* can cause chronic bacterial prostatitis and related recurrent bacteriuria.

Chronic idiopathic prostatitis

Chronic idiopathic prostatitis/chronic pelvic pain syndrome or prostatodynia is the most common but least understood form of the disease. It is a relapsing disease, found in men of any age, and may be inflammatory or non-inflammatory. In the inflammatory form, urine, semen, and prostatic secretions show no evidence of a known infecting organism but do contain white blood cells. In the non-inflammatory form, white blood cells are not found and there is no evidence of inflammation. Recently, the application of molecular techniques and the use of special culture media suggest that this syndrome may be due to a cryptic bacterial infection that is usually missed or undetected by routine conventional cultures. A number of organisms have been reported: *Trichomonas vaginalis, Chlamydia trachomatis*, genital mycoplasmas, staphylococci, coryneforms, and genital herpes viruses. However, these data are controversial, and interpretation is complicated by the presence of contaminating indigenous microbes during collection of specimens such as urine, urethral swabs and expressed prostatic secretions.

Asymptomatic inflammatory prostatitis

Asymptomatic inflammatory prostatitis may be diagnosed when the patient does not complain of pain or discomfort but has seminal leukocytosis. This type of prostatitis is usually diagnosed incidentally following semen analysis for investigations of infertility or suspected cancer of the prostate.

Female upper GU infections

Salpingitis

Infections of the fallopian tubes (salpingitis) can cause adhesions, as well as damage to the tubal endothelium. Adhesions or endothelial damage may result in tubal obstruction, and/or effects on the tubal transport mechanisms that are necessary for a fertilized egg to reach the uterus. Salpingitis increases the risk of ectopic pregnancy, and tubal abscesses formed during an episode of salpingitis may eventually resolve with formation of hydrosalpinges. Damaged tubes also become prone to recurrent infection, causing recurrent pelvic inflammatory disease. The risk of both infertility and ectopic pregnancy increases dramatically following PID: 50% of ectopic pregnancies are associated with PID, and PID increases the risk of a subsequent ectopic pregnancy by 8-fold. One episode of PID is associated with a 12–15% incidence of tubal occlusion, increasing to 35% after two episodes, and 75% of patients with recurrent PID have tubal occlusion. Chronic pelvic pain secondary to adhesive disease is also a possible long-term consequence of PID.

Oophoritis

Oophoritis, or 'inflammation of the ovary', is a condition that is often associated with pelvic inflammatory disease. Infection can ascend from bacterial colonization of the cervix, affecting the uterus, fallopian tubes and the ovary. *Neisseria gonorrhoeae* and *Chlamydia trachomatis* typically are colonized from the cervix in cases of oophoritis, but these pathogens are rarely isolated in ovarian tissue. Salpingitis and PID may be due initially to a single organism, but the disease quickly becomes polymicrobial because the initial infection facilitates superinfection by other organisms. Those that have been identified as causative agents include *Chlamydia trachomatis*, *Actinomyces israelii*, *Neisseria gonorrhoea*, *Mycoplasma hominis*, *Mycoplasma genitalium*, anaerobes (especially *Bacteroides* species), and rarely, herpes simplex. If left untreated, an abscess may form around the fallopian tubes and ovary, known as a **tubo-ovarian abscess** (TOA). Rupture of a TOA is a surgical emergency with high mortality.

Endometritis

Endometritis, inflammation of the endometrial lining of the uterus, can occur as a result of acending infection that reaches the non-pregnant uterus, or as a post-partum complication following delivery of a baby. In both cases, inflammation can also involve the myometrium and occasionally the parametrial tissues.

Endometritis not related to pregnancy is usually associated with pelvic inflammatory disease, often with accompanying salpingitis, oophoritis and pelvic peritonitis. Risk factors are similar to those that predispose to female pelvic infections in general, in particular uterine instrumentation (abortion, dilatation, curettage) and the presence of an intrauterine device, as well as those that present a risk for cervicitis, salpingitis, oophoritis and PID. The etiology is commonly polymicrobial, and history, clinical presentation, investigations and treatment are equivalent to those described for PID, or for the particular causative agent (e.g. chlamydia, gonococcus, tuberculosis etc.). In teenagers, post-abortion endometritis may be caused by the same organisms that cause PID, and initial treatment usually includes intravenous cefoxitin and doxycycline.

Post-partum infection of the endometrium can also involve the decidua, with possible extension into the myometrium and parametrial tissues. Risk factors for post-partum endometritis include the duration of labour, time of rupture of membranes prior to delivery, caesarean section, number of vaginal examinations during labour, extremes of patient age, low socio-economic status, and post-partum anemia. As with non-pregnancy related endometritis, the infection is usually polymicrobial, with a mixture of aerobic and anaerobic organisms found on culture. Chlamydia has been associated with late-onset post-partum endometritis. Patients present with fever and chills (usually within 36 hours of delivery), lower abdominal pain and foul-smelling lochia; systemic toxicity can result if initiation of broad-spectrum antibiotic therapy is delayed. The majority of cases should show clinical improvement within 48–72 hours of starting appropriate antibiotic treatment. In the USA, the incidence of post-partum endometritis is less than 3% after normal vaginal delivery, but this increases to 38.4% after emergency

Caesarean delivery: broad-spectrum prophylactic antibiotics significantly decrease the incidence of post-partum endometritis, and are indicated for caesarean deliveries.

Complications of both post-partum and non-pregnancy related endometritis include ascending infection, future infertility, salpingitis, oophoritis, localized peritonitis, tubo-ovarian abcess and chronic pelvic pain. Adolescents who develop endometritis after termination of pregnancy have an increased risk of future infertility and pregnancy complications; this group should be treated earlier and more aggressively. Complete aseptic technique in medical terminations of pregnancy can avoid episodes of post-abortal endometritis.

Pelvic inflammatory disease (PID)

Primary PID is usually caused by a sexually transmitted agent, but there can be superimposed infection that has spread from bowel or vaginal flora. **Secondary PID** is caused by a breach in the barrier that prevents spread of microbes from the lower genital tract; this can occur during termination of pregnancy, after childbirth, and during insertion of an intrauterine contraceptive device (IUCD). The infection may then be due to an existing STD, or to aerobic and anaerobic bowel and vaginal flora. Although PID is usually an ascending infection, it can also result from direct spread of organisms from appendicitis, diverticulitis, or hematogenous spread in cases of tuberculosis. Some of these organisms can cause endometritis in passing through the endometrial cavity, or spread beyond the fallopian tubes to cause oophoritis, or even pelvic peritonitis. Organisms may apparently also be transmitted via peritubal lymphatics.

Diagnosis

Diagnosis of PID is notoriously difficult, as symptoms may be vague or minimal. There may be a history of abdominal pain, pelvic pain, mucopurulent vaginal discharge, dyspareunia, fever, chills, nausea/vomiting, associated lower quadrant abdominal tenderness, rebound tenderness on pelvic examination, cervical motion tenderness, adnexal tenderness and palpable mass if a tubo-ovarian abscess is present. The disease is associated with unprotected sexual intercourse, multiple sexual partners, high-risk sexual behaviour, immunosuppression and recent instrumentation of the genital tract, e.g. endometrial biopsy, hysteroscopy, IUCD placement.

Tests may include wet film for microscopy and gram staining from the cervix and urethra to detect gonoccocci, cervical and urethral swabs for culture of gonococci and chlamydia, rectal and throat swabs as appropriate and blood tests for syphilis and hepatitis serology. However, positive microbiology from these sites cannot be directly extrapolated to the upper genital tract. Ultrasound may identify a pelvic mass, and the diagnosis can be confirmed by laparoscopy. PID is often a sexually transmitted disease, and the partner must therefore always be considered for testing and treatment.

Chlamydia trachomatis frequently causes asymptomatic ('silent') infection: it can be isolated from the genital tract of approximately 50% of patients with PID in Europe, and is now recognized as a major causative factor in infertility. The organism is discussed in detail in Chapter 10. *Actinomyces israelii* can cause unilateral disease, as well as oophoritis.

Pelvic anaerobic actinomycetes

Pelvic actinomycosis may be seen in association with all types of IUCDs. The risk of colonization is associated with the length of time the instrument is in place, rather than the composition of the IUCD or the presence, absence or morphology of an IUCD 'tail'. Incubation periods of from 2 months to 2 or more years have been reported before a presentation of symptomatic disease. Overall, studies summarize the incidence of pelvic actinomycosis to range from 3–25% in the presence of an IUCD, but the causal agent can be identified by culture in less than 10% of patients. *Actinomyces israelii* is the most common organism isolated or identified serologically (Mali *et al.*, 1986), although cases of *A. bovis*

(Henderson, 1973) and other non-*A. israelii* actinomycetes have also been described (Bhagavan & Gupta, 1978).

The anaerobic actinomycetes are natural inhabitants of the human mouth, tonsillar crypts and colon, and they occur only infrequently and intermittently as part of the normal flora of the vagina and cervix. The majority of infections are seen in the head and neck region, primarily in men, with occasional cases due to aspiration in the lung or secondary to seeding from a ruptured or inflamed appendix in the abdomen. In contrast, genital infections with the anaerobic actinomycetes are uncommon, almost exclusively seen in women. From 1883–1933 a series of 71 cases of pelvic actinomycosis had been described in the literature, with primary infection in the intestines that spread to the ovaries and fallopian tubes. The right ovary was most often involved, and the anatomic proximity of the right ovary with the appendix, an important site for intestinal actinomycosis, suggested that inflamed or ruptured appendices were the probable source of infection in these cases. The first cases of pelvic actinomycosis associated with foreign bodies in the genital tract were described in the German literature in 1928 and 1930 (Barth, 1928; Tietze, 1930). The women in these cases were using sterling silver pessaries known as 'Sterilittes'. Because of the infectious disease complications associated with these early devices, their use as a method of birth control lost favour for several decades. It was not until modern IUCDs were introduced into active use in the 1960s and 1970s that a resurgence in genital actinomycosis was documented in the literature by Gupta *et al.* (1976).

Life cycle

The anaerobic actinomycetes are slow-growing gram-positive bacteria that multiply by binary fission. Most are fastidious anaerobes and may require other anaerobes and facultative anaerobes to maintain an adequate growth milieu. *Staphylococcus* spp., *Streptococcus* spp. and facultative gram-negative organisms have also been identified in the

majority of patients where cultures were performed (Weese & Smith, 1975). Colonization in the female genital tract is stimulated greatly by the presence of a foreign body.

Transmission

The anaerobic actinomycetes are not transmitted sexually and are not generally considered as part of the normal vaginal flora. They are thought to be acquired in the female genital tract either by transfer from the gut across the perineum, or via oral genital contact. The oral route of infection is more likely, since the actinomycetes are normally found in the oral cavity but are rarely recovered from stool. Infection of the right ovary as a result of inflamed or ruptured appendices is also possible.

Clinical presentation

Genital actinomycosis is seen most often in women with foreign bodies present in the genital tract. Although IUCDs serve as the predominant foreign bodies to stimulate colonization, other foreign bodies such as hairpins (Giordano, 1895), pessaries (Barth, 1928; Tietze, 1930) and even surgical sutures (Tiamson, 1979) or staples (Gupta, 1982) have been described as the focus of infection. Colonization may be asymptomatic or minimally symptomatic, presenting only as shedding of actinomycotic granules into the vaginal fluid. Vaginal discharge is the most common symptom, and intermittent pelvic pain and abnormal bleeding are also commonly reported. IUCDs removed from these women may show signs of breakdown and may have inflammatory changes together with adherent bacterial elements. On the more symptomatic end of the disease spectrum, women may present with pelvic abscesses of the ovary, fallopian tubes and/or uterus. These abscesses are often unilateral, involving a single fallopian tube and ovary; bilateral ovarian abscesses are uncommon. Single or multiple abscesses may form in the uterine wall, usually surrounding an embedded IUCD. This type of invasive disease is accompanied by pain and fever, often with a copious foul-smelling vaginal discharge. Involved tissues become very hard and swollen, and may later undergo suppuration. The most extensive disease may present with a frozen or 'woody' pelvis demonstrating extensive adhesions and scarring as part of the inflammatory response. Infection usually proceeds by direct extension to adjacent tissues, and may also spread to contiguous spaces as a result of draining sinuses.

Clinical diagnosis

Cervical motion tenderness, the presence of one or more pelvic masses and a foul-smelling discharge suggest invasive disease. Imaging techniques such as ultrasound and pelvic computerized tomography (CT) may demonstrate the presence of an abscess. Since symptoms may be minimal or non-specific, and there may be actual asymptomatic colonization, the diagnosis can easily be missed on the basis of clinical presentation and physical examination alone. Definitive diagnosis requires additional diagnostic testing, most importantly a PAP smear or tissue examination.

Laboratory diagnosis

The majority of genital actinomycosis cases will present with some abnormalities of cervical exudates or vaginal fluids on PAP smear. The most sensitive method of diagnosis and screening is a PAP-stained preparation that identifies characteristic clumps of filamentous rod-shaped bacteria (Gupta bodies) and an acute inflammatory cell exudate (Fig. 11.1). The organisms are gram-positive, with clumps described as 'spidery', dark and irregular after Gram staining. A variety of other features may also be seen, such as the classic 'sulphur granule' of actinomycosis identified in pelvic infections. These sulphur granules are composed of filamentous bacteria radiating around a central core of neutral glycoproteins, lipids, and calcium (Bhagavan *et al.*, 1982).

Fluorescence staining using species-specific sera can be used to speciate actinomyces appearing in vaginal or cervical discharge. These antibody reagents are not commonly available for use in the

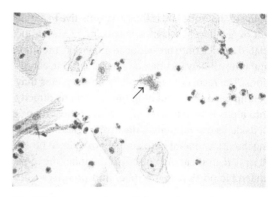

Fig. 11.1. Actinomycotic granule in a vaginal exudate. This PAP smear demonstrates a gnarled granule of actinomyces (arrow) together with a brisk acute inflammatory exudate. These findings in a genital specimen are most commonly seen in women who have had intrauterine devices in place for several years, with the foreign body serving as a nidus of infection. In this patient, the focus of infection was probably a post-hysterectomy surgical suture.

clinical laboratory and are of limited value in the overall identification of disease beyond PAP and Gram staining. The precipitin test used to detect antibody production has good performance characteristics (Persson & Holmberg, 1984b) but this assay is not widely used today.

Anaerobic actinomycetes are successfully cultured in only about 10% of those cases investigated, due to the type of specimens submitted for culture and the fastidious nature of the organism's growth requirements. Since anaerobes are part of the normal flora of the vagina, any specimens collected through the vagina (vaginal swabs, cervical swabs or endometrial swabs obtained across the cervix) are not appropriate for anaerobic culture, and thus will be rejected in most clinical laboratories. If specimens are to be submitted for anaerobic culture of actinomycetes, they must be obtained through more invasive methods that exclude contamination of the tissue with vaginal and cervical secretions. Laparotomy or laparoscopic samples of necrotic or inflamed tissue or abscess fluids are suitable for culture.

Actinomyces israelii, the organism most often implicated in this disease process, is a fastidious obligate anaerobe and is thus very sensitive to ambient oxygen levels. Diagnostic specimens should be plated at once onto pre-reduced anaerobic medium and immediately incubated under anaerobic conditions. The recovery rate for the actinomycetes may be improved by inoculating the specimens directly into a pre-reduced anaerobic broth at the patient's bedside, as this minimizes the toxic effects of exposing the strict anaerobes to ambient oxygen. In broth, *A. israelii* grows at the bottom of the tube (the most anaerobic portion of the tube) and produces tufts of very pleomorphic gram-positive branching rods that may appear either granular or as tufts of fluffy material. *A. israelii* grows very slowly, and two different colony morphologies may be seen on solid medium. Under a dissecting microscope, young colonies (2–3 days old) are 'spidery', with thin filaments of bacteria radiating out from a rough centre. After 1–2 weeks of growth, the colonies take on a smooth and lobulated morphology, resembling a 'molar tooth'.

Biochemically the actinomycetes are catalase, indole, H_2S, lecithinase and lipase negative, and do not hydrolyse starch or gelatin. More than 90% of strains ferment glucose and hydrolyse esculin. Although the majority of strains are negative for milk proteolysis, lactose fermentation and rhamanose fermentation, occasional colonies may produce positive reactions. *A. israelii* demonstrates variable growth on bile-containing agar and variably ferments mannitol. When grown in peptone yeast extract glucose (PYG) broth for 48 hours at 35 °C, *A. israelii* produces acetic, lactic and succinic acids as the major by-products of fermentative growth. *A. israelii* can be identified readily using commercially available anaerobic identification kits such as the Anaerobic Crystal, RANA, Presumpto Plate and MIDI fatty acid analyser systems.

Treatment

Treatment of pelvic actinomycosis may require several types of intervention. There is some dispute as to whether or not removal of the foreign body that stimulated colonization is required. Women wearing IUCDs have been successfully followed for several years, with detectable shedding of actinomyces into the cervical and vaginal fluids without the development of invasive disease or abscesses. After removal of the IUCD, the majority of women will resolve their colonization without any further intervention and require no antibiotic therapy. Removal of the IUCD is generally recommended and required for individuals with active, symptomatic disease. Draining, cleaning or removal of abscessed tissues help to eliminate infection. Late-stage disease may require extensive surgical intervention, with removal of one or both ovaries and/or total hysterectomy. These unfortunate outcomes were seen commonly in the early articles describing IUCD related actinomycosis (Schmidt *et al.*, 1980). The anaerobic actinomycetes are considered universally susceptible to penicillin, which is the drug of choice if antibiotic therapy is needed. In patients with extensive disease where surgical removal of involved tissues is not performed to salvage possible fertility, oral penicillin therapy may be required for 1–2 years.

Vaccine availability

No vaccine is available for actinomycosis.

Genital tuberculosis (GUTB)

Mycobacterium tuberculosis (MTB)

Epidemiology

Genital tuberculosis is a significant cause of female infertility in regions where pulmonary TB is prevalent, such as Southeast Asia, Africa and Eastern Europe. In India, genital tuberculosis occurs in 10% of cases of pulmonary TB, and 5% of all female pelvic infections are due to tuberculosis (Arora *et al.*, 2003). Populations of infertile women in India have been found to have an incidence of genital TB as high as 39% (Parikh *et al.*, 1997; Tripathy & Tripathy, 2002).

In the USA and Europe, the number of new active cases of primary (pulmonary) TB declined significantly from the 1950s to mid-1980, but between 1985 and 1991 this trend came to an abrupt end. The increase is thought to be due to multidrug-resistant (MDR) tuberculosis among HIV-infected individuals and in situations of over crowding, such as correctional institutions, homeless shelters, etc., or where host resistance may be compromised. The World Health Organization (WHO) reported an increase in global TB prevalence from 22 million cases in 1995 to 1.86 billion cases in 1997, and current reports indicate that at least one-third of the world's population (2 billion people) is infected with tuberculosis bacteria (Dye *et al.*, 1999). Approximately 10% of HIV-infected patients will develop co-existing *M. tuberculosis* infection, and 40% of those exposed develop active and rapidly progressive disease that is fatal in 72 to 89% of cases due to multiple drug resistance (MDR). This population acts as a source for new MDR infection; a WHO report released in 2004 estimated that 8 million new cases of TB develop each year globally, of which around 300,000 are new cases of MDR-TB. An individual with a healthy immune system infected with *M. tuberculosis* will develop active tuberculosis during their lifetime in about 10% of cases: 2 million people die of the disease annually, and another 1 million die of the combination of HIV and TB.

Genitourinary TB occurs in 15–20% of extra-pulmonary cases of *Mycobacterium tuberculosis* infection, reaching the pelvic region by hematogenous spread, in the same manner that it reaches other extra-pulmonary sites such as bones and joints. The kidneys, ureter, bladder or genital organs may be involved; the fallopian tubes are affected in the majority of cases, with the endometrium also a frequent site of infection. The ovaries are affected in 10–20% of cases, the cervix in approximately 5%, and vagina and vulva in <1%. Pelvic disease can also be secondary to *M. bovis* infection of bowel, peritoneum or lymph nodes. Ingestion of contaminated raw milk or dairy products from an *M. bovis*-infected cow causes intestinal tuberculosis.

Life cycle

Tubercle bacilli are non-motile, non-encapsulated rods that are facultative intracellular parasites. Primary infection occurs when aerosol droplets containing tubercle bacilli are inhaled into the terminal alveolae, causing an early exudative response. The organisms are phagocytosed and multiply within polymorphonuclear leukocytes, destroying them. As the infection enters a chronic phase, granulomas are formed. These are composed of collections of epithelioid histiocytic cells together with giant cells (Fig. 11.2). As the disease progresses with time, the centres of the granulomata may undergo caseous necrosis, characteristic of infections with TB (Figure 11.2b). At this stage the infection has generally spread to the hilar lymph nodes through lymphatic channels, and may further disseminate hematogenously to virtually every organ and tissue (military tuberculosis), producing a similar granulomatous response with caseous necrosis, fibrosis and calcification in the affected tissues. If the patient has an adequate immune response, these early lesions will heal with fibrosis and possibly also calcification. The presence of a calcified peripheral lung nodule together with a calcified mediastinal lymph node is often visible on X-ray, and is known as the Ghon complex. Approximately 95% of patients will have no further evidence of TB infection and will have microbiologic clearance of the organism from the body. A small proportion of patients with primary TB may still harbour viable organisms, and these patients will enter into a quiescent phase known as latent TB.

Reactivation disease occurs in an estimated 5–10% of individuals who have been infected with MTB. Post-primary reactivation disease generally evolves years after the primary infection, if a waning cell-mediated immunity allows reactivation of quiescent primary foci. Factors that can influence reactivation include malnutrition, alcoholism, diabetes, immunosuppression and increased age. Clinical features of genital tuberculosis usually develop 10 to 15 years after a primary infection.

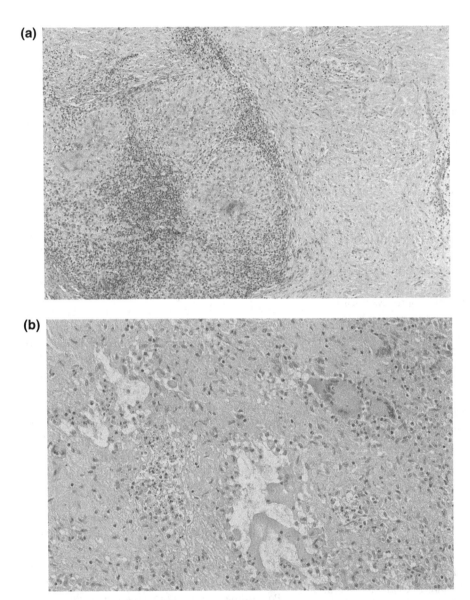

Fig. 11.2. H&E section of tissue with MTB. (*a*) Granulomatous inflammation, low power magnification. MTB infections produce this typical granulomatous infiltration seen at 10× magnification. The right hand portion of the image demonstrates extensive fibrosis surrounding the inflamed area, while the left hand portion of the image demonstrates several round granulomata composed primarily of epithelioid histiocytes admixed with occasional lymphocytes and plasma cells (round pale staining areas) surrounded by chronic inflammatory cells (lymphocytes and plasma cells, seen as the dark cellular components surrounding this inflammatory response). Several giant cells are seen in the granulomata. (*b*) Necrotizing granuloma, 20× magnification. Necrotizing granulomata are often seen in MTB infections. The areas of necrosis in this image are seen as the open spaces in the center and left-hand side of the image surrounded by the lightly coloured amorphous material representing dead tissue. Giant cells are seen in the upper right-hand portion of the Figure. (*c*) Langhans' Giant cells, high power(40×). This high power image demonstrates the typical morphology of the Langhans' giant cells produced during an inflammatory response to MTB. The cells are large, with many nuclei distributed around their periphery. The surrounding inflammatory cells represent a mixture of small lymphocytes, plasma cells and epithelioid histiocytes typically composing the granulomata.

(c)

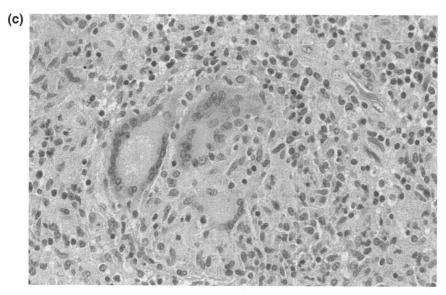

Fig. 11.2. (cont.)

Transmission

Exogenous transmission of *M. tuberculosis* occurs in adults and children via inhalation of aerosol cough or sneeze droplets from an infected individual. Crowded conditions and impaired host resistance enhance the probability of acquiring infection or disease. Certain ethnic groups, such as Asians, American Indians, Eskimos and Blacks are more likely to develop disease as opposed to infection, and an association has been found with HLA-Bw 15 histocompatibility antigen.

Endogenous reactivation disease occurs when quiescent primary foci are reactivated, usually within the respiratory tract, although any site to which MTB spreads during the primary infection may serve as the site of reactivation. Ninety percent of genital infections arise via hematogenous spread from a primary focus of lung, lymph nodes, urinary tract, bones and joints, and reflects reactivation disease rather than a manifestation of acute infection with MTB. Infection can also reach the pelvic organs by direct lymphatic spread from infected adjacent organs such as the peritoneum, bowel and mesenteric nodes. Tubercle bacilli can also be directly inoculated via vulva or vagina during sexual intercourse with a partner suffering from tuberculous lesions of the genitalia.

Clinical presentation

Clinical signs and symptoms for genitourinary TB (GUTB) are variable, and clinical diagnosis is difficult. A genital infection can be acute and rapidly extending, but the majority of cases are indolent: the disease can remain silent for more than 20 years. There may not be an obvious past history of TB or a history of contact, and there may be no obvious evidence of any tuberculous lesions elsewhere. Abdominal and vaginal examination may be normal: bimanual examination can reveal normal pelvic organs in around 50% of confirmed cases. The commonest symptom of pelvic tuberculosis is primary infertility, or secondary infertility after an ectopic pregnancy or miscarriage.

The classical presenting symptoms of TB such as malaise, weight loss, night sweats and fever are rarely seen in individuals with urogenital TB. Pelvic pain and menstrual disorders are the usual presentation, but menstrual function can remain normal in almost 50% of cases, and some patients may be asymptomatic. Menstrual disturbance can include abnormal uterine bleeding, amenorrhea, oligomenorrhea, menorrhagia, or post-menopausal bleeding. Some patients may suffer intermittent chronic lower abdominal pain, and this can be mistaken for appendicitis. Sixty to 70% of cases present with infertility due to pathology in the endometrium and fallopian tubes. The fallopian tubes are diseased in at least 90% of cases, and are probably the primary site for infection due to hematogenous spread, starting with distal endosalpingitis and progressing towards endometritis. Endometrial tuberculosis invariably indicates tuberculous salpingitis, but the tubes may be infected without associated endometritis.

Tuberculosis of the vulva and vagina usually presents with shallow, superficial indolent ulcers. The ulceration tends to spread slowly, healing in some areas with the formation of scar tissue. Inflammatory induration and edema due to fibrosis and lymphatic obstruction can lead to vulvar hypertrophic lesions. Vulvar lesions are usually painful and tender, vaginal ulcers are painless unless situated at the introitus. Bloodstained and purulent discharge may be seen with both. Tuberculosis of the cervix can be ulcerative, but often appears as a red papillary erosion that bleeds easily, resembling a carcinoma. It is generally painless, causing a bloodstained discharge and post-coital bleeding.

In the uterus, an endometrial biopsy can show tuberculous endometritis. A tuberculous ulcer may (rarely) be seen in the endometrium, and extensive involvement can lead to collections of caseous material to form pyometra. The myometrium is involved in 2.5% of cases, with abscess formation. The disease can also cause adhesions and partial obliteration of the uterine cavity. In the presence of endometrial disease, the tubal lumina are obliterated in 50% of cases.

Disease in the fallopian tubes begins in the distal submucosa and gradually progresses towards the cornua. Disease that has spread via the bloodstream starts as endosalpingitis, and direct spread from bowel or peritoneum causes an exosalpingitis with tubercles on the peritoneal surface of the tubes that may be surrounded by adhesions. Local distal obstruction can result in the formation of a hydrosalpinx or pyosalpinx, which can become calcified. A tuberculous pyosalpinx is often free from adhesions, and may present as an abdominal tumour. In some cases, symptoms and exacerbation of disease is due to secondary infection by other organisms.

The ovaries are infected in approximately 30% of cases of tuberculous salpingitis; ovarian TB without tubal involvement is rare. There may be surface tubercles, adhesions and thickening of the capsule, retention cysts, and occasionally caseating abscess cavities within the ovary, but in many cases the ovaries have a normal macroscopic appearance, diagnosis being made after ovarian biopsy.

Pelvic tuberculosis should be suspected if a pelvic infection is slow to respond to standard antimicrobial therapy, shows exacerbation after curettage or tubal patency test, or is not accompanied by peripheral polymorphonuclear leukocytosis. Pelvic ultrasound and hysterosalpingography (HSG) may be helpful in making a diagnosis, but the variety of possible pathology gives an equally varied appearance on HSG. There may be an irregular distribution of contrast around the tubes, resembling a "cotton wool" plug, considered a characteristic feature of TB. Focal strictures can give the tube a beaded appearance, and calcifications within the tubal lumen may be seen as a characteristic feature. In the fibrotic stage of disease, the tubes are rigid, no peristalsis is detected, and the tube resembles a pipe-like conduit. Within the endometrial cavity, there may be adhesions varying from thin to very thick synechiae, and, in the end stages of the disease, obliteration of the uterine cavity and marked irregularity of its contour. Calcifications of the pelvic lymph nodes and ovaries may be observed in the pelvis.

Mantoux test

The PPD (purified protein derivative) test is used to determine if a patient has an immune response to the tubercle bacillus. The test most commonly used is known as the Mantoux test, in which the protein solution is injected to form a bubble intradermally. Between 48 and 72 hours following inoculation, the reaction is read as the number of millimetres (mm) of palpated induration at the site of inoculation. The PPD test is non-specific for the diagnosis of GUTB, indicating only prior inhalation of MTB and may not reflect currently active disease. It is found to be positive in 62–100% of active cases, and may be negative (0 mm of induration) in active primary and reactivation TB, especially if the patient is immunocompromised. A chest X-ray may show calcification in 10–66% of cases, but a normal X-ray does not rule out the diagnosis of GUTB.

Urogenital disease can only be diagnosed with certainty after culture of menstrual blood or endometrial curettings, or after laparoscopic biopsy of affected tissue for histopathology to eliminate other causes of pelvic pathology such as tubo-ovarian mass of gonococcal or pyogenic origin, pelvic endometriosis, ovarian cyst or pelvic hematocoele.

Laboratory diagnosis

Direct detection of MTB

Waxes and long-chain fatty acids in the mycobacterial cell wall make the *M. tuberculosis* organisms resistant to the uptake of most stains. Although they are considered to be gram-positive bacilli in the Gram's stain classification, uptake of Gram's violet stain is incomplete, producing a 'beaded' or 'granular' appearance after staining. The organisms are slender, straight or slightly bent and may appear to be snapping apart. Very few organisms are generally present, even if there is extensive granulomatous inflammation, and the smear prepared from the clinical specimen must therefore be carefully reviewed in order to make a diagnosis. Concentrated urine samples or a tissue homogenate can be used to make the diagnosis of MTB from genital sources. An acid-fast stain is considered the standard of care for the direct detection of MTB. The College of American Pathologists further recommends the use of a fluorescent acid-fast stain for direct detection: Auramine O with or without rhodamine

as a second fluorochrome is used in the majority of institutions. Facilities lacking a fluorescent microscope may use carbolfuchsin-based stains such as the Ziel–Nielsen hot stain or the Kinyoun cold stain. These stains bind to the mycolic acid in the waxy cell walls of the mycobacteria. After stringent acid alcohol destaining, only mycobacterial organisms will remain stained. Auramine O stained mycobacteria appear yellow by fluorescence microscopy, while the auramine–rhodamine stained mycobacteria will appear orange–red. Fluorescently stained slides may be scanned at 40x, and mycobacterial morphology confirmed under oil (100×). Both forms of the carbolfuchsin-based stain produce bright pink-red rods on staining and the slides must be scanned under oil (100×). Approximately $1 \times 10^{4-5}$ organisms per ml are required before a single organism can be detected on a smear and, for this reason, specimens are usually concentrated prior to direct examination for mycobacteria. It should be noted that both dead and living mycobacteria will stain with these dyes.

Histology

Biopsy tissues demonstrate granulomatous inflammation on direct examination after Hematoxylin-Eosin (H&E) staining. Figure 11.2 demonstrates these characteristic findings on H&E. Collections of epithelioid histiocytes cluster together to form granulomata (Fig. 11.2(*a*)) that are surrounded by chronic inflammatory cells and fibrosis. In larger granulomata, central caseous necrosis may be present (Fig. 11.2(*b*)). Giant cells are seen in varying numbers, as demonstrated by the morphology seen in Fig. 11.2(*c*). The tubercle bacilli can only be visualized using a tissue acid-fast stain. The carobolfuchsin-based Fite stain can be used, but some laboratories use a form of Auramine O staining with Evans Blue dye as a fluorescence quencher. If the carbolfuchsin stain is used, the slides must be reviewed under oil (100×). Even if extensive granulomatous inflammation is present, acid-fast stains from tissue sections are often negative due to the small numbers of organisms present.

Culture

Mycobacteria can be cultured by a variety of methods, which fall into one of two general categories: broth enrichment cultures or direct inoculation cultures. Mycobacterial generation time is very slow, and therefore it is important to eliminate any non-mycobacteria from the clinical specimens suspected of containing normal flora. For respiratory specimens such as sputa, or genital specimens likely to be contaminated with vaginal flora, the specimens must be decontaminated with a mixture of 2–4% NaOH prior to culture. After 15 minutes of treatment with the NaOH solution, the specimen is neutralized back to a pH of 7.0. The specimen is then generally inoculated into both a broth enrichment medium and onto a solid medium for culture. Specimens taken from normally sterile sites such as tissue biopsies do not require decontamination. Endometrial specimens should be taken in the premenstrual phase, preferably from the cornua, and if collected correctly, should not require decontamination before homogenisation and culture.

Both liquid and solid media used to culture mycobacteria contain the bacterial inhibitor malachite green in varying concentrations, in order to inhibit normal flora. The standard broth enrichment culture, BACTEC 460 (Becton Dickenson Diagnostic Instruments, Sparks, MD) utilizes C^{14}-radiolabelled palmitic acid as a food source for the mycobacteria in a defined chemical Middlebrook medium (7H9, 7H10, 7H11, or 7H12) (Fig. 11.3). The organisms utilize this fatty acid for cell wall synthesis, and C^{14}-radiolabelled CO_2 is liberated into the bottle. Radioactivity is detected by the BACTEC instrument in air samples aspirated from within each bottle. The MB/BacT Mycobacteria Detection System utilizes the BacT Alert instrumentation (Organon Technika, Durham, NC) to identify mycobacterial growth by detecting CO_2 with a gas permeable sensor that changes from dark green to yellow when CO_2 is produced by the mycobacteria. This system does not require radiolabelled CO_2. Similarly, The ESP MYCO system (Difco Laboratories, Detroit, MI) utilizes the ESP blood culture instrumentation to

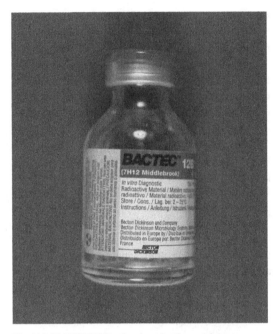

Fig. 11.3. BACTEC 12B broth culture bottle containing Middlebrook 7H12 medium (Becton Dickenson Diagnostic Instruments, Sparks, MD) for the support of mycobacterial growth. Liquid medium for MTB culture provides an amplified and more rapid culture system for the detection of mycobacterium than the direct culture onto solid medium. Decontaminated and concentrated specimens are inoculated directly into the liquid medium and incubated at 37 °C. This system uses the BACTEC 460 system to measure the production of C^{14}-radiolabelled CO_2 that is produced as the mycobacteria utilize the radiolabelled palmitic acid supplement in the medium. This bottle is uninoculated.

monitor Middlebrook 7H9 medium-containing bottles. These bottles are continuously monitored to detect changes in gas pressure, a sign of mycobacterial growth. The Mycobacteria Growth Indicator Tube system (BBL, Becton Dickinson Microbiology Systems, Hunt Valley, MD) utilizes modified Middlebrook 7H11 medium containing oleic acid supplements and the PANTA antibiotic mixture to suppress the growth of contaminating non-mycobacterial organisms. A fluorescent compound embedded in the silicone at the bottom of each tube is used as the indicator for mycobacterial growth. Free oxygen in the medium quenches the fluorochrome activity, and bottles that have no growth will not fluoresce when exposed to long-wave UV light. Mycobacterial growth uses oxygen in the tubes, and the indicator will fluoresce when illuminated with the UV light source. In each of these systems, bottles that are found to be positive are then stained with an acid-fast stain to confirm that a mycobacterium has been cultured. A pellet of mycobacterial growth is subsequently tested using the GenProbe system (San Diego, CA) to detect MTB. These rapid and very specific probe assays allow laboratories to efficiently and safely identify MTB in clinical specimens. This not only provides a definitive diagnosis weeks earlier than performing biochemical identification, but also decreases the laboratory risk for technologist exposure. Non-tuberculous mycobacteria require subculture onto solid media and either biochemical characterization or detection with specific probes, if available.

Several solid media are commonly used to culture mycobacteria in the clinical laboratory. These are divided into chemically defined media (Middlebrook 7H10 or 7H11 media) or coagulated egg-based media (Lowenstein–Jensen, American Thoracic Society, or Petragnaní media). Chemically defined media have the benefit of being clear, so that mycobacterial growth can be more rapidly recognized. However, they are usually used in Petri dishes, which pose a risk to technologists if the unsealed plates are dropped. Coagulated egg media are opaque, and are generally used in screw-top tubes (Fig. 11.3). These are safer to work with and are generally used for all amplified subcultures, biochemical tests and for all strains that are used for quality control. Egg-based media contain malachite green inhibitor at a concentration 10–20 times greater than that of the Middlebrook recipes. On solid medium, MTB produces dry, crumbly, buff coloured, slow growing colonies (Fig. 11.4). MTB grows best at 37 °C with 3–11% CO_2.

Biochemical identification may still be required in some laboratories that do not have probe technology, and three tests are required for a definitive diagnosis of MTB. In the light test, cultures of MTB will

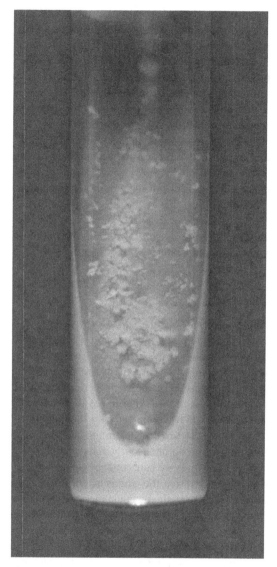

Fig. 11.4. MTB growth on Lowenstein–Jensen Medium. Note the characteristic dry and crumbly heaped-up colony morphology. The presence of buff-coloured colonies of this morphology in culture gives a very high index of suspicion that the organism is MTB, and appropriate precautions should be taken with these cultures.

produce no carotene pigment before or after inoculation of the colonies in the light. To perform this test, a Lowenstein–Jensen slant of MTB growth is cultured in the dark (wrapped in aluminium foil). The colour of the colonies is recorded when sufficient visible growth is detected; the microbial growth on the slant is then exposed to light for 30 minutes, and the tube is rewrapped, incubated for 1–3 days and then re-evaluated for pigment production. MTB colonies are dry and crumbly, buff coloured in the dark and remaining buff after exposure to light.

MTB is the only non-pigment producer that is positive for nitrate production and accumulates niacin in the culture medium. A positive result for both of these assays is diagnostic. Additional biochemical characteristics that may be helpful in identifying MTB include a relative lack of catalase activity, and inhibition of growth by *p*-nitro-acetylamino-hydroxy-propiophenone (NAP) reagent.

Treatment

Medical: Current standard treatment regimes for GUTB last from 6 to 8 months, and a strategy that includes an adherence plan that emphasizes directly observed therapy (DOT, patients are observed to ingest each dose of medication), is recommended whenever possible. This maximizes the likelihood that therapy will be completed over the long duration of time. Standard drug treatment includes multiple drugs given simultaneously, and recommended treatment regimes are constantly being updated to monitor and prevent the emergence of drug resistance. Current treatment guidelines are available from the Centers for Disease Control and Prevention (CDC, 2003), and are published on their website: http://www.cdc.gov/.

International recommendations and guidelines have also been developed by the World Health Organization (WHO, 1996) and the International Union Against Tuberculosis and Lung Disease (IUATLD, http://www.tbrieder.org/).

Four drugs are administered for 2 months followed by administration of two drugs (INH and Rifampicin) for a further 4 months unless resistance to either agent exists. If the patient is HIV positive, drug treatment should be continued for 9 months. First-line drugs include Isoniazid (INH), Rifampin (RIF), Pyrizinamide (PYA) and Ethambutol (EMB). Rifabutin may be used as a substitute for RIF in patients who are receiving medication that may interact with RIF, or who are intolerant to RIF. Rifapentine may be used with INH in the continuation phase. Combined preparations are available in some countries, and these formulations minimize the number of pills that must be taken daily. Different regimes are used, according to the site and extent of disease, and each individual treatment must be based upon full clinical assessment and culture results. Second-line drugs used to treat drug-resistant tuberculosis include Cycloserine, Ethionamide, Streptomycin, Amikacin and kanamycin, Capreomycin, *p*-aminosalicylic acid (PAS) and fluoroquinolones (levofloxacin, moxifloxacin and gatifloxacin).

Surgical intervention either as ablation or reconstruction is often required during the course of drug treatment, and is indicated in the presence of the following:

- persistent or recurrent pelvic mass following 6 months of chemotherapy;
- persistent or recurrent disease following medical treatment;
- persistent recurrent symptoms;
- non-healing fistulas;
- multiple drug-resistant disease.

Any surgery should be preceded by 3 to 6 months of anti-tuberculous drugs in full dosage, and followed by the full course of treatment. Surgery is contraindicated if there is active tuberculosis in any site, and in the presence of plastic peritonitis and dense adhesions around the pelvic organs, due to the risk of injury to bladder, ureter or bowel.

Infertility and GUTB

Restoration of fertility is rare in cases of genital TB. Ectopic pregnancy following antituberculous drug therapy for pelvic TB is a recognized clinical syndrome, and miscarriage is also common. The indication for tubal reconstructive microsurgery depends on the stage of the disease, but has an overall success of no more than 22%. The majority of patients are referred for assisted reproduction treatment with IVF.

Vaccine availability

The vaccine used against TB today was developed in the early 1900s, BCG (Bacille Calmette-Guerin). It is widely administered to infants throughout the world, but not in the USA. and parts of Europe where TB is mainly controlled with drugs. BCG appears to reduce the risk of serious childhood forms of TB (meningeal and milliary), but has not been shown to protect against long-term respiratory disease in children or adults who were vaccinated as children. The degree that protective immunity extends into adulthood is unknown. BCG vaccination in adults is controversial, with numerous studies providing conflicting results. The high incidence of TB in developing countries where infant BCG immunization is widely practised indicates that BCG is not highly efficacious over the long duration of time that individuals are at risk for contracting the disease, and clearly there is a need for better vaccination strategies. The BCG vaccine is not used in most countries that are not endemic for MTB infection, for several reasons. First, there are many contraindications to vaccinating with BCG. As a live vaccine, the potential for disseminated disease is not insignificant, especially in patients who are immunocompromised. Patients with primary immunodeficiency and those with AIDS may develop disseminated disease after vaccination with the organism. Secondly, vaccination with BCG may interfere with the routine PPD screening of populations at risk for acquiring MTB infections. Although many BCG recipients (particularly adults with a remote history of vaccination) will have zero mm of induration (negative PPD interpretation), others may have 1–10 mm of induration around the PPD site. These small reaction sizes make interpretation difficult in these patients, especially in the presence of HIV infection or other situations of immune compromise. Patients with this range of induration require additional evaluation including chest X-rays, and if this is suspicious, culture and staining of at least three sputa to rule out active MTB infection. Prophylaxis may also be required. In the USA, these individuals are treated prophylactically with isoniazid, as are recent immigrants with abnormal PPD findings. The presence of a large area of induration (>10 or 15 mm depending upon immune status) is generally considered evidence of a current or past infection with MTB, and these patients should be managed accordingly. Several new vaccine candidates for TB using live recombinant bacilli have recently been developed, with promising results when tested in animals. A new clinical trial with one of these vaccines, BVG03, was begun in the USA in February 2004. This live vaccine over-expresses the major protein secreted by *M. tuberculosis*, and uses the BCG (Bacille Calmette–Guérin) as a delivery vehicle.

FURTHER READING

PATHOLOGY OF THE UPPER GENITAL TRACT

Alcamo, I. E. (ed.). (1998). *Schaum's Outline of Theory and Problems in Microbiology*. New York: McGraw-Hill.

Baron, E. J., Chang, R. S., Howard, D. H., Miller, J. N. & Turner, J. A. (eds). (1994). *Medical Microbiology – A Short Course*. New York: Wiley-Liss.

Domingue, G. D. & Hellstrom, W. J. G. (1998). Prostatitis. *Clinical Microbiology Reviews*, 11(4): 604–13.

Egger-Kruse, W. (1999). Genital tract infection and infertility, Preface. *Human Reproduction Update*, 5(5): 391–2.

Holmes, K. K., Sparling, P. F., Marsh, P. *et al.* (1999). *Sexually Transmitted Diseases*, 3rd edn. New York: McGraw-Hill.

Paavonenen, J. & Eggert-Kruse, W. (1999). *Chlamydia trachomatis*: impact on human reproduction. *Human Reproduction Update*, 5(5): 433–47.

Spagna, V. A. & Prior, R. B. (eds) (1985). *Sexually Transmitted Diseases: A Clinical Syndrome Approach* New York and Basel: Marcel Dekker, Inc.

Weidner, W., Krause, W. & Ludwig, M. (1999). Relevance of male accessory gland infection for subsequent fertility with special focus on prostatitis. *Human Reproduction Update*, 5(5): 421–32.

REFERENCES

ACTINOMYCOSIS

Barth, H. (1928). Uber parametritis Actinomycotica und ihre Entstehung & *Archiv Gynaekologie*, 134: 310–21.

Bhagavan, B. S. & Gupta, P. K. (1978). Genital actinomycosis and intrauterine contraceptive devices. *Human Pathology*, 9: 567–78.

Bhagavan, B. S., Ruffier, J. & Shinn, B. (1982). Pseudoactinomycotic radiate granules in the lower female genital tract: relationship to the Splendore–Hoeppli phenomenon. *Human Pathology*, **13**: 898–904.

Giordano, D. (1895). Un caso di actinomicosi dell'utero. *Clinica Chirurgica*, **3**: 237–9.

Gupta, P. K. (1982). Intrauterine contraceptive devices: vaginal cytology, pathologic changes and clinical implications. *Acta Cytologica*, **26**: 571–613.

Gupta, P. K., Hollander, D. H. & Frost, J. K. (1976). Actinomycetes in cervico–vaginal smears: an association with IUD usage. *Acta Cytologica*, **20**: 295–7.

Henderson, S. R. (1973). Pelvic actinomycosis associated with an intrauterine device. *Obstetrics and Gynecology*, **41**: 726–32.

Mali, B., Joshi, J. V., Wagle, U. *et al.* (1986). Actinomyces in cervical smears of women using intrauterine contraceptive devices. *Acta Cytologica*, **30**: 367–71.

Persson, E. & Holmberg, K. (1984). Clinical evaluation of precipitin tests for genital actinomycosis. *Journal of Clinical Microbiology*, **20**: 917–22.

Schmidt, W. A., Webb, J. A., Bedrossian, C. W. M., Bastian, F. O. & Ali, V. (1980). Actinomycosis and intrauterine contraceptive devices: the clinicopathologic entity. *Diagnosis in Gynecology and Obstetrics*, **2**: 165–77.

Tiamson, E. M. (1979). Genital actinomycosis. *Human Pathology*, **10**: 119–20.

Tietze, K. (1930). Sieben Salle Schwerster Schabigung deurich intrauterine pessare (ein von isoliestes Genitalaktinomy Kase) *Deutsche Medikalische Wochenschrift*, **56**: 1307–9.

Weese, W. C. & Smith, I. M. (1975). A study of 57 cases of actinomycosis over a 36-year period. *Archives of Internal Medicine*, **135**: 1562–8.

FURTHER READING

ACTINOMYCOSIS

Aubert, J. M., Gobeaux-Castadot, M. J. & Boria, M. (1980). Actinomyces in the endometrium of IUD users. *Contraception*, **21**: 577–83.

Buckley, J. W. & Tolanai, G. (1976). An alert to genital actinomycosis. *Canadian Medical Association Journal*, **115**: 1193.

Cornell, V. H. (1933). Actinomycosis of tubes and ovaries. *American Journal of Pathology*, **X**: 519–30.

Curtis, E. M. & Pine, L. (1981). Actinomyces in the vaginas of women with and without intrauterine contraceptive devices. *American Journal of Obstetrics and Gynecology*, **140**: 880–4.

Gupta, P. K. & sWoodruff, J. D. (1982). Actinomyces in vaginal smears. *Journal of the American Medical Association*, **247**: 1175–6.

Hagar, W. D., Douglas, B., Majmudak, B. *et al.* (1979). Pelvic colonization with actinomyces in women using intrauterine contraceptive devices. *American Journal of Obstetrics and Gynecology*, **135**: 680–4.

Jones, M. C. & Dowling, E. A. (1979). The prevalence of actinomycetes-like organisms found in cervicovaginal smears of 300 IUD wearers. *Acta Cytologica*, **23**: 282–6.

Paalman, R. J., Dockerty, M. B. & Mussey, R. D. (1949). Actinomycosis of the ovaries and fallopian tubes. *American Journal of Obstetrics and Gynecology*, **58**: 419–31.

Persson, E. & Holmberg, K. (1984). A longitudinal study of *Actinomyces israelii* in the female genital tract. *Acta Obstetrica Gynecologica Scandinavica*, **63**: 207–16.

Petitti, D. A., Yamamoto, D. & Morgenstern, N. (1983). Factors associated with actinomyces-like organisms on Papanicolaou smear in users of intrauterine contraceptive devices. *American Journal of Obstetrics and Gynecology*, **145**: 338–41.

Schiffer, M. A., Elguezabal, A., Sultana, M. & Allen, A. C. (1975). Actinomycosis infections associated with intrauterine contraceptive devices. *Obstetrics and Gynecology*, **45**: 67–72.

REFERENCES

GENITAL TUBERCULOSIS

Arora, V. K., Gupta, R. & Arora, R. (2003). Female genital tuberculosis – need for more research. *Indian Journal of Tuberculosis*, **50**, 9–11.

Centers for Disease Control and Prevention (2003). Treatment of tuberculosis. *Morbidity and Mortality Weekly*, **52**(RR11), 1–77 http://www.cdc.gov/.

Dye, C., Scheele, S., Dolin, P., Pathania, V. & Raviglione, M. C. (1999). Consensus statement. Global burden of tuberculosis: estimated incidence, prevalence, and mortality by country. WHO Global Surveillance and Monitoring Project. *Journal of the American Medical Association*, **18**, 282(7), 677–86.

International Union Against Tuberculosis and Lung Disease (IUATLD, http://www.tbrieder.org/.

Parikh, F. R., Nadkarni, S. G., Kamat, S. A., Naik, N., Soonawala, S. B. & Parikh, R. M. (1997). Genital tuberculosis – a major pelvic factor causing infertility in Indian women. *Fertility and Sterility*, **67**(3), 497–500.

Tripathy, S. N. & Tripathy, S. N. (2002). Infertility and pregnancy outcome in female genital tuberculosis. *International Journal of Gynaecology and Obstetrics*, **76**(2), 159–63.

World Health Organization (1996). Treatment of tuberculosis: guidelines for national programmes. Geneva: WHO/TB/ 96.199. Available at: http://www.who.int/gtb/publications

FURTHER READING

GENITAL TUBERCULOSIS

Koneman, E. W., Allen, S. D., Janda, W. M., Schreckenberger, P. C. & Winn, W. C. (1997). Mycobacteria. In *Color Atlas and Textbook of Diagnostic Microbiology*, 5th edn., pp 893–952. Philadelphia, PA: J. B Lippincott Co.

http://www.eurekalert.org/pubnews.php

http://www.sunmed.org/pelvictb.html

12

Cytomegalovirus and blood-borne viruses

Although cytomegalovirus (CMV), hepatitis B, C, D viridae (HBV, HCV, HDV), human T-lymphotrophic virus (HTLV) and human immunodeficiency virus (HIV) are not associated with genital tract manifestations, they may be considered as sexually transmitted diseases. These agents pose a particular risk in assisted reproductive technologies because of their potential for transmission to staff, to other patients, and to children born as a result of treatment, particularly via cycles that involve the use of donor gametes. They are responsible for a wide spectrum of clinical illnesses involving multiple organ systems, and all have been recognized to be more prevalent in populations attending STD clinics than in the general population.

The infectious agents of CMV, HIV, HTLV, HBV, HCV and HDV can persist in the blood unknown to the carrier, who may be asymptomatic; they can also be transmitted via other body fluids, including:

- cerebrospinal fluid (CSF)
- pleural fluid
- breast milk
- amniotic fluid
- peritoneal fluid
- pericardial fluid
- synovial fluid
- vaginal secretions
- semen
- any other fluid containing visible blood, as well as all unfixed tissues, organs, and parts of bodies.

Blood-borne virus (BBV) transmission can occur via:

- sexual intercourse
- sharing needles/syringes
- re-use of unsterilized or inadequately sterilized injection equipment
- skin puncture by blood-contaminated sharp objects such as needles, instruments or glass
- childbirth – before or during birth, or through breast feeding
- blood transfusion

The viruses are also transmitted, less commonly, through:

- contamination of open wounds and skin lesions such as eczema, etc,
- splashing the mucous membranes of the eye, nose, or mouth,
- human bites when blood is drawn.

BBV are not known to be transmitted by the respiratory route, although this possibility cannot be dismissed when there is an abnormally high level of exposure, under laboratory conditions. Unless adequate precautions are taken, they may be transmitted to workers or patients/clients in the course of many medical and para-medical procedures, and the IVF clinic poses a particular risk in this respect. Transmission has been documented in association with clinical procedures, and cases of nosocomial HCV infection have been reported (Levy *et al.*, 2000).

Cytomegalovirus (CMV)

Cytomegalovirus is an enveloped icosahedral double-stranded DNA virus, a member of the

Herpesviridae that shares their feature of interacting with human DNA to establish chronic, recurrent or latent infections. It was first recognized as a human pathogen in 1947, associated with fulminant congenital infections. In 1965 it was identified in association with a disease resembling infectious mononucleosis in young adults and it is now known to be ubiquitous, common in both the perinatal period and in young adult life. Virtually all CMV infections in immunocompetent people are subclinical and asymptomatic. Active (generally subclinical) infection is systemic, and during infection the virus is widely disseminated throughout the body: CMV can be found in urine, saliva, milk, semen, and cervical secretions. The development of CMV immunity results in latency, but the virus can be reactivated intermittently throughout life, including during pregnancy and during periods of immunosuppression. It is one of the most common causes of intrauterine infections during pregnancy and primary CMV infection in the mother can result in severe fetal disease with perinatal death or congenital malformations. CMV is a major cause of opportunistic infection in organ transplant recipients, in patients undergoing treatment for malignancy and in patients with HIV infection or AIDS.

CMV does not directly affect fertility, but it has become a virus of interest and concern in ART practice because of its potential transmission through the use of donor gametes. The introduction of guidelines and regulations regarding CMV screening has made a considerable impact on availability of donor semen, since it is estimated that around 60% of the population in the USA and Western Europe has acquired CMV infection by the age of 40.

Humans are the only reservoir for CMV infection; prevalence of the virus varies worldwide from 50% in rural populations to 90–100% in an urban environment. In general, CMV infection is acquired earlier in life among populations with a lower socio-economic status: by the age of 6, 90% of the population in developing countries is seropositive, as compared to approximately 30% in the USA and Europe. There is a higher prevalence of antibodies in women and

virus shedding as well as antibody titres are higher in women under evaluation for venereal disease. Shedding of virus and antibody titres are positively correlated with number of sex partners and with current or past STD. Antibody prevalence is also higher in homosexual men (94–100%). Co-infection with multiple strains of CMV has been demonstrated in semen of homosexual men, suggesting that reinfection of the genital tract and possibly other sites is relatively common in promiscuous populations.

CMV structure

The virus has 208 predicted open reading frames (ORF), 33 of which have substantial amino acid homologies with HSV-1, VZV and EBV; it carries seven conserved sequence blocks that are also found in the other herpesviruses, but in a different order. These conserved sequences regulate DNA replication and repair, nucleotide metabolism and virion structure. CMV has an icosahedral capsid, with a simple core of DNA associated with polyamines (spermine and spermidine). The major capsid protein (MCP) is structural and a minor capsid protein (mCP) anchors DNA. Other assembly and associated proteins play a role in virus maturation. The phospholipid envelope is involved in mediating adhesion to host cell receptors and cell–cell transmission and fusion. There are at least 20 tegument proteins, many of which are phosphorylated. Some of these proteins are strongly immunogenic and act as targets in antigenaemia assays.

Life cycle

The kinetics of human CMV infection are very slow, with an incubation period of from 7 to 14 days before symptoms may be seen. In vitro, the virus attaches to widely distributed specific receptors on the cell membrane and attachment is rapid and efficient in a variety of cell lines. However, CMV replicates and grows well only in a restricted range of human cells, due to a post-penetration block to viral gene expression. The virus enters by direct fusion of the viral envelope with the plasma membrane of a mucosal cell and the process of viral replication follows a pattern similar to that already described for herpes simplex viruses (Chapter 7). After entry, the virus can either replicate and destroy the cell, or it can be incorporated into the host cell DNA. Once infection is established, it cannot be cleared, due to absence of induced specific immunity; infected individuals carry CMV for life. The virus may enter latency by integrating its genome into a cell line or by continuing to replicate at a low level. Direct reactivation of latent virus from monocytes or granulocyte–macrophage progenitor cells has not been reported, but this cell population is suspected to be the major reservoir of latent virus.

Host cell RNA polymerase II transcribes CMV DNA in the nucleus of infected cells and transcription of the viral genome occurs in three phases:

(i) immediate early (alpha): does not require *de novo* protein synthesis. The gene products act as stimulators and repressors of alpha gene expression, as well as transactivators of beta and gamma gene expression.

(ii) delayed early (beta): divided into two subclasses, with transcription occurring 4–8 hours after infection (beta-1) and 8–24 hrs after infection (beta-2). The products of these genes are necessary for DNA replication and nucleotide metabolism.

(iii) late (gamma): divided into two subclasses, with transcription occurring 12–36 hours after infection (gamma-1) and 24–48 hours after infection (gamma-2). The products of these genes are necessary for the synthesis of structural proteins and for virus maturation.

This time sequence is complicated by three factors.

(i) Translation of viral mRNA does not always occur.

(ii) Transcription continues and peaks late in infection, regardless of when expression begins.

(iii) CMV replication and expression of various gene products are sensitive to any conditions that decrease cell viability, i.e. CMV grows well only in healthy active cells.

The process of DNA replication is similar to that of HSV, with large concatomeric units cleaved and

packaged into mature capsids. The viral membrane contains lipids derived from the host cell nuclear and cytoplasmic membranes; virus maturation probably starts during budding at the inner nuclear membrane and the particles then find their way out of the cell in vesicles or through a complex process of fusion into the cytoplasm and re-envelopment at the plasma membrane.

After initiating infection via a mucosal surface, the virus spreads locally to lymphoid tissue and then circulates systemically in lymphocytes and monocytes to involve lymph nodes and the spleen. Infection then localizes in ductal epithelial cells of organs such as salivary glands, kidney tubules, cervix, testes and epididymis. Infected cells are frequently swollen and may contain large intranuclear inclusions surrounded by a clear halo, which can be identified as inclusion bodies under electron microscopy.

CMV enters latency in mononuclear blood cells. Latently infected cells will circulate in the peripheral blood or become localized in normal tissues or exudates containing white blood cells. Virus replication may be intermittently reactivated leading to mucosal shedding of CMV into urine and oral and genital secretions. Although reactivation of active replication is generally asymptomatic, it may cause active disease in an immunocompromised host. Much of the disease transmission seen with this virus is based upon asymptomatic reactivation.

Transmission

After primary infection, infectious virus is produced for long periods and can be transmitted through contact with oropharyngeal secretions (saliva), urine, cervical and vaginal secretions, semen, breast milk, tears, feces and blood. Day-care centres are a notorious source of CMV in the USA – surveys have shown that over 25% of children in day-care centres can actively transmit the virus. It is also readily transmitted by sexual contact: both primary and secondary CMV may be spread to additional hosts. The virus is vertically transmitted from mother to fetus or neonate, and transmission is seen during first, second and third trimesters of pregnancy, as well as at parturition. In the USA, about 0.5% of all infants have congenital CMV infections (Revello *et al.*, 2002). Vertical transmission may occur if a CMV seronegative mother develops an acute infection, secondary to reactivation of a CMV seropositive mother's infection with CMV, or secondary to a new CMV infection in a previously infected mother. Severe fetal disease is more commonly associated with vertical transmission from the mother during her primary infection than with secondary reactivation. Breast milk is the most common mode of transmission in some parts of the world.

Parenteral exposure, transfusion and transplant in particular represent a high risk for virus transmission: hospital acquired infections can result from organ allografts or blood transfusions from seropositive donors or virus-infected unscreened blood products. The risk for acquiring CMV post-transfusion is highest for those products containing large numbers of white blood cells (platelet concentrates, white blood cell products and unfiltered red blood cell products). The risk for acquiring infections through blood transfusion diminishes greatly if leukodepleted products are used.

CMV in semen

The potential risk of viral transmission via gamete donation continues to be a subject of concern, controversy and debate. Fertility societies in the USA and the UK have created guidelines that advise the use of gametes from CMV seropositive donors only for seropositive recipients. Samples should be re-tested after quarantine in order to identify seroconversion of donors that initially test as seronegative. In 2003, the French CECOS Federation published the results of a prospective multicentric study that involved 16 different French medical teams, evaluating tests used to screen for CMV in relation to the risk of viral infection due to donor sperm (Bresson *et al.*, 2003). Serum samples were collected from sperm donors for anti-CMV IgM and IgG antibody testing at the onset of the study, and 6 months later, and the frozen donor sperm samples were tested for CMV by rapid and conventional cultures and by PCR. A total of

635 semen samples from 231 donors were tested: overall 10 of the 635 samples were culture and/or PCR positive (1.57% of samples, 3.05% of donors, 5.3% of seropositive donors, 1.75% of initially seronegative donors). Of the positive samples, one donor was IgG and IgM negative both initially and after quarantine. Two donors were IgG positive and IgM negative in both tests, three were IgG and IgM positive at the first test, and one donor showed evidence of seroconversion from IgG and IgM negative in the first test to IgG positive IgM $+/-$ (borderline) after quarantine. There was excellent correlation between cultures and PCR results for the 541 negative samples of 190 donors. However, the positive samples did not show 100% correlation between the two techniques: six ejaculates from three donors were culture negative/PCR positive, and, surprisingly, three ejaculates from one donor were culture positive/PCR negative. The authors suggest that molecular methods for detection of infectious CMV in semen are not yet completely reliable, and require further development and standardization. A strict application of serology testing, in particular IgM, with repeat testing after a 180-day quarantine is recommended as the the most effective means of preventing potential CMV transmission by sperm donation. Semen samples from donors who are initially IgM positive, or who exhibit IgG and/or IgM seroconversion during quarantine should not be used for assisted reproduction procedures.

Clinical presentation

Immunocompetent host

In the absence of immunocompromise, primary CMV infections are generally subclinical and asymptomatic. Viral replication takes place in a large range of ductal epithelial cells such as the salivary glands and kidneys, as well as in endothelial and fibroblast cells. Although the virus is lytic, provided there is normal cellular and antibody immune response, clinical evidence of infection is minimal because of its slow replication, restricted cell tropism and limited cell to cell spread. Overall, cell-mediated immunity mechanisms and antibody responses eventually control the virus, although infected cells remain in the body throughout life and can be a source of reactivation and disease when cell-mediated immunity (CMI) defences are impaired. Occasionally, an acute mononucleosis-like syndrome may be seen in healthy young adults, similar to the infectious mononucleosis caused by the Epstein–Barr virus, with fever, abnormal liver function tests, mild lymphadenopathy and fatigue; pharyngitis is unusual. In rare cases, a disseminated CMV mononucleosis syndrome may develop, with potential complications that include pneumonia, hepatitis, meningitis, retinitis and autoantibody production. Risk factors for developing symptomatic disease include a primary infection during teen or adult ages, engaging in intercourse at a young age, many sexual partners, homosexuality and a history of other STDs. Smaller amounts of virus may initiate more severe disease and persistent infection in individuals who are immunodeficient, immunosuppressed or of young age.

Congenital CMV disease

CMV is one of the most common causes of intrauterine infection and the most common congenital viral infection in humans, affecting 0.4–2.3% of all live births worldwide. Severity of disease ranges from inapparent asymptomatic infection to fetal death. Fetal CMV infection can be modulated by the presence of maternal antiviral antibodies and cellular antiviral responses prior to conception, and these may reduce, but not eliminate intrauterine transmission. Severe disease classically presents as a small, microcephalic neonate with psychomotor retardation, hepatosplenomegaly, chorioretinitis, hemolytic anemia, jaundice and purpura due to thrombocytopenia. About one-third of all infected neonates will manifest severe to moderate symptoms; a congenitally infected neonate may be asymptomatic at birth, or may subsequently develop hearing or visual difficulties over several months following birth.

The most severe fetal disease is seen when a previously CMV seronegative mother experiences primary infection in early pregnancy; transmission occurs at a rate of 30–40%. Although transmission may occur late in the pregnancy or from a mother during asymptomatic reactivation, these infections are much less likely to produce symptomatic disease in the neonate.

Immunocompromised host

Impaired cellular immunity allows the virus to escape control and the effects of infection are more serious. In renal transplant patients, infection can lead to renal dysfunction and graft rejection. Bone marrow or heart–lung transplant patients can develop severe viral pneumonia. CMV is a particular threat to HIV patients, causing lesions and even perforation of the gut, CNS infections with encephalitis, retinitis and possible damage to the cochlea, as well as viral pneumonia.

Laboratory diagnosis

Direct detection

CMV may be detected directly in cytologic and tissue specimens through the identification of intranuclear and cytoplasmic viral inclusions in infected cells (Fig. 12.1). The intranuclear inclusions in CMV are similar to those seen in HSV infections, large and blot-like, occupying much of the infected cell's nucleus. These large inclusions contain viral capsids and the viral DNA. The host cellular DNA appears on the periphery of the nuclear membrane. Cytoplasmic inclusions containing completed CMV virions are also commonly seen, along with the nuclear inclusions. Electron microscopy effectively demonstrates intracellular viral inclusions, but does not distinguish among the various Herpesviridae. Monoclonal antibody stains may be used to stain tissue sections for a definitive diagnosis.

Viral burden can be assessed with an antigenemia assay that demonstrates the number of infected white blood cells in a blood buffy coat preparation. Fluorescently labelled anti pp65 antigen is used to stain white cells infected with CMV. This may detect low numbers of infected cells reflecting latent

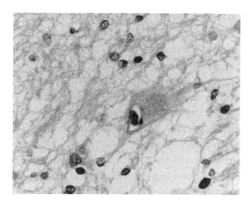

Fig. 12.1. Cytomegalovirus infected neuron with the characteristic intranuclear and cytoplasmic inclusions seen in a patient with CMV encephalitis. The large, blot-like inclusion occupies the centre of the nucleus, and the cellular DNA is seen at the periphery of the nuclear membrane, surrounding the viral inclusion as a dark staining ring in this H&E stained slide. The cytoplasm contains pale inclusions typical of the CMV infection.

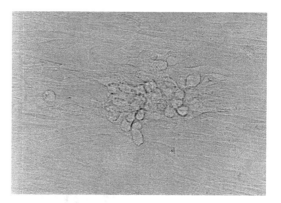

Fig. 12.2. Tube culture of CMV in MRC-5 cells. CMV, similar to the Herpes simplex viruses, grows best in a fibroblast cell line such as MRC-5 cells. Plaques or clusters of infected cells are produced slowly in the standard tube culture, and may take up to 21 days for detection. Plaques are generally small and well defined, with round and granular infected cells.

infection, or increased numbers of infected cells seen during active disease. This assay requires a relatively high white blood cell count and is therefore not useful in patients with severe neutropenia. The specimen has very limited stability, a further disadvantage for the assay.

Culture

CMV cultures are commonly performed on fibroblast cell lines such as MRC-5 cells. Culture rates vary from several days to 3–4 weeks for the standard tube culture. Plaques of approximately 10 rounded and refractile infected cells develop near the butt of the tube, and CMV is detected after the characteristic cytopathic effect develops (Fig. 12.2).

Since detection of CMV in this type of culture requires extensive cellular changes caused by the very slow-growing virus, the test is generally supplemented with a spin amplified culture technique such as the shell vial assay (Fig. 12.3).

The shell vial assay linked with monoclonal antibody staining for the immediate early antigen can detect infection 1 to 3 days after inoculation. Fluorescence antibody staining demonstrates the character-

istic nuclear distribution of the immediate early antigen before a cytopathic effect can be seen in the cell monolayer. However, the tube culture remains the more sensitive of the two culture techniques. CMV culture of urine or sputum will be positive in most cases of congenital CMV disease where virus is shed in large numbers, but culture will detect less than half of the cases of central nervous system disease or viremia.

Serum antibody assays (*serology*)

Serology may be used to detect past or current infection. IgM antibodies are first detected early in the primary infection; IgG anti-CMV antibodies are produced within a few weeks of infection and will generally remain as a life-long marker of past infection. Acute infection may be diagnosed by detecting IgM anti-CMV, by demonstrating seroconversion from negative to positive or by demonstrating a four-fold or greater rise in CMV-specific IgG titre. However, antibody response to CMV infection is very inconsistent – IgM antibodies can persist for weeks or months following primary infection and may increase in concentration during reactivation of viral replication. Immunocompromised hosts may fail to mount

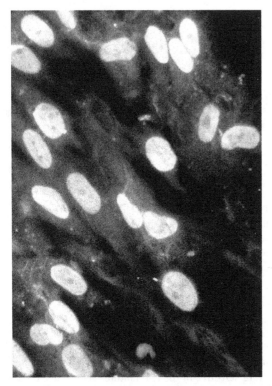

Fig. 12.3. Shell vial culture of CMV. Shell vial culture shortens detection time for CMV from several weeks to several days. MRC-5 cells are grown on a cover slip in the bottom of a straight-sided vial. The specimen is inoculated into the vial and this is then centrifuged to enhance infection. After 1–2 days, the cover slip is removed from the vial, fixed and stained with fluorescently labelled antibodies against CMV's immediate early antigen. Nuclear staining seen under fluorescence microscopy indicates the presence of CMV in the specimen.

adequate antibody responses. Exogenous anti-CMV antibodies can also confound serologic diagnosis in patients receiving serum-containing transfusion products or antibody concentrates.

Molecular detection

PCR assays for CMV have been available experimentally for several years. Earlier qualitative assays are of questionable efficacy since PCR efficiently detects even the low level of viremia seen in asymptomatic latent infections. Quantitative PCR has become popular in recent years and has largely replaced antigenemia assays as the marker for CMV viral load. Quantitative PCR is useful even in situations of profound cytopenias and therefore may be used in severely immunocompromised patients with suspected CMV disease. The correlation of increased viral load with active disease makes this assay much more useful than the qualitative assays.

In immunocompetent adults, virus excretion follows acute infection, but the duration and quantity of virus varies enormously. People with past infection can also excrete virus and therefore in the absence of clinical symptoms, virus detection is unreliable for diagnosis of acute infection: serology is more appropriate. Congenital CMV can be diagnosed by detecting virus and/or viral nucleic acids from specimens obtained during the first two weeks of life, usually urine or saliva.

CMV infection is nearly universal in allograft recipients of kidneys, bone marrow, heart–lung, etc. Serology is not useful for diagnosis, since post-transplant immunosuppression will suppress IgM. Blood and tissue cultures for CMV are of limited use since they are frequently negative even in the face of invasive desease. Most transplant services now use quantitative PCR for CMV to assess risk of CMV disease in the transplant recipient.

CMV infection is also nearly universal in HIV patients and the diagnosis in this population suffers from the same limitations as that in allograft recipients. The most direct evidence of infection is identification of CMV in biopsies. Blood cultures and antigenemia assays can be used to estimate viral load, but quantitative PCR to detect CMV DNA in plasma of HIV patients is probably the most useful assay for viral load estimation.

Treatment

Ganciclovir

Ganciclovir (GCV, dihydroxypropoxymethylguanine), an analogue of deoxyguanosine with a similar mode of action to acyclovir, is effective in killing

CMV. It interferes with nucleic acid chain termination, inhibiting viral DNA polymerase. Treatment may predispose to bacterial and fungal infections; side effects of GCV include leukopenia, thrombocytopenia, rash, CNS abnormalities, GI symptoms, abnormal spermatogenesis and teratogenesis. Acyclovir (used for HSV-1 and HSV-2 treatment) is not effective against CMV. GCV is used prophylactically immediately following bone marrow, liver, heart or lung transplants.

Foscarnet

Foscarnet (phosphonoformic acid) inhibits CMV DNA polymerase directly; it also inhibits many herpesvirus polymerases and has some antiretroviral activity. Renal toxicity as a side effect precludes its prophylactic use in transplant patients.

GCV and forscarnet in combination have been shown to have strong in vitro activity against CMV and are also used in the treatment of AIDS patients; however, resistance to both agents is becoming common, especially in AIDS patients. A combined course of therapy for 14–21 days is used to control established disease (pneumonitis, hepatitis, oesophagitis, colitis) in allograft recipients. Retreatment is sometimes necessary if symptomatic infection recurs. The combination is also efficient in controlling CMV retinitis, but viral replication will resume after withdrawing the drugs and therefore therapy, including intraocular delivery, must be continued. Long-term therapy may lead to the development of resistant viral strains.

There is a relative lack of data regarding the efficacy of either foscarnet or GCV in treating congenital CMV infection. Interpretation of case reports is difficult, due to natural variation in disease severity. Anecdotal information, however, does not support the use of antiviral therapy in fetal infections despite treatment during pregnancy or immediately after birth. Fetal death or disease progress have been noted in several cases. One controlled clinical trial using GCV to treat infants with CMV infection was stopped due to toxicities, particularly neutropenia. Treatment of the mother and prenatal prevention approaches (such as maternal vaccination) are the preferred approaches to preventing fetal disease.

Vaccine availability

Even natural immunity does not necessarily prevent re-infection with a different strain of CMV, and therefore attempts to produce a CMV vaccine have been difficult. Since the major focus of vaccine development is to decrease the incidence of fetal infection, inducing a primary immune response in the pregnant woman may be all that is required; severe fetal disease is rarely seen in a child whose mother already has CMV antibodies. Vaccine development has included live attenuated and recombinant virus vaccines, viral subunit vaccines, peptide vaccines and DNA vaccines. A strain of CMV known as Towne strain has been attenuated by in vitro culture. When administered to seronegative volunteers, it induces neutralizing antibodies and cell mediated immunity, but it produces only a limited protective immune response. In three trials on vaccinated renal transplant recipients, patients had a significant reduction in the CMV disease severity, although there was no decrease in the number of cases of CMV infection seen between the vaccinated and unvaccinated groups. The Towne strain has also been used to create genetically engineered strains containing large inserts from a low-passage reference CMV strain (Toledo) that are seen as potential vaccine candidates. Many viral envelope and matrix proteins (gB, gH, and pp65) are strongly immunogenic, and these may be useful as vaccines to prevent congenital infection, as well as in allograft recipients. Subunit vaccines have also been developed, particularly since CMV is potentially teratogenic and vaccination might pose a risk to pregnant women. Recombinant gB CMV molecule, derived from a transmembrane protein has been shown to induce a significant antibody response at mucosal surfaces. Whether this vaccine will produce a sufficient immune response capable of preventing fetal infection or significant disease is not known. Initial trials investigating the introduction of pp65 viral subunits into a canary-pox vector have been inconclusive. Peptide and DNA vaccines are also in early stages of development.

Hepatitis B virus (HBV)

Hepatitis B infections are common and widespread; it has been estimated that 1 out of 3 people worldwide have been infected with HBV. HBV infection causes acute and chronic hepatitis and approximately 10% of chronic cases may progress to cirrhosis and hepatocellular carcinoma. Chronic carrier state is common: it is estimated that around 10% of healthy adults and at least 85% of young infants infected by HBV become chronic carriers, maintaining an infected state for 6 months or more. In some communities the carrier rate may be as high as 20% in the adult population. Current figures suggest that there are approximately 400 million chronic carriers worldwide, over 75% of them in the Asia-Pacific region. Prevalence is higher in populations attending STD clinics, in prostitutes, homosexual men and in drug addict populations. One million people die each year from acute and chronic liver disease due to HBV infection, making it the ninth leading cause of death worldwide. The virus is 100 times more infectious than HIV, and in the US, approximately two healthcare workers are infected each day with HBV. Despite its role as a sexually and vertically transmitted pathogen, HBV has no direct impact on infertility.

Life cycle

HBV genome

The HBV genome consists of two strands of DNA of unequal length:

(i) The long strand is constant and carries all the protein-coding capacity of the virus. It is negative-sense (not equivalent to mRNA) and has four open reading frames that code for viral DNA polymerase, envelope protein, precore protein (processed to viral capsid) and a fourth protein that may be involved in the activation of host cell genes.

(ii) The short strand is variable in length.

HBV replication

(i) After uncoating, viral DNA polymerase repairs the DNA short strand, forming a double-stranded DNA.

(ii) Host RNA polymerase transcribes the long strand into mRNA copies.

(iii) mRNA is transcribed into viral proteins.

(iv) mRNA + the products of transcription are packaged into core structures in the cytoplasm.

(v) Viral DNA polymerase reverse transcribes pregenomic mRNA into long strand DNA.

(vi) The same enzyme replaces pregenomic RNA with short strand DNA.

(vii) Core antigen acquires an outer shell of surface antigens.

Three major antigens are referred to in discussing hepatitis infections:

(i) virus proteins on the outer shell = *s*urface antigens: **HepBsAg**;

(ii) capsid proteins = *c*ore antigen, surrounds the viral DNA: **HepBcAg**;

(iii) an alternatively processed subunit of the pre-core gene that is only synthesized under conditions of high viral replication is secreted into the plasma, and provides a useful *e*arly marker for infectivity: **HepBeAg**.

Transmission

The majority of cases seen in developed countries are acquired as sexually transmitted diseases, by injecting drug use, re-use of inadequately sterilized injection equipment or by occupational exposure (needle stick injuries). Viral titres can be very high in the blood of infected persons; saliva and semen contain lower concentrations. Blood and plasma supplies in developed countries have been screened for HBV for many years, and transmission by blood transfusion is now rare in these countries. Other less common causes of HBV transmission include blood exchange during tattooing or body piercing with inadequately sterilized instruments, and other non-specific household exposures. Risk factors associated with even minimal exposure to blood, such as sharing toothbrushes and razors have been identified with HBV transmission. The risk of HBV infection is high in promiscuous homosexual men and can probably be prevented by correct use of condoms. Healthcare workers and patients receiving hemodialysis are also at increased risk of infection. The virus can also be transmitted to the neonate during delivery, with very high risk of developing chronic HBV infection; if a mother is HbeAg positive, the risk of transmission to her baby may be as high as 70%. Twenty to thirty per cent of patients report no known exposure.

Clinical presentation

HBV infection is asymptomatic in about 50% of cases. Infection without symptoms and illness without jaundice occurs, particularly in children and the immunocompromised.

In symptomatic cases, the mean incubation period for acute HBV infection is 75 days, but it may range from 45 to 180 days. The degree of illness is variable, clearly influenced by host response to the virus. Following the incubation period of several weeks, the prodromal phase lasts 1–2 weeks. During this phase there may be flu-like symptoms including malaise, low-grade fever, fatigue, muscle or joint pain, loss of appetite, nausea and vomiting, weight loss and right upper quadrant pain. About 1–2% of infections lead to life-threatening acute fulminant hepatitis, with sudden and acute onset of jaundice, increased liver function tests and abdominal swelling. Fulminant hepatitis is more likely to develop in a patient who has concomitant alcohol abuse or superimposed HDV (delta virus) infection. The severity of illness and the extent and duration of jaundice is variable – dark urine and hyperbilirubinemia can persist for a month in the acute phase. Liver function tests such as aspartate aminotransferase (AST), alanine aminotransferase (ALT) and alkaline phosphatase are generally markedly elevated, reflecting active hepatocyte destruction. This phase can be fatal.

Approximately 90 to 95% of acutely infected adults will develop neutralizing antibodies and recover without sequelae; the remaining 3–5% will become chronically infected. Continued viral replication leads to an inflammatory cell response in these patients and a subsequent cytokine response causes

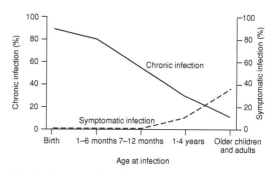

Fig. 12.4. Outcome of hepatitis B virus infection by age of infection. The highest proportion of infections with HBV that progress to become chronic are those acquired early in life. These infections are often asymptomatic in the neonate. Infections acquired in older children and adults are more likely to be symptomatic and are less likely to become chronic (Centers for Disease Control and Prevention data, http://www.cdc.gov/ncidod/diseases/hepatitis/slideset/index.htm).

hepatocyte cell lysis. Transaminases are generally elevated, and this may be the only indication that a patient is infected. Some patients may also experience decreased hepatic metabolism, detected by an increase in the prothrombin time and hypoalbuminemia. In patients with acute infection this period resolves after several weeks, but it may persist for decades in patients with chronic infections. The probability of developing chronic infection depends largely upon the individual's age when infection is acquired, the highest rate being with infections acquired very early in life. Almost 90% of neonates, 50% of young children and approximately 10% of adults infected by HBV go on to develop chronic infection (Fig. 12.4).

Repeated episodes of inflammation ultimately lead to advanced stages of fibrosis and cirrhosis. As cirrhosis develops, less viable liver parenchyma remains and this is reflected in decreasing transaminase levels. Cirrhosis predisposes to the development of hepatocellular carcinoma, probably related to the chronic inflammatory response with repeated cycles of hepatocyte regeneration. No HBV-specific oncogene has been identified. Hepatocellular carcinoma rarely develops before 25–30 years of HBV infection.

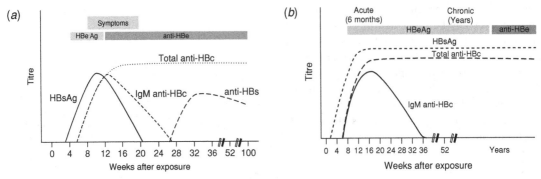

Fig. 12.5. Typical serologic time course for (*a*) acute and (*b*) chronic infections with hepatitis B virus. (*a*) In the acute HBV infection, both symptoms and viremia occur about a month following exposure and last for several weeks to months. Viremia as measured by HbsAg disappears by approximately 6 months following infection. IgM anti-HBc is produced during the acute phase of infection, and is ultimately replaced by the production of IgG anti-HBc and anti-HBs; these remain as markers of past infection and immunity, respectively. (*b*) In the chronic infection, viremia persists beyond 6 months. IgM anti-HBc and IgG anti-HBc follow the same time course as in the acute infection, but IgG anti-HBs is not produced in the chronic infection. The patient remains infectious and intermittently symptomatic in the chronic phase of infection with HBV (Centers for Disease Control and Prevention data, http://www.cdc.gov/ncidod/diseases/hepatitis/slideset/index.htm).

Laboratory diagnosis

Serology and antigen detection remain the gold standard for diagnosis of both acute and chronic HBV infections (Fig. 12.5(*a*), (*b*)). Patients with acute, chronic and recovered infections are identified by sequential detection of IgM antibodies and viral antigens, followed by the development of IgG antibody and the disappearance of viral antigens. The following antibody and antigen markers are important in the diagnosis of HBV infection:

- infective marker for acute and chronic infections: HBsAg;
- infective marker for chronic infections: HBeAg;
- antibody to the core antigen, Anti-HBc:

   (i) anti-HBc IgM titres rise in acute infection;
   (ii) anti-HBc IgG is retained for life after HBV infection.

- HBe, the e antigen, correlates with HBV DNA and DNA polymerase activity during viral replication.
- Anti-HBs, antibody to the surface antigen is seen after infection and after vaccination.

In newly diagnosed symptomatic HbsAg positive patients, a monthly blood test is recommended to assess the potential change in HBV markers. Patients who are HbsAg positive and asymptomatic should be assessed six months later, followed by yearly blood tests if they are persistently HbsAg positive. Chronic HBs carriers who are also positive for Hbe antigen are potentially highly infectious via the blood-borne or sexual route. Chronic HbsAg carriers with anti-Hbe are less infectious.

Figure 12.5(*a*) demonstrates the time course for acute infection. The first laboratory indicator of infection with HBV is the appearance of viremia, generally detected with an assay for HbsAg. Viremia can also be detected using a molecular assay such as PCR or an assay to detect HBeAg. Measurable levels of anti-HBc IgM antibodies can be detected within a month or more following the detection of circulating virus. IgM antibodies will continue to be produced for several months, and IgG antibodies are also produced. HbsAg will generally remain detectable for 4–6 months, but the patient may still be infectious even after the levels of HbsAg are below detectable levels. During the 'window period' between the fall in HBsAg level and the production of measurable neutralizing anti-HBs antibody, antibodies to HBc may be the only routinely tested indicator of infection. Although anti-HBe and PCR for HBV may also detect current infection, these are not usually included in routine testing panels for Hepatitis B. As the infection is cleared, measurable levels of anti-HBs appear in the patient's serum. Patients who have recovered from HBV infection will have both anti-HBs and anti-HBc detectable in serum for years following disease resolution.

Patients who progress to chronic HBV infection (Fig. 12.5(b)) continue to be infective and viremic, with HbsAg and HbeAg persistently detectable for years or for life. As is seen in acute infection, IgM anti-HBc is transiently produced followed by IgG anti-HBc. No detectable levels of the neutralizing anti-HBs are produced during the chronic infection, but patients may produce anti-HBe late in the time course of infection.

Molecular diagnostic assays are increasingly used to detect HBV infection, both for clinical and for research purposes. Qualitative and quantitative PCR assays are commercially available, although neither are currently FDA approved for use in patient testing. Quantitative HBV PCR viral load may be used to supplement biopsy in predicting patient prognosis, as disease severity appears to correlate with viral load. The Hepatitis B surface antigen (HbsAg) has three major antigenic determinants, which allow at least four subtypes. Subtype determination may be useful in detecting viral transmisssion in an outbreak investigation, but is not routinely ordered as part of the normal evaluation of a patient with HBV infection. However, genomic analysis has provided evidence for intrafamilial non-sexual transmission.

Histological diagnosis of Hepatitis B and prognosis may also be assessed by liver biopsy (Fig. 12.6). Acute hepatitis is characterized histologically by necrosis of individual hepatocytes with an inflammatory infiltrate seen primarily in the tissues surrounding the portal tracts (Fig. 12.6(a)). Eosinophilic necrotic hepatocytes (councilman bodies) may be seen scattered throughout the parenchyma of the liver (Fig. 12.6(b)). Inflammation is more extensive in chronic HBV infections; this may include significant necrosis involving more of the portal tracts, ultimately progressing to extensive bridging fibrosis

(Fig. 12.6(c)), cirrhosis and hepatocellular carcinoma (Fig. 12.6(d)).

Treatment

Alpha interferon has been approved in the USA for the treatment of chronic hepatitis B, and is recommended for patients who have Stage 2 chronic disease (HBeAg positive). HBeAg will become undetectable in about 40% of these patients after 16 weeks of treatment with interferon-alpha, and this correlates with an improved prognosis. A few patients (less than 10%) may be apparently 'cured', as assessed by loss of HBsAg. Patients with severe decompensated liver disease are not appropriate for interferon alpha treatment; those to be treated should be selected on the basis of:

- documented evidence of serum HBsAg for 6 months or more;
- evidence of HBeAg as a marker of viral replication
- elevated serum aminotransferase as evidence of ongoing liver inflammation;
- liver biopsy to detect the grade of inflammatory response and necrosis, and to determine the stage of fibrosis and cirrhosis present prior to treatment.

Recommended dose of interferon-alpha-2b for the treatment of chronic HBV infection is 5 000 000 units daily by subcutaneous or IM injection, for a total of 16 weeks. The patient must be monitored carefully for side effects during the treatment period.

The nucleoside analogue lamivudine (3TC), also effective against HIV, has been approved for treatment of chronic hepatitis B patients who are HBeAg positive. The recommended treatment regime is 100 mg/day orally, taken for one year. In comparative studies, lamivudine improved liver biopsy results and was as effective as interferon-alpha in reducing serum HBeAg. In August 2002, the US FDA also recommended approval for adevofird-pivoxil in HBV treatment, another nucleoside analogue also effective against HIV. Other nucleoside analogues, as well as combinations of analogues and combinations of interferon/analogues are being studied in clinical trials. Liver transplantation is

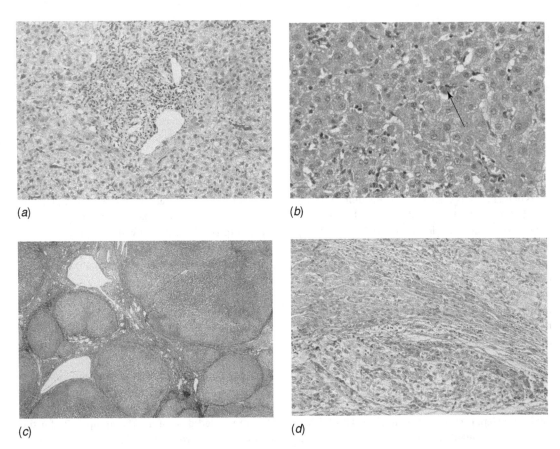

Fig. 12.6. Hepatic tissue response to infection with hepatitis B virus. In the acute phase of HBV infection, hepatic inflammation is limited to the portal triad (the areas surrounding the two large veins in the frame (*a*) image). The remainder of the tissue demonstrates relatively normal liver morphology. (*b*) Occasional hepatocyte death is seen as pink and shrunken 'councilman bodies', also seen in acute HBV infections (arrowed object). This represents piecemeal necrosis of HBV infected hepatocytes. (*c*) In chronic HBV infections, repeated episodes of inflammation and recovery eventually produce extensive fibrosis and regenerative nodularity in the liver. (*d*) Extensive fibrosis and cirrhosis predispose individuals with chronic HBV infections to hepatocellular carcinoma.

the last resort available to patients who develop decompensated HBV-related cirrhosis. Reinfection of the donor liver may be seen in some patients post transplantation.

Vaccine availability

Hepatitis B infection is the most preventable STD, since effective vaccines are available. The vaccine is given in a series of three injections, at 0, 3, and 6 months. All individuals at risk for infection should

be vaccinated, and children are now offered HBV vaccination as part of their routine immunization series. This childhood vaccination for HBV is important even in low prevalence populations, since it is directed at preventing infection in the patient population at highest risk for developing chronic HBV infection and its sequelae. The vaccine provides immunity in about 90% of adults who complete the series, and in about 95% of children who are vaccinated. Post-exposure prophylaxis with hepatitis B immune globulin is also effective for non-immune individuals after a known exposure (e.g. needle stick, see Chapter 14).

Hepatitis C virus (HCV)

Hepatitis C virus was identified as the causative agent of parenterally transmitted 'non-A, non-B' hepatitis in 1989. HCV was the first virus to be identified entirely by the use of molecular techniques, without growing the virus in tissue culture or using it to infect small laboratory animals. The complete genomes of several HCV isolates have subsequently been cloned and sequenced. Although its discovery and characterization led to an understanding of post-transfusion hepatitis, the lack of tissue culture systems that permit HCV infection and replication hinder understanding of its pathogenesis. HCV is a major cause of acute hepatitis and chronic liver disease, and can lead to end stage liver disease with cirrhosis and hepatocellular carcinoma.

At the end of 2002, it was estimated that 200 000 people in England and 4 million in the USA were infected with Hepatitis C, many of them undiagnosed. An estimated 170 million people are chronically infected globally, with 3 to 4 million newly infected each year. The prevalence of HCV varies around the world: in the USA, approximately 1.8% of the current population are chronically infected, while Egypt has the highest prevalence for HCV (22%), probably linked to parenteral anti-schistosomal therapy in that population. People infected 20–30 years ago are now progressing to serious liver disease.

Life cycle

HCV is a single-stranded enveloped RNA virus in the flaviviridae family. The virus is a slightly pleomorphic sphere of 40–60 nm diameter, with a lipid envelope. Small surface projections on the envelope can be seen as 'fringes' in negative staining procedures for electron microscopy. The nucleocapsid is a symmetrical 25–30 nm polyhedron. Virions contain 15–20% lipid, and are sensitive to heat, organic solvents and detergents; infectivity is destroyed by organic solvents that destroy its envelope.

The **HCV genome** is a single strand of linear positive sense ssRNA of 9401 nucleotides. The genome contains a 5′ untranslated region, a large open reading frame encoding for a polyprotein of 3011 amino acids and an untranslated 3′ end. There are 3 structural proteins encoded at the N-terminal end of the RNA and the C-terminal portion codes for four proteins that function in viral replication. Several of these proteins are responsible for stimulating the immune response seen in some patients. The ability of the virus genome to undergo mutations is an important feature, as it leads to significant genetic heterogeneity. This, in turn, is probably related to its high propensity (80%) for inducing chronic infection. The proteins coding for envelope proteins E1-and E2/NG1 are the most variable, while the untranslated 5′ region is highly conserved. Based on nucleotide sequence data, HCV has been divided into 6 genotypes, with 11 subtypes commonly identified (Simmonds *et al.*, 1993). Humans and chimpanzees are the only known species susceptible to infection, with both developing similar disease. Despite the fact that the entire genome has been sequenced, a permissive cell culture system has not been established. This, together with the fact that a non-primate model does not exist, has hindered further studies of the viral life cycle and the development of specific drugs against HCV.

Transmission

HCV is spread primarily by direct contact with human blood. The major causes of HCV infection worldwide are unscreened blood transfusions, reuse of needles, syringes and medical equipment that have not been adequately sterilized, or needle-sharing among drug users. Sexual and perinatal transmission may occur, although less frequently. Percutaneous procedures such as ear and body piercing, circumcision and tatooing can also transmit the virus if inadequately sterilized equipment is used. In both developed and developing countries, high risk groups include injecting drug users, recipients of unscreened blood, hemophiliacs, dialysis patients and persons with multiple sex partners who engage in unprotected sex. In developed countries, it is estimated that 90% of persons with chronic HCV infection are current and former injecting drug users or have a history of transfusion (prior to 1992) of unscreened blood or blood products. A recent prevalence study in US veterans has demonstrated a high rate of infection in this patient population. HCV has been identified in saliva, in semen, follicular fluid aspirated during IVF procedures (Devaux *et al.*, 2003), and associated with human zona-intact oocytes collected from infected women for IVF and ICSI (Papenthos-Roche, 2004). Patient-to-patient transmission of HCV virus has been reported during assisted conception treatment (see Chapter 14).

Clinical presentation

The incubation period of HCV infection ranges from 15 to 150 days; the acute phase of infection is asymptomatic in 60–70% of cases, or may have only mild symptoms. The most common symptoms associated with acute infection include fatigue and jaundice. In rare cases, an acute infection may present with significant clinical disease and even liver failure. HCV infection will occasionally be self-limiting, but the majority of these patients remain viremic. Between 50% and 85% of patients with acute HCV infection proceed to chronic disease; chronic infections are generally asymptomatic, with little or no clinical evidence of disease. Progression is usually indolent, with fatigue as the most common complaint. Once chronic disease develops, the virus is almost never cleared without treatment. Liver enzymes may fluctuate or persist and the degree of liver damage is variable: cirrhosis develops in 10–20%, and about 20% of those with cirrhosis will develop end-stage liver disease. Hepatocellular carcinoma develops in 1–5% of patients with chronic infection over a period of 20 to 30 years. It is difficult to predict the course of disease in any individual, but HCV genotype and concomitant alcohol use are major factors that influence the severity of aggressive disease. Alcohol abuse,

particularly binge drinking, is associated with rapid progression to cirrhosis and the onset of fulminant liver failure. HCV 1b has been associated with severe liver disease, more frequent progression to hepatocellular carcinoma and lack of response to interferon therapy.

Laboratory diagnosis

The diagnosis of HCV infection relies primarily on detecting abnormal liver function and HCV-specific antibodies; molecular techniques are used to detect circulating virus in the peripheral blood (Fig. 12.7(*a*), (*b*)). Viremia, indicated by HCV RNA in the peripheral blood, can be detected after an incubation period of several weeks. If symptoms appear, their onset will be several weeks after detectable viremia. Liver function tests such as AST, ALT, gamma glutamic transpeptidase (GGT) and bilirubin will all be elevated during this phase of infection; anti-HCV antibodies may take several months to appear. Although many patients will have demonstrable levels of antibody by 3–6 months, in about 10% of patients, seroconversion may require 9–12 months, or may not occur at all. Therefore, diagnosis of an acute infection with HCV should not rely exclusively on seroconversion. For a small proportion of patients, viremia may be cleared following the acute infection. In those patients, HCV RNA will no longer be detectable, liver function tests will return to normal (Fig. 12.7(*a*)) and serology serves as the only marker of past infection. The majority of patients, however, will not clear the virus but will proceed instead to chronic HCV infection. The disease course in these patients is characterized by periods of exacerbation and remission, with the accompanying inflammatory response that follows the acute syndrome (Fig. 12.7(*b*)). Liver function tests are intermittently elevated, with periods of normalization. Viremia may be intermittent or persistent. Liver biopsy during this active phase of infection will demonstrate a chronic inflammatory response, often accompanied by fatty changes. The liver may become cirrhotic with time.

Several assays are commercially available for the detection of HCV-specific antibodies. HCV antigens

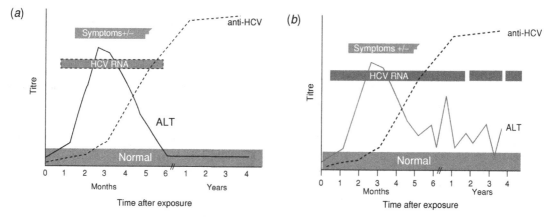

Fig. 12.7. Pattern of serology in (*a*) acute and (*b*) chronic HCV infection. Acute infection with HCV has a similar time course to that of HBV infection. After an incubation period of several weeks, the patient becomes viremic and may develop symptoms. A relatively small proportion of patients will clear the infection. Anti-HCV is produced late in the disease process, and some individuals may not demonstrate serologic evidence of infection for up to a year. (*b*) The majority of patients with HCV infection will develop a chronic infection. The disease course is marked by periods of disease progress and remission. Liver function tests (here represented by ALT) show a sawtooth pattern of elevation and normalization. Symptoms may be intermittent (fatigue, jaundice etc.), but these may not be recognized as HCV infection. The patient remains viremic despite the production of anti-HCV antibodies, and will often progress to cirrhosis and liver failure (Centers for Disease Control and Prevention data, http://www.cdc.gov/ncidod/diseases/hepatitis/slideset/index.htm).

have been produced by recombinant technology that are apparently specific and sensitive in detecting anti-HCV. Enzyme immunosorbent assays (EIA) can be used to detect anti-HCV for screening: current EIAs are very sensitive and relatively specific. EIAs can detect more than 95% of chronically infected patients but can detect only 50% to 70% of acute infections; additional testing is required to confirm a positive EIA result. The CDC recommends the use of either a recombinant immunoblot assay (RIBA) for confirmation of serology, or a reverse transcriptase PCR assay to detect viral RNA from serum specimens. The RIBA assay identifies antibodies that react with individual HCV antigens. These are the same antigens used in the EIA test and thus do not detect different viral epitopes: at least two bands must be detected by RIBA to confirm the positive EIA. The qualitative RT-PCR is a more sensitive assay that detects a different viral marker. This qualitative assay can detect as little as 50 copies/ml, and may detect infection prior to the development of anti-HCV antibodies.

Quantitative molecular assays have been used to assess relative prognosis: viral loads of over 2 000 000 have been linked to worse prognosis and failure to respond to therapy. HCV exhibits considerable genetic variability, with six known genotypes and over 50 subtypes that differ markedly based upon geography. Genotype assays identify the most common genotypes and subtypes by detecting differences in the RNA sequence. HCV genotype should be assessed at the time of initial diagnosis, since this is linked not only to overall prognosis, but also to the predicted response to therapy. Individuals with genotypes 2 and 3 are overall most likely to benefit from aggressive therapy, while patients with genotype 1b are unlikely to derive benefit from treatment. INNO-LIPA is a line probe assay that features 19 different HCV-specific DNA probes attached to nitrocellulose strips. Products from RT–PCR are allowed to bind to the specific probes and then identified by a biotin–streptavidin–alkaline phosphatase staining procedure. This assay can identify all six genotypes and their most common subtypes. The INNO-LIPA

HCV II line probe assay uses the RT-PCR product from the Roche Amplicore HCV monitor assay to determine HCV genotype. Nucleic acid sequencing likewise uses RT–PCR products from the viral NS5 region. Although this assay is labor intensive and costly, the original Simmonds Classification (Simmonds *et al.*, 1993) was based on this data and it therefore remains the gold standard for HCV genotype determination. Restriction endonuclease cleavage and cleavage fragment length polymorphism (CFLP) assays may also be used to assess genotype. A CFLP assay using Amplicore RT-PCR products as the DNA source is available from Third Wave Technologies Inc (Madison, Wi).

Treatment

Antiviral drugs such as interferon taken alone or in combination with ribavirin can be used to treat chronic hepatitis C, but the cost of treatment is very high. Treatment with interferon alone is effective in about 10% to 20% of patients. Interferon combined with ribavirin is effective in about 30% to 50% of patients in inducing initial responses to treatment, but less than half have a sustained response. Ribavirin does not appear to be effective when used alone. These early treatments had relatively poor response rates with high relapse following discontinuation of therapy. Newer regimens currently in trials with slow-release pegylated-interferon-alpha have shown dramatic improvement, particularly in long-term maintenance of virus clearance following the discontinuation of therapy. Genotypes 2 and 3 overall have better response to therapy, while 1a and 1b tend to be more refractory to treatment. Liver transplantation is the last resort for patients with decompensated HCV-related cirrhosis, but transplantation is often complicated by re-infection of the new graft with the patient's original strain of HCV. Patients awaiting transplant must discontinue high-risk hepatotoxic activities such as alcohol consumption/abuse, often seen in HCV positive patients with end stage disease.

Since treatment for chronic hepatitis C is too costly for use in developing countries, the greatest impact on hepatitis C disease burden globally is likely to be achieved by reducing the risk of HCV transmission from nosocomial exposures, with implementation of:

- screening and testing of blood and organ donors,
- virus inactivation of plasma derived products;
- implementation and maintenance of infection control practices in healthcare settings, including appropriate sterilization of medical and dental equipment;
- promotion of behaviour change among the general public and healthcare workers in order to reduce overuse of injections and promote safe injection practices;
- risk reduction counselling for persons with high-risk drug and sexual practices.

Vaccine availability

No vaccine is currently available to prevent hepatitis C. Although research is in progress, vaccine development is complicated by the high mutation rate of the HCV genome and by lack of information about protective immune response following HCV infection. Some studies have shown the presence of virus-neutralizing antibodies in patients with HCV infection, but it is not known whether the immune system is able to eliminate the virus. Despite the production of an antibody response in the majority of chronically infected patients, less than one-quarter of patients are able to clear the infection. The burden of disease and the high rate of progression to chronic hepatitis makes HCV the perfect candidate for vaccine development.

Hepatitis D virus (HDV)

Hepatitis D virus (also known as Delta virus or Delta agent) was first described in 1977, when it was identified as an important blood-borne pathogen that causes acute, chronic and fulminant hepatitis syndromes in infected patients. HDV is an enveloped, small circular defective ssRNA virus, 35–37 nm in size, with a morphology similar to the HBV Dane particle. HDV RNA is one of the shortest viral genomes known to infect humans. This piece of RNA codes for only one known product, HDAg, and a single cell must be simultaneously infected with both HDV and HBV in order for HDV to replicate. HDV is therefore seen most often in areas of the world where HBV is also common, but with a more limited distribution of extensive prevalence. Endemic pockets are seen in southern Italy, parts of Africa, the Amazon River Basin in South America and some Middle Eastern countries. Risk factors for acquiring infection with HDV are similar to those for HBV infection.

Life cycle

The Delta agent is a defective RNA virus that requires HBV co-infection to carry out its complete replication cycle. Overall, approximately 4% of acute infections with HBV have HDV co-infection. The vast majority (approximately 80%) represent superinfection of HDV in a previous chronic HBV infection. HDV depends upon HBV to produce surface antigen for the assembly of infectious HDV virions. In the absence of HBV, new infective HDV virions cannot be produced, the infection is non-productive and there is no inflammatory response in the liver.

The HDV ssRNA genome has a negative strand orientation. Inside the hepatocyte, RNA with both positive and negative strand orientation is seen. There are six open reading frames: one of these lies on the positive strand and codes for the only known HDV-specific protein produced, the 24 kD HDV Ag protein. Within the hepatic cells, HDV RNA appears to circularize and anneal together for replication as a 'double rolling' circle. The ss negative sense RNA circularizes using self-complementing sequences, HDV Ag coats the RNA, and this is then coated with HBsAg capsid produced by the co-infecting HBV. The viral particles are enveloped with host cell nuclear membrane to produce the infective HDV virion.

Transmission

HDV is transmitted in the same manner as HBV, through sexual contact, contact with contaminated blood or blood products and through the exchange of infected body fluids. Individuals at increased risk for acquiring infection include IV drug abusers who share needles, hemophiliacs receiving pooled human-derived coagulation factors, transfused patient populations, hemodialysis patients, male homosexuals (particularly those with large numbers of sexual contacts) and the sexual partners of these high risk groups. Intrafamilial transmission of HDV has been described, suggesting that this virus may be spread by a means of casual transmission that has not yet been characterized. HDV transmission is more likely in high prevalence HDV–HBV areas of the world, including the Amazon River Basin, Equatorial Africa, the Mediterranean and Middle East and Asiatic regions of what was previously the USSR. So far it is uncommon in South east, Asia and China, although these regions have a high prevalence of HBV; the recent introduction of HDV into the population could make this area an additional source of virus transmission. Rapid spread of HDV is anticipated in a population practicing intravenous drug abuse (IVDA) and sharing needles, the most common risk factor for acquiring HDV infection. In the USA and in most of Europe, HDV infections are extremely rare, found mainly in IV drug users and their sexual contacts.

Clinical presentation

Clinical presentation with HDV infection depends upon the time course of HBV infection. Patients may be acutely co-infected with both HBV and HDV simultaneously, or HDV superinfection may be superimposed on a chronic HBV infection. The disease outcome for these two scenarios is quite different (see Fig. 12.8).

In the case of HDV–HBV co-infection, previously healthy patients generally present with an acute hepatitis syndrome 4 to 26 weeks following infection. During the 4–12-week period jaundice generally develops, with abnormal liver function tests and transient HBV and HDV viremia. The vast majority of patients (>90%) will recover from the dual infection in about 6 months and will develop complete

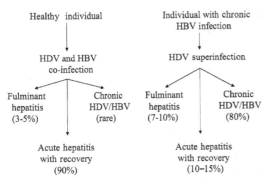

Fig. 12.8. Outcomes for HDV co-infection and superinfection with HBV. The outcome for HDV infection varies considerably depending upon the timing of HBV infection. Simultaneous co-infection with both viruses resolves completely after acute infection in the majority of patients, but 3–4% will develop fatal fulminant hepatitis. In contrast, the vast majority who survive HDV superinfection in chronic HBV develop chronic HBV and HDV infections.

immunity to both viruses. Following recovery, the only markers of infection generally seen in these patients are IgG anti-HBs and IgG anti-HBc antibodies. An HDV-specific antibody response is not usually detected. Three to five per cent of patients will develop a fulminant hepatitis syndrome. In these cases, dramatic hepatocyte lysis destroys most of the liver, which becomes soft. Liver function tests are extremely elevated and fulminant hepatitis is invariably fatal without attempted liver transplant. Chronic HDV and HBV infection following coinfection with the two viruses is extremely rare.

Superinfection of HDV in the presence of HBV infection presents quite differently. Hepatitis D superinfection should be suspected in a patient with chronic hepatitis B whose condition suddenly worsens, with an acute hepatitis characterized by jaundice, elevated liver function tests, malaise, anorexia and abdominal discomfort. Ten to 15% of patients will recover completely from both acute HDV and chronic HBV infections; 7–10% will develop fulminant hepatitis and die. In contrast to co-infection, over 80% of patients with superinfection will progress to chronic HDV and HBV infection. Individuals with the dual infection usually develop

rapidly progressive disease and cirrhosis at an earlier age than those with HBV infection alone.

Laboratory diagnosis

Laboratory diagnosis of HDV infection is not straightforward. Unlike the HbsAg, the Delta antigen circulates for a relatively short period of time during the late incubation period. EIAs available for the detection of Delta antigen are relatively insensitive, often negative even in the presence of a true HDV infection. Northern blot analysis can be used to detect the Delta antigen, but this assay is not widely available. The diagnosis of HDV infection therefore relies on serology as the gold standard (Fig. 12.9(*a*), (*b*)).

Diagnosis is confirmed by the presence of HBsAg and anti-HDV in the serum. In acute coinfection with HBV (Fig. 12.9(*a*)) IgM anti-HDV antibodies are transient and produced at only low levels. IgM anti-HDV antibodies usually fall to below detectable levels before HBsAg is cleared and before anti-HBsAg is produced. In these acute infections, the levels of IgG anti-HDV similarly drop off to undetectable levels shortly after the resolution of infection, and anti-HBsAg will remain the only antibody detected following infection. Symptoms and abnormal liver function tests will peak around the time of HBV viremia, usually between 1 and 6 months after initial infection. In chronic infections with HDV and HBV (Fig. 12.9(*b*)), IgM anti-HDV antibodies peak and fall in the first 6 months of infection. Both IgM and IgG anti-HDV antibodies are produced by 4–5 months after infection, along with IgG anti-HBc. Both HBsAg and HDV viral RNA will continue to circulate in the peripheral blood as indicators of persistent hepatic infection. Liver function tests peak during the acute infection and remain elevated during the chronic phase of infection.

Diagnostic tests available for HDV infection are relatively limited. IgM and IgG anti-HDV antibodies are detected by EIA assays. Patients with fulminant hepatitis should be tested for IgM anti-HDV, and patients with chronic HBV infection may be tested for total anti-HDV antibodies (representing both IgG

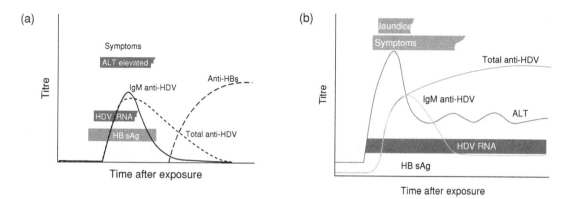

Fig. 12.9. Typical serologic time course for (*a*) co-infection and (*b*) superinfection in HDV and HBV infections. (*a*) HDV and HBV co-infection produces a severe acute infection during which both HBV and HDV may be detected. IgM anti-HDV is initially produced, but the levels fall after the infection resolves, and no delta-specific antibodies are generally detected following convalescence. Anti-HBs and Anti-HBc are usually the only markers of past infection and recovery seen following co-infection with HBV and HDV.

(*b*) HDV infection superimposed upon a previous chronic HBV infection leads to an acute exacerbation of hepatitis that is usually symptomatic. If the patient survives the acute infection, both HDV and HBV viremia are generally seen on entering into a chronic phase. Liver function tests remain intermittently elevated and the chronic infection often progresses rapidly to cirrhosis. Total anti-HDV remains elevated as a marker of current infection throughout the chronic infection (Centers for Disease Control and Prevention data, http://www.cdc.gov/ncidod/diseases/hepatitis/slideset/index.htm).

and IgM). IgM antibodies are known to remain elevated even after the acute infection has progressed to a chronic phase. Since antibody titres will be high in chronic infections, this assay is relatively sensitive in detecting the chronic phase. However, antibody levels tend to be low in acute infections, and several determinations may be necessary. Antigen assays and molecular tests to detect HDV viremia are available experimentally only and are not considered to be necessary for patient care.

Treatment

Although interferon-alpha has been used to treat patients with chronic hepatitis B and hepatitis D infection, the response rate is only 40%. Some studies suggest that doses higher than those used for hepatitis B infection may be beneficial. Lamivudine, which has been shown to be active in preventing HBV replication, has little or no activity in preventing HDV replication and is not effective in treating HBV and HDV dual infections. Similarly, famcyclovir is not

effective in HDV infections. Liver transplant carries the risk of transplanted organ reinfection with both HDV and HBV. Prophylactic treatment with HBIg (immunoglobulins against HBsAg) may diminish the risk of reinfection; the best response to this strategy is seen in patients with very low levels of HBV viremia prior to transplantation.

Vaccine availability

Since HDV requires co-infection with HBV to produce a productive infection, HDV infections are prevented by adequate response to the HBV vaccine. Individuals at high risk for developing HDV infection should therefore be vaccinated to prevent dual infection with HDV and HBV.

HIV and AIDS

Acquired immune deficiency syndrome (AIDS) was first described in the USA in 1981 as a syndrome of diseases characterized by compromised cell-mediated immunity that allowed the development of life-threatening opportunistic infections. In retrospect, cases of AIDS were seen as early as 1978, and it was through clusters of cases in New York and California that the new and unusual disease phenomenon was recognized between 1980–1981. A retrovirus, human immunodeficiency virus (HIV) was identified as the causative agent in 1983; recent evidence suggests that the virus may have emerged during the 1950s (Gao *et al.*, 1999), probably from a primate retroviral ancestor. Two species are well characterized, classified in the lentivirus subfamily of retroviruses: HIV-1 and HIV-2. The nucleic acid of these two viruses have 50% homology and their p24 antigens cross-react in serologic tests. HIV-2 is found mostly in West Africa, tends to produce less severe disease and spreads less efficiently than does HIV-1. HIV-2 is genomically and antigenically related to Simian Immunodeficiency Virus (SIV) and seroconversion against SIV has been reported in laboratory personnel working with this virus. AIDS is now seen worldwide, with the fastest growing numbers of cases in Africa and Southeast Asia. By 1992, over 12 million people were infected globally, 8 million in Africa, and the pandemic then became most volatile in Thailand, Burma and India. In the USA, the epidemic is growing rapidly among minority populations and is a leading killer of African-American males aged 25 to 44. According to the US Centers for Disease Control and Prevention (CDC), AIDS affects nearly seven times more African-Americans and three times more Hispanics than Caucasians.

Life cycle

HIV-1 and -2 are enveloped viruses, variable in size and shape, but with an approximate diameter of 100 nm. Each virion contains two identical molecules of single-stranded positive sense RNA, with a 5′cap and 3′ polyA (like mRNA). These RNA strands are physically linked as a dimer by hydrogen bonds. Retroviruses have four properties that make them unique as pathogens.

(i) They are the only viruses which are truly diploid.
(ii) Positive sense RNA does not serve directly as mRNA immediately after infection.
(iii) Their genome is produced by cell transcription machinery.
(iv) Their genome requires a specific tRNA for replication.

These properties allow retrovirus infection to disturb cellular DNA metabolism by at least four different mechanisms.

(i) The virus can pick up a host oncogene after integration and transduce it into a host cell during the next cycle of replication; this transduced gene may no longer be under the host cell's usual control, leading to excess expression of the oncogene.
(ii) The provirus can integrate into a DNA sequence which is close to a host regulatory gene, and may increase expression of host regulatory genes.
(iii) It may inactivate a host gene through insertion mutation, and if these inactivated genes are suppressor genes, this can lead to excess expression of other genes.
(iv) A virus-specified transactivating gene may transactivate cellular genes and stimulate the growth of uninfected cells.

Integration of the viral genome into host cell DNA is an important factor in the aetiology of the disease and in its resistance to effective treatment.

The HIV genome contains only nine genes:
- three structural genes: **5′gag, pol and env-3′**
- four regulatory genes: **tat, rev, nef and vif**
- two more genes of as yet unknown function.

The genes are flanked by regulatory sequences, lateral terminal repeats (LTRs) that contain enhancer and suppressor sequences.

Stuctural genes

A virus-specified protease enzyme cleaves the **gag** gene product to produce three core proteins:
p24 is the main capsid protein and is a key antigen in diagnosis of infection.
p17 – a matrix protein
nc7 (6/9) – a nucleocapsid protein

The **pol** gene product produces three enzymes: reverse transcriptase, protease, and integrase.

The **env** gene product produces two envelope antigens: gp120, and gp41 (the latter is a peplomer).

- Antibodies against p120 neutralize the virus.
- gp41 is a key antigen in diagnosis of infection.

Regulatory genes

- **Tat** protein transactivates HIV expression
- **Rev** protein up-regulates virus expression
- **Nef** protein down-regulates virus expression
- **Vif** protein is necessary for the production of infectious virions

Susceptible helper T-cells are infected through a series of steps.

(i) Surface glycoprotein (SU) on HIV binds to a specific receptor on the host target cell. This interaction is specific and dictates cell tropism, i.e. the primary receptor for HIV is the CD4 molecule on the surface of Helper T-cell lymphocytes. A second receptor that loops through the cell membrane seven times is also required for infection to occur, the '7 transmembrane receptor'. HIV must bind to both of these receptors in order to infect the cell. Some lymphocytes have a different '7 transmembrane receptor', and these cells may avoid infection.

(ii) The SU-CD4 complex undergoes a conformational change that reveals a fusion domain, and the virus envelope fuses with the host cell membrane and enters the cell.

(iii) Inside the cell the virus is partially uncoated, releasing its core particle (NC) in the cytoplasm.

(iv) Viral RNA is reverse transcribed into DNA inside the core particle.

Reverse transcription

Reverse transcription occurs in the cytoplasm, resulting in synthesis of the double stranded DNA product known as the provirus. This is longer than viral RNA by one U3, R, U5 sequence, and there are LTRs of this sequence at each end of the provirus genome. When the process is completed, the provirus DNA migrates to the nucleus for integration. Reverse transcription is highly error-prone, the RNA sequence is often 'mis-read', so that viruses produced in a single infected cell may have a variety of subtle molecular differences in surface coat and enzymes – HIV surface molecules are continually changing throughout the course of infection.

Integration of the HIV provirus is catalysed by the IN (integrase) polypeptide. This process is highly specific with respect to the provirus, but random with respect to host cell DNA. A linear DNA form (probably the direct product of reverse transcription (RT) is believed to be the substrate for IN: the ends of the LTRs are brought together and cleaved to form a staggered cut and this molecule is inserted into host cell DNA. The integrated provirus contains one or two fewer bases at the ends of the LTRs, and the ends of integrated LTRs always have the same sequence: 5'-TG . . . CA-3'. Four to six base pairs of host cell DNA flanking the provirus are duplicated.

Once integrated, the provirus is present for the lifetime of the cell – there is no excision mechanism and the cell cannot be 'cured'.

Gene expression

Transcription of viral DNA begins if the cell is activated. Retroviruses use cellular transcriptional machinery for expression and therefore they are expressed like cellular genes. Both HTLV and HIV encode additional transcriptional and post-transcriptional regulatory factors: in order to compress maximal information into a small genome, they use 'tricks', such as splicing and ribosomal frameshifting, as well as complex transcription patterns that are regulated by the host cell apparatus. Viral RNA is translated into a polypeptide chain that must be cleaved by viral protease to produce the functional products. This process can be blocked by protease inhibitors, interfering with continued infection, and multiple-drug therapies now normally include the use of a protease inhibitor.

Virus assembly

Viral RNA and its associated proteins are packaged into their capsid and nucleocapsid in the cell cytoplasm and released from the lymphocyte surface by budding, incorporating lymphocyte membrane components with viral surface proteins. These surface proteins then bind to receptors on other T-helper cells, facilitating continued infection.

HIV mutates at a very high frequency during its replication, and a large number of genomically distinct isolates can be found in the same person at any time. Mutations affecting the p120 site are very frequent – this affects the virus's susceptibility to neutralizing antibody. Mutations in the **pol** gene (codes for reverse transcriptase) are also frequent, and these mutations are responsible for making the virus resistant to zidovudine.

Transmission

HIV is sexually transmitted in semen and vaginal fluids and the most common route of transmission is through unprotected sex with an infected partner. The virus can enter the body through epithelial tissue of the vagina, vulva, penis, rectum, or mouth during sex, and virus entry is greatly facilitated by mucosal trauma, especially in the presence of genital ulcer disease. Transmission is most efficient from men to women and from men to receptive male partners. Efficient female-to-male transmission is seen in Africa and in sex-for-money or sex-for-drugs populations, probably linked to the incidence of genital ulcer disease in these groups. Although HIV has been identified in the saliva of infected people, there is no evidence of spread through saliva during kissing. However, it can be spread during oral sex, especially in the presence of mouth ulcers or bleeding gums. HIV is not spread through sweat, tears, urine or feces, and inter-family studies have shown that it is not spread through casual contact such as sharing food utensils, towels, bedding, swimming pools, telephones or toilet seats. The virus is also spread via infected blood: blood transfusions and blood-derived products previously carried a risk, but this has been minimized by stringent screening

criteria for blood donors and heat treatment of blood products. Prior to the introduction of HIV testing for semen donors, cases of HIV transmission were reported following artificial insemination with fresh semen (Araneta *et al.*, 1995). HIV is readily spread among injection drug users by needle or syringe sharing. Although the virus may be transmitted iatrogenically via accidental sticks with contaminated needles or other medical instruments, the efficiency of such transmission is estimated to be only 0.3%. Infection and seroconversion in the needlestick recipient are probably influenced by the contact person's viral load. HIV can also be spread through direct contact with blood-contaminated body fluids, particularly via conjunctival mucosa or skin that is not intact. Transplacental transmission occurs in approximately 15–35% of untreated infected women during pregnancy; babies can also be infected during birth and via infected breast milk. HIV is not believed to be spread by biting insects such as mosquitoes or bedbugs.

Risk factors for transmission of the virus include:

- the presence of other STDs, particularly genital ulcer diseases;
- other risk factors generally seen with STDs: prostitution, consorting with a prostitute, increased numbers of sex partners, sex at an early age;
- engaging in unprotected intercourse. Barrier methods – male and female condoms provide the best protection. Diaphragms and oral contraceptives provide no protection;
- receptive partners. Anal intercourse is particularly efficient in transmission, probably on the basis of mucosal trauma. Oral intercourse is less often associated with transmission, but is still a risk factor;
- male homosexual sex practices;
- IVDA, based on sex-for-drugs or sharing infected needles;
- birth to an infected mother.

Clinical presentation

Initial infection is usually asymptomatic, or it may be accompanied by flu-like symptoms within 1 to 2 months of exposure to the virus (fever, headache,

Table 12.1. AIDS defining opportunistic infections

AIDS defining illness	Site of infection	Usual CD4 count at presentation ($\times 10^6$/l)
Candidiasis	Esophageal, bronchial, tracheal or pulmonary	<300
HPV-related cancer	Cervical	<200
Coccidioidomycosis	Pulmonary or extrapulmonary	<200
Cryptosporidiosis	Chronic intestinal disease, >1 month in duration	<100
Cytomegalovirus disease	Brain, eye, pulmonary and other sites not including liver spleen or lymph nodes	<50
HIV-related encephalopathy	Brain	<200
Herpes simplex	Chronic ulcers >1 month duration, or bronchial, esophageal, pulmonary infections	<100
Histoplasmosis	Pulmonary or disseminated	<200
Isosporiasis	Chronic intestinal disease, >1 month in duration	<100
Kaposi's sarcoma	Any location including skin lesions and lesions in any solid organs	<200
Lymphoma, Burkitt's	Any location	<50, but some with CD4 >200
Lymphoma, immunoblastic	Any location	<50, but some with CD4 >200
Lymphoma, not otherwise specified	Primary disease of the brain	<50, but some with CD4 >200
Mycobacterium avium intracellulare complex or *M. kansasii*	Pulmonary, extrapulmonary and disseminated infections	<100
M. tuberculosis	Pulmonary or extrapulmonary sites	<350
Other *Mycobacertium* spp.	Extrapulmonary or disseminated	<100
Pneumocystis carinii	Pulmonary	<200
Bacterial pneumonia, recurrent	Pulmonary	<400, with four-fold increased risk <200
Progressive multifocal leukoencephalopathy	Brain	<200
Salmonella spp.	Septicemia	<400
Toxoplasmosis	Brain	<100
HIV wasting disease	Systemic	<200

tiredness, muscle/joint pains, skin rash, enlarged lymph nodes). HIV viral load in the peripheral blood may be very high during this time. These symptoms usually disappear within a week to a month, and are often attributed to another viral infection. A long period of latent infection then follows, during which the virus multiplies in lymphocytes and in the monocyte/macrophage scavenger system that has phagocytized infected CD4+ cells. This macrophage scavenger system serves as a huge virus reservoir even when treatment has reduced circulating HIV to undetectable levels. Although the person is asymptomatic, he/she is highly infectious, with HIV present in high titres in genital fluids – this period

is described as 'HIV infected'. The virus actively multiplies, infects and kills cells of the immune system, but the duration of this asymptomatic period is highly variable and individual. Some patients develop symptoms within a few months, whereas others may be symptom-free for 10 years or more. Children usually experience symptoms within 2 years of infection. With time, the helper-T cell lymphocyte (CD4+) count drops, inducing a state of immunodeficiency in the patient. The drop in helper T-cell count to below 400×10^6/l (healthy adult count is 1000 or more) then allows the onset of a series of opportunistic infections, listed in Table 12.1.

With the drop in lymphocytes, these opportunistic infections bring a variety of complications, characterized initially by lymphadenopathy. Other symptoms during this period may include lack of energy, weight loss, frequent fevers and sweats, persistent or frequent yeast infections (oral or vaginal), persistent skin rashes or flaky skin, pelvic inflammatory disease in women that does not respond to treatment, short-term memory loss, recurrent and frequent severe herpes simplex or herpes zoster infections. These may be present for months or years before the onset of recognizable opportunistic infection. The patient is defined as having AIDS when opportunistic infection is recognized. The CDC has defined AIDS as HIV infection resulting in a blood CD4+ T-cell count of less than 200/ml. The definition also includes 26 clinical conditions whose onset heralds the conversion from HIV infection to the AIDS syndrome. These are known as AIDS defining illnesses and include, in addition to opportunistic infections, some of the AIDS related malignancies (summarized in Table 12.1). The onset of these AIDS defining illnesses correlates approximately to the degree of immunosuppression or CD4+ helper T-cell count. Symptoms of opportunistic infections are common in people with AIDS, related to the site of infection (Table 12.1). Children with AIDS are susceptible to the same opportunistic infections as adults with the disease, and they may also have severe forms of common childhood bacterial infections, such as conjunctivitis (pink eye), ear infections, and tonsillitis.

There is usually a gradual decline in CD4+ T-cell count during the course of infection, but abrupt and dramatic drops may be seen in some individuals. However, manifestation of symptoms is not necessarily *directly* related to T-cell count; some individuals will experience early symptoms with counts >200, and some patients may avoid opportunistic infections even if the CD4+ count is <200. A relatively small number of patients experience no progression from HIV to AIDS. These individuals have no symptoms of AIDS even after a period of 10 years or more, and ongoing research is directed towards determining whether this is a feature of their genetics, their immune system or of the virus strain.

The period of decreasing natural immunity is also associated with tumour formation, especially those caused by viruses, such as Kaposi's sarcoma, cervical cancer and B-cell lymphomas of the central nervous system. These conditions are more aggressive and refractory to treatment in the presence of AIDS. With effective antiretroviral therapies and antibiotics to prevent opportunistic infections, an increasing number of patients are now presenting with tumours as their AIDS defining illnesses.

HIV infection has no direct effect upon reproductive health: there is no decrease in fertility or impairment of reproductive capacity. Since early infection may be asymptomatic, normal sexual activity allows the opportunity for sexual spread. Infection may be transmitted to the fetus during pregnancy or at birth.

Laboratory diagnosis

Diagnosis of HIV infection relies on several different diagnostic tests. Investigations usually begin with serologic evaluation, although the virus and its related antigens (p24) can be detected using molecular techniques such as PCR, bDNA testing, or nucleic acid amplification test (NAT). The choice of initial test will depend upon the stage of infection under investigation and the level of sensitivity required for the screening process. Only approved HIV tests should be used for diagnostic testing, carried out by laboratory personnel who are appropriately trained, following the kit manufacturer's directions for test performance and specimen requirements. The detectable levels of antibody, antigen and viral load vary over the course of the disease, as summarized in Fig. 12.10 (time course of HIV diagnostic marker evolution).

During the first month of HIV infection, which is usually asymptomatic or presents flu-like symptoms only, HIV viremia may be detected by molecular techniques or by HIV culture in referral laboratories with special research facilities. HIV can be cultured from blood as early as 4–11 days following infection, but virus culture is not routinely used for patient diagnosis. Molecular assays are very sensitive, and

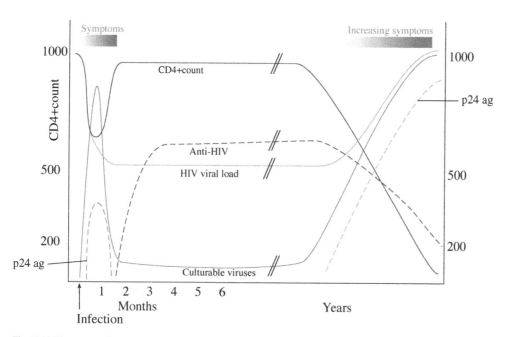

Fig. 12.10. Time course for serologic and antigenic diagnosis of HIV infection. Viremia is the first marker for HIV, detectable within 4–7 days of infection. P24 antigen may be transiently detected during the acute infection, but this falls as anti-HIV antibodies first become detectable approximately 1–3 months following infection. The patient will remain viremic for months or years, with detectable anti-HIV antibodies. As the CD4+ count falls, viral load, culturable virus, and p24 antigen all increase. Patients may manifest increasing symptoms during this phase of infection, corresponding to the conversion from HIV to AIDS.

can detect very low HIV numbers (<100 copies/ml). Many laboratories validate quantitative PCR assays to detect a range that is less than the manufacturer's reported dynamic range for the assay. Quantitation is less reliable at the lower cut-off limits, and a repeat assessment yielding a result within one log of the first assay is generally accepted as an accurate result for these molecular assays.

The Roche Diagnostics PCR-based Amplicor HIV-1 Monitor standard test assay measures from 200 to 800 000 copies of HIV RNA per mL (Amplicor Roche, Basel, Switzerland). These assays are generally positive within 10 days of infection; blood donors are screened by using a nucleic acid amplification test in order to detect viremia prior to the development of antibody or antigen responses. The HIV p24 antigen becomes positive around 15 days following infection (5 days later than HIV RNA detection by molecular techniques). Although not

recommended for patient diagnosis, the p24 antigen assay was previously used for screening blood donors because it was the earliest indicator of infection, before the NAT test became available. Initial studies showed that p24 antigen is generally positive in patients with acute HIV infection, when the EIA for HIV antibodies is still negative. The level of p24 falls relatively rapidly after the resolution of symptoms and becomes negative within 1–2 weeks. Antibodies to the virus generally do not reach detectable levels in the blood until at least 21 days following infection, and therefore an EIA used for routine patient and blood donor screening is the last test to become positive. Three months after infection, antibodies can be detected in 95% of patients; a small proportion of patients will not demonstrate detectable levels until 6 months after infection. For needle stick exposures and rape cases, generally EIA or ELISA testing should be carried out at baseline exposure and then again intermittently for at least 12 months.

EIA/ELISA testing is both highly sensitive and specific, but some false-positive tests do occur. A positive result should be repeated on the same sample. If it is positive a second time, a more specific test should be performed. The Western blot is the 'gold standard' confirmation for diagnosis of HIV infection. This assay detects patient antibodies to specific HIV proteins that have been separated by electrophoresis and transferred onto a solid nitrocellulose strip. The strips are incubated with patient sera so that antibodies, if present, will bind to the separate proteins. Positive Western blots are defined as those in which antibody binding is demonstrated for at least two of the three major HIV bands (gp 160/120, gp 41, and p24) with a staining intensity at least comparable to that seen on the positive control for gp 41. An indeterminate result is one in which an insufficient number of bands can be seen, or the staining intensity is inadequate to consider the specimens positive. A negative result is one in which no HIV-specific bands are detected on Western blotting.

Inexpensive tests for the detection of antibodies to HIV are widely available, and these are sensitive and specific at least 3 months post-infection. Rapid (10-min) serum tests, home collection systems and tests for HIV antibody in oral secretions and urine are useful in some situations, but they require confirmation by standard serum testing because of concerns about their sensitivity. Newer assays that collect oral mucosal transudates are becoming available, and these have a higher sensitivity (99.9%) compared to EIA and Western blot using serum (Gallo *et al.*, 1997). The CDC guidelines still recommend confirmation of both positive and negative test results. These assays are further limited by the fact that they detect only HIV-1, and the patient population needs to be screened for potential exposure to HIV-2.

Molecular diagnostic tests are used not only for early detection of infection, but are also helpful when used quantitatively to determine viral load. Viral load is generally assessed at the time of initial diagnosis and is then repeated intermittently to follow disease progress and/or response to therapy. Several different plasma RNA assays are sensitive and accurate over a wide range of viral concentrations (up to 1 000 000 copies/ml of plasma). The reverse-transcription polymerase chain reaction (RT–PCR) amplifies viral nucleic acids, and the branched DNA (bDNA) assay amplifies the signal of the labelled probe that specifically binds to viral RNA, e.g. Quantiplex (bDNA) Assay for HIV-1 RNA (Chiron Corporation, 4560 Horton St., Emeryville, CA, USA). The current lower limits of detection are about 400 copies/ml for RT-PCR and 50 copies/ml for bDNA, but the sensitivity of these tests is still being improved.

Other methods for nucleic acid amplification with increased sensitivity of HIV RNA quantitation are also under development, such as transcription-mediated amplification (TMA), nested PCR techniques and nucleic acid sequence-based amplification (NASBA, Organon Technika, Research Triangle Park, NC, USA). The NASBA assay detects a range of $50-5 \times 10^6$ copies of HIV RNA per ml. HIV genotyping can use sequence data to predict response to therapy. Culture methods are not used routinely, but may be used for phenotyping in order to predict response to therapy. Microbiology is also crucial in identifying the various opportunistic infections seen in AIDS. A CD4/CD8 lymphocyte count and ratio is used to predict onset of opportunistic infections and to define AIDS conversion. CD4+ counts may also be used to assess whether an individual requires prophylactic antibiotic treatment. An HIV-infected person's risk of developing AIDS or dying can be estimated by combining CD4+ lymphocyte counts and levels of plasma RNA. The CD4+ count provides information on immediate vulnerability to opportunistic infections, and the plasma HIV RNA level predicts future CD4+ levels. Reduction of plasma RNA levels by antiretroviral therapy often increases CD4+ lymphocyte counts and reduces the risk of complications and death.

Treatment

Treatment protocols continue to evolve as newer antiviral agents become available. The initial azathioprine (AZT) monotherapy protocols that were thought to provide adequate treatment led to the emergence of drug-resistant HIV strains. Combination therapy is now favoured, in order to overcome the problem of rapid virus resistance. New drugs continue to be introduced for trials, with ever-changing complicated regimens. The combination of RT inhibitors + protease inhibitors is referred to as highly active antiretroviral therapy (HAART). Although this is not a cure for AIDS, viral loads can be reduced to nearly undetectable levels, significantly reducing the number of deaths and improving the general prognosis for AIDS patients. Conversion from HIV to AIDS can be delayed for many patients and subsequent immune reconstitution allows them to discontinue some prophylactic drugs for opportunistic infections when the CD4 + count rises above $200 \times 10^6 - 400 \times 10^6/l$. However, integration of the provirus makes the virus latent, and cure is therefore very difficult.

HAART protocols use multiple drugs that target different aspects of HIV replication, including nucleoside and non-nucleoside reverse transcriptase inhibitors and protease inhibitors. Other classes of drugs that interfere with target cell binding are also in development. HAART drug combinations are selected to minimize side effects, optimize therapy and provide the easiest dosing schedule possible in order to improve quality of life for the patients.

Nucleoside analogues that inhibit reverse transcriptase may slow virus spread in the body and delay the onset of opportunistic infections. This group includes the following.

Zidovudine (AZT, azathioprine)	Didanosine
Zalcitadine	Stavudine (D4T)
Lamivudine (3TC)	Abacavir (Ziagen)
Tenofovir (Viread)	

Non-nucleoside reverse transcriptase inhibitors (NNRTIs) are also used in combination with the RT inhibitors. This class includes the following.

Delvaridine (Rescriptor)
Nevirapine (Viramune)
Efravirenz (Sustiva)

More recently, protease inhibitors that interrupt virus replication have also been FDA approved for treatment.

Ritonavir (Norvir)	Abacavir (Ziagen)
Indinavir (Crixivan)	Amprenivir (Agenerase)
Nelfinavir (Viracept)	Lopinavir (Kaletra)

Single drug therapy with AZT is still used in pregnancy to diminish the risk of transmission to the fetus. Treatment throughout pregnancy, labour, and delivery (by caesarean section), and for the first 6 weeks of the baby's life can reduce the chance of HIV transmission to around 1%. Studies addressing the time frame that is important for administration of AZT therapy during pregnancy indicate that maternal–fetal transmission occurs most significantly late in the third trimester. This allows the risk of fetal infection to be dramatically reduced by a short course of targeted therapy. In developing countries where the cost of AZT may be prohibitive, mothers can be treated at one-third of the cost of treating throughout pregnancy. A recent study in Uganda suggests that a single oral dose of nevirapine (NVP) given to an HIV-infected woman during labour and another to her baby within 3 days of birth can significantly reduce the transmission rate: this may be more affordable and practical than AZT therapy in many parts of the world.

Antibiotics/antivirals are also used prophylactically to prevent the onset or recurrence of opportunistic infections. The CDC has issued revised guidelines for prophylactic treatment of opportunistic infections seen in AIDS, with recommendations for 19 AIDS-related diseases. These are summarized in Table 12.2.

Over the past 10 years, management of HIV has changed dramatically. Infectious disease experts now classify AIDS as a chronic illness: antiretroviral therapy yields higher life expectancy, individuals remain asymptomatic without treatment for more than 10 years, and vertical transmission from mother to infant is reduced. Whether assisted conception treatment should be offered to seropositive patients is a complicated issue that has become one of current concern, and this needs to be evaluated from

Table 12.2. Prophylaxis to prevent first episode of opportunistic infections in adults and adolescents

Pathogen	Indication for prophylaxis	First choice prophylactic
Prophylaxis strongly recommended as standard of care		
Pneumocystis carinii	CD4+counts <200/μl or the presence of oropharyngeal candidiasis	Trimethoprim-sulfamethoxazole daily
Mycobacterium tuberculosis (MTB)	PPD reaction ≥5 mm or exposure to a person with active TB	Isoniazid (INH) plus pyridoxine for 9 months
INH resistant MTB	Exposure to a patient with INH resistant MTB	Rifampin or rifabutin for 4 months
Multidrug resistant MTB	Exposure to a patient with multidrug resistant MTB	Treatment depends upon the susceptibility pattern of the MTB isolate to which the patient was exposed
Toxoplasma gondii	IgG antibody to *T. gondii* and CD4 count of <100/μl	Trimethoprim-sulfamethoxazole daily
Varicella zoster virus (VZV)	Exposure to a patient with shingles or chicken pox and no demonstrable antibody to VZV	VZV immune globulin administered within 96 hours of exposure
Prophylaxis usually recommended		
Streptococcus pneumoniae	CD4+count ≥200/μl	Pneumococcal 23-valent vaccine
Hepatitis B virus	All non-immune patients	3 doses of HBV vaccine
Influenza virus	All patients yearly	Inactivated trivalent vaccine
Hepatitis A virus	All non-immune patients at increased risk for infection with HAV and patients with chronic liver disease	2 doses of HAV vaccine
Effective, but not routinely administered prophylaxis		
Bacterial infections	Neutropenia	Granulocyte-colony-stimulating factor (GCSF)
Cryptococcus neoformans	CD4+count <50/μl	Fluconazole
Histoplasma capsulatum	CD4+count of <100/μl	Itraconazole
Cytomegalovirus	CD4+count of <50/μl and CMV antibody positive	Ganciclovir

PPD; purified protein derivative.

several different viewpoints, including the rights of the individual, safe handling of specimens to avoid risk of transmission and welfare of the child.

Vaccine availability

Significant effort has been invested in the development of an anti-HIV vaccine, as the only viable way to limit the spread of disease worldwide. Unfortunately, despite many trials, no effective vaccines have yet been developed. Early in 2003 a promising vaccine trial was discontinued due to lack of efficacy in preventing disease compared to the placebo control. Healthcare providers are so far left with only advice

to offer: avoidance of high risk activities, use of efficient barrier forms for birth control and STD prevention (condoms). Blood, semen and tissue donors must continue to be screened for HIV infection and for all high risk activities that serve as markers for HIV infection.

Human T-lymphotrophic viruses (HTLV)

The human T-lymphotrophic viruses, HTLV-I and HTLV-II are closely related viruses in the oncornavirus subfamily of retroviruses, first described in the early 1980s. These retroviruses can transform lymphocytes to produce stable clones that proliferate in vitro and in vivo. The two viruses have a dramatically different geographic prevalence.

HTLV-I

Up to 15% of the population in Japan, the Caribbean, Malaysia and parts of Africa show evidence of HTLV-I infection. Serologic evidence of infection increases with age, seen more often in women than in men. In non-endemic regions of the world such as the United States, seroprevalence is reported to be only 0.016% in the healthy blood donor population; positive donors generally report a connection with an endemic region of the world or close contact with a person from one of these areas.

HTLV-II

The worldwide seroprevalence of HTLV-II has not been well delineated. In the United States, Europe and Asia, HTLV-II is seen primarily in injecting drug users. It also appears to be endemic in some American Indian populations of North, Central and South America, as well as in pygmy tribes in Central Africa.

Life cycle

HTLV-I and HTLV-II both demonstrate CD4+ (T-helper cell) tropism, and the steps in viral infection are the same as those seen with HIV. The virus binds to the CD4 receptor on T-helper lymphocytes and is internalized. Viral RNA is reverse transcribed in the cytoplasm to produce the DNA provirus, which migrates to the cell nucleus where the DNA is incorporated into the cell's genomic DNA. Viral particles may be produced after gene expression, causing cell lysis, or the viral genome may remain latent in the cellular genome. T-cells with latent infection may be transformed 20–30 years after the primary infection, causing adult T-cell leukaemia/lymphoma (ATLL). Malignant transformation appears to be related to the viral *Tax* gene that codes for a regulatory protein. This protein enhances the transcription of both viral and cellular genes, leading to uncontrolled

proliferation of an infected T-helper cell clonal population.

Transmission

Although generally considered to be blood-borne pathogens, HTLV-I and HTLV-II can also be transmitted via a number of other routes. HTLV-I can be transmitted from mother to child, primarily through breast feeding; approximately 25% of children breast fed by HTLV-I-positive mothers acquire the infection compared to only 5% of children who are not breast fed. The 5% of infants who were not breast fed acquired the infection either transplacentally (vertically) or during parturition. HTLV-I may also be transmitted sexually. In a study of married couples in Japan, sexual transmission from an infected male to his partner occurred in over 60% of couples over a 10-year period. Transmission from females to their male partners was not as efficient; less than 1% of the males seroconverted over the same 10-year period. Sexual transmission appears to be enhanced in the presence of genital ulcer disease. Efficient transmission has been well documented through transfusion of cellular products from infected donors and through other percutaneous exposure such as sharing needles or healthcare worker needle stick exposures.

HTLV-II can be transmitted via transfusion and via sharing of infected needles in IV drug abuse. Sexual transmission is suggested by the observation that many of the women in the USA infected with HTLV-II have sexual contact with an infected injecting drug user as their only risk factor. The majority of studies suggest that transmission via sexual contact is from males to females, and not the reverse. There is some evidence for transmission of HTLV-II from infected mother to infant via breast milk, particularly in populations where infection is endemic.

Clinical presentation

HTLV-I is associated with two diseases, adult T-cell leukaemia/lymphoma (ATLL) and HTLV-I associated myelopathy/tropical spastic paresis (HAM/TSP). Clinical features of ATLL include lymphadenopathy, leukocytosis, hepatosplenomegaly, microabscesses in the dermis and epidermis and hypercalcemia. ATLL is a malignancy of HTLV-I immortalized T-lymphocytes. The infected T-cells undergo a monoclonal expansion; malignant lymphocytes have flower-shaped nuclear contours, and these 'flower cells' may be found in the peripheral blood. A broad clinical spectrum is seen with HTLV-I related disease, and ATLL has been divided into four subtypes: acute, lymphomatous, chronic and smoldering. Approximately 55% of patients present with acute leukaemia, 20% with the lymphomatous form, 20% with the chronic and 5% with the smoldering form.

Acute ATLL is seen most frequently in Japan, presenting with lymphadenopathy, skin lesions and involvement of the bone marrow and spleen. Leukemic cells can be detected in peripheral blood, and lactic dehydrogenase (LDH), bilirubin and calcium levels are often dramatically elevated. The incidence of disease is greatest in individuals between 40 and 60 years of age and survival from the time of acute ATLL diagnosis is generally less than one year. Although the lifetime risk for an infected individual to develop ATLL is only 2–4%, this translates to a significant disease burden in endemic areas. In Japan, HTLV-I infection is the leading cause of acute leukemias. In endemic areas, the viral infection is usually acquired early in life, and this presents an increased risk for developing ATLL.

The **lymphomatous ATLL** subtype is characterized by bulky lymphadenopathy and organomegaly, and this clinical syndrome is seen predominantly in the Caribbean, where it represents about one-third of ATLL cases. Although these patients have increased LDH and hypercalcemia, the leukemic cells are not seen at significant levels circulating in the peripheral blood. Patients with chronic ATLL generally have few circulating ATLL cells, mild lymphadenopathy, organomegaly, skin involvement and no hypercalcemia. These patients may eventually develop an acute leukemic syndrome. The smoldering form of disease represents a 'pre-ATLL'. These patients are asymptomatic and approximately half of them may have a leukocytosis that spontaneously resolves. The other half progress to an acute leukemia.

HAM/TSP is a progressive neurologic disease that is characterized by permanent lower extremity weakness, spasticity and hyper-reflexia. Symptoms may also include lower back pain and sensory disturbances such as tingling and burning sensations, as well as impaired vibratory sense, urinary incontinence and impotence. HAM/TSP develops in <1% of HTLV-I infected individuals, with women affected more frequently than men.

HTLV-II has not been definitively associated with any disease. Case reports suggest an association with some neurologic syndromes similar to HAM/TSP and possibly to hairy cell leukaemia.

Laboratory diagnosis

HTLV-I and HTLV-II infections are detected initially by testing for antibodies with an FDA-approved or licensed EIA. These assays are generally more sensitive in detecting antibodies against HTLV-I than HTLV-II. The CDC recommends that all repeatedly positive specimens should be confirmed by another method such as Western immunoblot or radioimmunoprecipitation assays that distinguish between HTLV-I and HTLV-II. These tests identify antibodies against HTLV-I/II p24 core protein and an envelope protein (gp 21, gp46 and gp61/68). Positive samples should show antibodies against p24 and either gp46 or gp61/68, or both. If immunoreactivity to either core protein or envelope protein, but not both, is present, the test is interpreted as intermediate. If there is no reactivity to any HTLV-I/II related antigens, the EIA result is considered a false positive. Newer EIA and Western blot assays containing a recombinant p21e envelope protein may enhance the sensitivity of HTLV-I/II detection, but there is concern about the specificity of this antigen. The viruses can be detected by PCR assays available for research purposes; these are more sensitive in detecting HTLV-I than HTLV-II. A line immunoassay (INNO-LIA, Immunogenetics, Belgium) has been developed that uses a recombinant viral protein embedded strip to identify HTLV-I and HTLV-II specific antibodies. This assay is more sensitive for confirming HTLV-II than HTLV-I infections. Viral culture is available only in a limited number of reference laboratories.

Lymph node biopsy shows a diffuse T-cell non-Hodgkin's lymphoma; evaluation of the ATLL cells demonstrates a malignant clone of T-helper cells that tend to be positive for CD4, CD3 and CD25. They are negative for CD1, CD8 and terminal deoxyribonucleotide transferase (TdT). Confirmation that the tumour is an ATLL lymphoma requires serologic identification of HTLV-1 infection. Peripheral blood containing cleaved lymphocytes from the clonal expansion 'flower cells' can suggest the diagnosis, but these are not specific for ATLL.

Treatment

Chemotherapy treatment can decrease or eliminate tumour bulk when AALT is diagnosed. Protocols include multiple drugs, and the CHOP protocol (cyclophosphamide, doxorubicin, vincristine and prednisone) has been reported to be effective in inducing remission. However, chemotherapy is not curative and relapse is common. Trials using Zidovudine and α-interferon treatment regimens have been attempted. Nearly half of patients who failed standard chemotherapy responded to this antiviral therapy with either complete remission or a greater than 50% reduction in tumour size. Patients diagnosed with ATLL, as well as individuals who have been identified as positive for HTLV-I and HTLV-II, should be counselled regarding methods to limit viral spread. Patients should not donate blood, semen, organs, or other tissues, should use latex condoms to prevent sexual transmission, and must avoid sharing needles for injecting drug use. HTLV-I and -II positive women are advised against breast feeding to prevent transmission to the neonate.

Vaccine availability

Although there is currently no human vaccine for the prevention of HTLV-I or HTLV-II, vaccines are under development in animal models. The major focus of prevention of disease with these viruses lies with testing blood supplies and deferral of donors from future donations, together with counselling measures as described above.

REFERENCES

Araneta, M. R. G., Mascola, L., Eller, A. *et al.* (1995). HIV transmission through donor artificial insemination. *Journal of the American Medical Association*, **273**: 854–8.

Bresson, J. L., Clavequin, M. C., Mazeron, M. C. *et al.* and for Fédération Française des CECOS (2003). Risk of cytomegalovirus transmission by cryopreserved semen: a study of 635 semen samples from 231 donors. *Human Reproduction*, **18**: 1881–6.

Gallo, D., George, J. R., Fitchen, J. H. *et al.* for the OraSure HIV Clinical Trials Group (1997). Evaluation of a system using oral mucosal transudate for HIV-1 antibody screening and confirmatory testing. *Journal of the American Medical Association*, **277**: 254–8.

Gao, F., Bailes, E., Robertson, D. L. *et al.* (1999). Origin of HIV-1 in the chimpanzee *Pantroglodytes troglodytes*. *Nature*, **397**: 436–41.

Levy, R., Tardy, J. C., Bourlet, T. *et al.* (2000). Transmission risk of hepatitis C virus in assisted reproductive techniques. *Human Reproduction*, **15**: 810–16.

Papaxanthos-Roche, A., Trimoulet, P., Commenges-Ducos, M., Hocke, C., Fleury, H. J. A., & Mayer, G. (2004). PCR-detected hepatitis C virus RNA associated with human zona-intact oocytes collected from infected women from ART. *Human Reproduction*, **19**: 1170–5.

Revello, M. G., Zavattoni, M., Furione, M., Lilleri, D., Gorini, G. & Gerna, G. (2002). Diagnosis and outcome of preconceptual and periconceptual primary cytomegalovirus infections. *Journal of Infectious Diseases*, **186**(4): 553–7.

Simmonds, P., Holmes, E. C., Cha, T. A. *et al.* (1993). Classification of hepatitis C virus into six major genotypes and a series of subtypes by phylogenetic analysis of the NS-5 region. *Journal of General Virology*, **74**: 2391–9.

FURTHER READING

GENERAL

Cotran, R. S., Kumar, V. & Collins, T. (eds.) (1999). *Robbins Pathologic Basis of Disease*, 6th edn. Philadelphia, PA: W. B. Saunders Company.

Holmes, K. K., Sparling, P. F., Mardh, P. A. *et al.* (eds). (1999). *Sexually Transmitted Diseases*, 3rd edn. New York: McGraw-Hill Health Professions Division.

Koneman, E. W., Allen, S. D., Janda, W. M., Schreckenberger, P. C. & Winn, W. C. (eds.) (1997). *Color Atlas and Textbook of Diagnostic Microbiology*, 5th edn. Philadelphia, PA: Lippincott.

Murray, P. R., Barton, E. J., Pfaller, M. A., Tenover, F. C. & Yolken, R. H. (eds). (1999). *Manual of Clinical Microbiology*, 7th edn. Washington, DC: ASM Press.

CYTOMEGALOVIRUS

Aitken, C., Barrett-Muir, W., Millar, C. *et al.* (1999). Use of molecular assays in diagnosis and monitoring of cytomegalovirus disease following renal transplant. *Journal of Clinical Microbiology*, **37**: 2804–7.

American Society for Reproductive Medicine (2002). 2002 guidelines for gamete and embryo donation: a practice committee report – guidelines and minimum standards. *Fertility and Sterility*, **77**(suppl. 5): S1-S8.

Berenberg, W. & Nankervis, G. (1970). Long-term follow-up of cytomegalic inclusion disease of infancy. *Pediatrics*, **46**: 403–10.

Boeckh, M. & Biovin, G. (1998). Quantitation of cytomegalovirus: Methodologic aspects and clinical applications. *Clinical Microbiology Reviews*, **11**: 533–54.

Boeckh, M., Gallez-Hawkins, G. M., Myerson, D., Zaia, J. A. & Bowden, R. A. (1997). Plasma polymerase chain reaction for cytomegalovirus DNA after allogeneic marrow transplantation: comparison with polymerase chain reaction using peripheral blood leukocytes, pp65 antigenemia, and viral culture. *Transplantation*, **64**: 108–13.

Bowden, R. A., Slichter, S. J., Sayers, M. *et al.* (1995). A comparison of filtered leukocyte-reduced and Cytomegalovirus (CMV) seronegative blood products for the prevention of transfusions-associated CMV infection after marrow transplantation. *Blood*, **9**: 3598–603.

British Andrology Society (1999). British andrology society guidelines for the screening of semen donors for donor insemination. *Human Reproduction*, **14**: 1823–6.

Chandler, S. H., Handsfield, H. H. & McDougall, J. K. (1987). Isolation of multiple strains of cytomegalovirus from women attending a clinic for sexually transmitted diseases. *Journal of Infectious Diseases*, **155**: 655–60.

Chou, S. (1986). Acquisition of donor strains of cytomegalovirus by renal-transplant recipients. *New England Journal of Medicine*, **314**: 1418–23.

Davis, L. E., Stewart, J. A. & Garvin, S. (1975). Cytomegalovirus infection: A seroepidemiologic comparison of nuns and women from a venereal disease clinic. *American Journal of Epidemiology*, **102**: 327–30.

Fowler, K. B., Stagno, S., Pass, R. F., Britt, W. J., Boll, T. J. & Alford, C. A. (1992). The outcome of congenital cytomegalovirus infection in relation to maternal antibody status. *New England Journal of Medicine*, **326**: 663–7.

Gleaves, C. A., Smith, T. F., Schuster, A. & Pearson, G. R. (1982). Rapid detection of cytomegalovirus in MRC-5 cells inoculated with urine specimens by using low speed centrifugation and monoclonal antibody to early antigen. *Journal of Clinical Microbiology*, **19**: 917–19.

Grundy, J. E., Lui, S. F., Super, M. *et al.* (1988). Symptomatic cytomegalovirus infection in seropositive kidney recipients: reinfection with donor virus rather than reactivation of recipient virus. *Lancet*, **ii**: 132–5.

Handsfield, H. H., Chandler, S. H., Caine, V. A. *et al.* (1985). Cytomegalovirus infection in sex partners: evidence for sexual transmission. *Journal of Infectious Diseases*, **151**: 344–8.

Hodinka, R. L. (1999). Human cytomegalovirus. In *Manual of Clinical Microbiology*, 7th edn., ed. P. R. Murray, E. J. Barton, M. A. Pfaller, F. C. Tenover & R. H. Yolken, pp. 888–99. Washington, DC: ASM Press.

Huang, E. S., Alford, C. A., Reynolds, D. W., Stagno, S. & Pass, R. F. (1980). Molecular epidemiology of cytomegalovirus infections in women and their infants. *New England Journal of Medicine*, **303**: 958–62.

Keating, M. R. (1999). Antiviral agents for non-human immunodeficiency virus infections. *Mayo Clinic Proceedings*, **74**: 1266–83.

Koneman, E. W., Allen, S. D., Janda, W. M., Schreckenberger, P. C. & Winn, W. C. (1997). Diagnosis of infections caused by viruses, chlamydia, rickettsia and related organisms. In *Color Atlas and Textbook of Diagnostic Microbiology*, 5th edn, pp. 1177–293. Philadelphia, PA: Lippincott.

Kumar, M. L., Nankervis, G. A. & Gold, E. (1973). Inapparent congenital cytomegalovirus infection: a follow-up study. *New England Journal of Medicine*, **288**: 1370–2.

Lang, D. J. & Kummer, J. F. (1972). Demonstration of cytomegalovirus in semen. *New England Journal of Medicine*, **28**: 756–8.

Lang, D. J., Kummer, J. F. & Hartley, D. P. (1974). Cytomegalovirus in semen: Persistence and demonstration in extracellular fluids. *New England Journal of Medicine*, **291**: 121–3.

Landry, M. L., Ferguson, D., Stevens-Ayers, T., de Jonge, M. W. & Boeckh, M. (1996). Evaluation of CMV Brite kit for detection of cytomegalovirus pp65 antigenemia in periph-eral blood leukocytes by immunofluorescence. *Journal of Clinical Microbiology*, **34**: 1337–9.

Li, H., Dummer, S., Estes, W. R., Meng, S., Wright, P. F. & Tang, Y. W. (2003). Measurement of human cytomegalovirus loads by quantitative real-time PCR for monitoring clinical inter-vention in transplant recipients. *Journal of Clinical Micro-biology*, **41**: 187–91.

Liesnard, C. A., Revelard, P. & Englert, Y. (1998). Is match-ing between women and donors feasible to avoid cytomegalovirus infection in artificial insemination with donor semen. *Human Reproduction*, **13**: 25–34.

Mansat, A., Mengelle, C., Chalet, M. *et al.* (1997). Cyto-megalovirus detection in cryopreserved semen samples collected for therapeutic donor insemination. *Human Reproduction*, **12**: 1663–6.

Pannekoek, Y., Westenberg, S. M., de Vries, J. *et al.* (2000). PCR assessment of *Chlamydia trachomatis* infection of semen specimens processed for artificial insemination. *Journal of Clinical Microbiology*, **38**: 3763–7.

Pass, R. F., Stagno, S., Myers, G. J. & Alford, C. A. (1980). Out-come of symptomatic congenital cytomegalovirus infec-tion: results of long-term longitudinal follow-up. *Pediatrics*, **66**: 758–62.

Preece, P. M., Blount, J. M., Glover, J., Fletcher, G. M., Peckham, C. S. & Griffiths, P. D. (1983). The consequences of primary cytomegalovirus infection in pregnancy. *Archives of Disease in Childhood*, **58**: 970–5.

Prior, J. R., Morroll, D. R., Birks, A. G., Matson, P. L. & Lieberman, B. A. (1994). The screening for cytomegalovirus antibody in semen donors and recipients within a donor insemination programme. *Human Reproduction*, **9**: 2076–8.

Przepiorka, D., LeParc, G. F., Werch, J. & Lichtiger, B. (1996). Pre-vention of transfusion-associated cytomegalovirus infec-tion: practice parameters. *American Journal of Clinical Pathology*, **106**: 163–9.

Rabella, N. & Drew, W. L. (1990). Comparison of conventional and shell vial cultures for detecting cytomegalovirus infec-tion. *Journal of Clinical Microbiology*, **28**: 806–7.

Revello, M. G. & Gerna, G. (2002). Diagnosis and management of human cytomegalovirus infection in the mother, fetus, and newborn infant. *Clinical Microbiology Reviews*, **15**: 680–715.

Reynolds, D. W., Stagno, S., Stubbs, K. G. *et al.* (1974). Inap-parent congenital cytomegalovirus infection with elevated cord IgM levels. *New England Journal of Medicine*, **290**: 291–6.

Stagno, S., Reynolds, D. W., Amos, C. S. *et al.* (1977a). Audi-tory and visual defects resulting from symptomatic and subclinical congenital cytomegalovirus and toxoplasma infections. *Pediatrics*, **59**: 669–78.

Stagno, S., Reynolds, D. W., Huang, E. S., Thames, S. D., Smith, R. J. & Alford, C. A. (1977b) Cytomegalovirus infection: occur-rence in an immune population. *New England Journal of Medicine*, **296**: 1254–8.

Stagno, S., Pass, R. F., Dworsky, M. E. *et al.* (1982). Congenital cytomegalovirus infection: the relative importance of pri-mary and recurrent maternal infection. *New England Jour-nal of Medicine*, **306**: 945–9.

Stagno, S., Pass, R. F., Cloud, G. *et al.* (1986). Primary cytomegalovirus infection in pregnancy: incidence, trans-mission to fetus, and clinical outcome. *Journal of the Amer-ican Medical Association*, **256**: 1904–8.

Strauss, R. G. (1999). Leukocyte-reduction to prevent transfusion-transmitted cytomegalovirus infection. *Pediatric Transplant*, **3**(Suppl.1): 19–22.

Vochem, M., Hamprecht, K., Jahn, G. & Speer, C. P. (1998). Trans-mission of cytomegalovirus to preterm infants through breast milk. *Pediatric Infectious Disease Journal*, **17**: 53–8.

HEPATITIS B VIRUS

Batts, K. P. & Ludwig, J. (1995). Chronic hepatitis: an update on terminology and reporting. *American Journal of Surgical Pathology*, **19**: 1409–17.

Blumberg, B. S. (1977). Australian antigen and the biology of hepatitis B. *Science*, **197**: 17–25.

Centers for Disease Control and Prevention (1996). Outbreaks of Hepatitis B virus infection among hemodialysis patients – California, Nebraska, and Texas, 1994. *Morbidity and Mor-tality Weekly Report*, **45**: 285–9.

(2002). Sexually transmitted diseases treatment guidelines 2002. *Morbidity and Mortality Weekly Report*, **51**(No. RR-6): 59–61.

Crawford, J. M. (1999). The liver and the biliary tract. In *Rob-bins Pathologic Basis of Disease*, 6th edn, ed. R. S. Cotran, V. Kumar & T. Collins, pp. 856–67. Philadelphia, PA: W. B. Saunders Company.

Fattovich, G., Giustina, G. & Schalm, S. W. (1995). Occurence of hepatocellular carcinoma and decompensation in western European patients with cirrhosis type B. *Hepatology*, **21**: 77–82.

Hendricks, D. A., Stowe, B. J. & Hoo, B. S. (1995). Quantitation of HBV DNA in human serum using a branched DNA (bDNA) signal amplification assay. *American Journal of Clinical Pathology*, **104**: 537–46.

Lee, W. M. (1997). Hepatitis B virus infection. *New England Jour-nal of Medicine*, **337**: 1733–45.

Liaw, Y. F., Tai, D. I., Chu, C. M. & Chen, T. J. (1988) The development of cirrhosis in patients with chronic type b hepatitis: a prospective study. *Hepatology*, **8**: 493–6.

Margolis, H. S., Coleman, P. J., Brown, R. E., Mast, E. E., Sheingold, S. H. & Arevalo, J. A. (1995). Prevention of hepatitis B virus transmission by immunization. *Journal of the American Medical Association*, **274**: 1201–8.

MacMahon, B. J., Alberts, S. R., Wainwright, R. B., Bulkow, L. & Lanier, A. P. (1990). Hepatitis B-related sequelae: prospective study in 1400 hepatitis B surface antigen-positive Alaska native carriers. *Archives of Internal Medicine*, **150**: 1051–4.

Sacher, R. A., Peters, S. M. & Bryan, J. A. (2000). Testing for viral hepatitis: a practice parameter. *American Journal of Clinical Pathology*, **113**: 12–17.

Williams, I., Smith, G., Kernan, D. *et al.* (1997). Hepatitis B virus transmission in an elementary school setting. *Journal of the American Medical Association*, **278**: 2167–9.

HEPATITIS C VIRUS

Bourlet, T., Levy, R., Maertens, A. *et al.* (2002). Detection and characterization of hepatitis C virus RNA in seminal plasma and spermatozoon fractions of semen from patients attempting medically assisted conception. *Journal of Clinical Microbiology*, **40**: 3252–5.

Choo, Q. L., Kuo, G., Weiner, A. J., Overby, L. R., Bradley, D. W. & Houghton, M. (1989) Isolation of a cDNA clone derived from a blood-borne non-A, non-B viral hepatitis genome. *Science*, **244**: 359–62.

Devaux, A., Soula, V., Sifer, C. *et al.* (2003). Hepatitis C virus detection in follicular fluid and culture media from HCV$^+$ women, and viral risk during IVF procedures. *Human Reproduction*, **18**: 2342–9.

Dos Santos, V. A., Azevedo, R. S., Camargo, M. E. & Alves, V. A. F. (1999). Serodiagnosis of hepatitis C virus: effect of new evaluation of cutoff values for enzyme-linked immunosorbent assay in Brazilian patients. *American Journal of Clinical Pathology*, **112**: 418–24.

Germer, J. J. & Zein, N. N. (2001). Advances in the molecular diagnosis of hepatitis C and their clinical implications. *Mayo Clinic Proceedings*, **76**: 911–20.

Germer, J. J., Heimgartner, P. J., Ilstrup, D. M., Harmsen, W. S., Jenkins, G. D. & Patel, R. (2002). Comparative evaluation of the Versant HCV RNA 3.0, Quantiplex HCV RNA 2.0, and COBAS AMLICOR HCV MONITOR version 2.0 assays for quantification of hepatitis C virus RNA in serum. *Journal of Clinical Microbiology*, **40**: 495–500.

Keating, M. R. (1999). Antiviral agents for non-human immunodeficiency virus infections. *Mayo Clinic Proceedings*, **74**: 1266–83.

Lauer, G. M. & Walker, B. D. (2001). Hepatitis C virus infection. *New England Journal of Medicine*, **345**: 41–52.

Lee, S. C., Antony, A., Lee, N. *et al.* (2000). Improved version 2.0 qualitative and quantitative AMPLICORE Reverse transcription-PCR tests for hepatitis C virus RNA: calibration to international units, enhanced genotype reactivity, and performance characteristics. *Journal of Clinical Microbiology*, **38**: 4171–9.

Podzorski, R. P. (2002). Molecular testing in the diagnosis and management of hepatitis C virus infection. *Archives of Pathology and Laboratory Medicine*, **126**: 285–90.

Saito, K., Sullivan, D., Haruna, Y., Theise, N. D., Thung, S. N. & Gerber, M. A. (1997). Detection of hepatitis C virus RNA sequences in hepatocellular carcinoma and its precursors by microdissection polymerase chain reaction. *Archives of Pathology and Laboratory Medicine*, **121**: 400–3.

Sulkowski, M. S., Ray, S. C. & Thomas, D. L. (2002). Needlestick transmission of hepatitis C. *Journal of the American Medical Association*, **287**: 2406–13.

Thomas, D. L., Astemborski, J., Rai, R. M. *et al.* (2000). The natural history of hepatitis C virus infection: host, viral, and environmental factors. *Journal of the American Medical Association*, **284**: 450–6.

WHO home page http://www.who.int: Fact sheet no 164, Hepatitis C (October 2000).

Zein, N. N. & Persing, D. H. (1996). Hepatitis C genotypes: current trends and future implications. *Mayo Clinic Proceedings*, **71**: 458–62.

HEPATITIS D VIRUS

Aragona, M., Macagno, S., Caredda, F. *et al.* (1987). Serological response to the hepatitis Delta virus in hepatitis D. *Lancet*, **i**: 478–80.

Crawford, J. M. (1999). The liver and the biliary tract. In *Robbins Pathologic Basis of Disease*, 6th edn, ed. R. S. Cotran, V. Kumar & T. Collins, pp. 856–67. Philadelphia, PA: W. B. Saunders Company.

Dalekos, G. N., Galanakis, E., Zervou, E., Tzoufi, M., Lapatsanis, P. D. & Tsianos, E. V. (2000). Interferon-alpha treatment of children with chronic hepatitis D virus infection: the Greek experience. *Hepatogastroenterology*, **47**: 1072–6.

Farci, P., Gerin, J. L., Aragona, M. *et al.* (1986). Diagnostic and prognostic significance of the IgM antibody to the hepatitis Delta virus. *Journal of the American Medical Association*, **255**: 1443–6.

Gaeta, G. B., Stroffolini, T., Chiaramonte, M. *et al.* (2000). Chronic Hepatitis D: a vanishing disease? An Italian multicenter study. *Hepatology*, **32**: 824–7.

Gudima, S., Chang, J., Moraleda, G., Azolinsky, A. & Taylor, J. (2002). Parameters of human hepatitis delta virus genome replication: the quantity, quality, and intracellular distribution of viral proteins and RNA. *Journal of Virology*, **76**: 3709–19.

Hoofnagle, J. H. (1989) Type D hepatitis. *Journal of the American Medical Association*, **261**: 1321–5.

Kuhns, M. C. (1995). Viral hepatitis: Part 1: The discovery, diagnostic tests, and new viruses. *Laboratory Medicine*, **26**: 650–9.

Lau, D. T., Doo, E., Park, Y. *et al.* (1999). Lamivudine for chronic delta hepatitis. *Hepatology*, **30**: 546–9.

Marzano, A., Salizzoni, M. & Rizzetto, M. (1999). Liver transplantation in viral hepatitis. New insights. *Acta Gastroenterologica Belgica*, **62**: 342–7.

Niro, G. A., Casey, J. L., Gravinese, E. *et al.* (1999). Intrafamilial transmission of hepatitis delta virus: molecular evidence. *Journal of Hepatology*, **30**: 564–9.

Sacher, R. A., Peters, S. M. & Bryan, J. A. (2000). Testing for viral hepatitis: a practice parameter. *American Journal of Clinical Pathology*, **113**: 12–17.

Yuraydin, C., Bozkaya, H., Gurel, S. *et al.* (2002). Famcyclovir treatment of chronic delta hepatitis. *Journal of Hepatology*, **37**: 266–71.

HIV AND AIDS

Allain, J. P., Laurian, Y., Paul, D. A. *et al.* (1987). Long-term evaluation of HIV antigen and antibodies to p24 and gp41 in patients with hemophilia. *New England Journal of Medicine*, **317**: 1114–21.

Busch, M. P. & Satten, G. A. (1997). Time course of viremia and antibody seroconversion following human immunodeficiency virus exposure. *American Journal of Medicine*, **102** (Suppl.2): 117–24.

Cao, Y., Qin, L., Zhang, L., Safrit, J. & Ho, D. (1995). Virologic and immunologic characterization of long-term survivors of human immunodeficiency virus type 1 infection. *New England Journal of Medicine*, **332**: 201–8.

Centers for Disease Control and Prevention (1992). 1993 revised classification system for HIV infection and expanded surveillance case definition for AIDS among adolescents and adults. *Morbidity and Mortality Weekly Report*, **41**(No.RR-17): 1–19.

(1996). Case-control study of HIV seroconversion in health-care workers after percutaneous exposure to HIV-infected blood in France, United Kingdom, and United States, January 1988–August 1994. *Morbidity and Mortality Weekly Report*, **275**: 929–33.

(1997). Transmission of HIV possibly associated with exposure of mucous membrane to contaminated blood. *Morbidity and Mortality Weekly Report*, **46**: 620–3.

(2001a). Updated US public health services guidelines for the management of occupational exposures to HBV, HCV and HIV and recommendations for postexposure prophylaxis. *Morbidity and Mortality Weekly Report*, **50**(RR-11): 1–42.

(2001b). Revised guidelines for HIV counselling, testing, and referral. *Morbidity and Mortality Weekly Report*, **50**(No. RR-19): 1–55.

(2001c). HIV and AIDS – United States 1981–2000. *Morbidity and Mortality Weekly Report*, **50**: 430–4.

(2001d). The global HIV and AIDS epidemic, 2001. *Morbidity and Mortality Weekly Report*, **50**: 434–9.

(2002). Guidelines for preventing opportunistic infections among HIV-infected persons – 2002. *Morbidity and Mortality Weekly Report*, **51**(no.RR-8): 1–52.

Dickover, R. E., Garratty, E. M., Herman, S. A. *et al.* (1996). Identification of levels of maternal HIV-1 RNA associated with risk of perinatal transmission: effect of maternal zidovudine treatment on viral load. *Journal of the American Medical Association*, **275**: 599–605.

Elbeik, T., Charlebois, E., Nassos, P. *et al.* (2002). Quantitiative and cost comparison of ultrasensitive human immunodeficiency virus type 1 RNA viral load assays: Bayer bDNA quantiplex version 3.0 and 2.0 and Roche PCR Amplicore Monitor version 1.5. *Journal of Clinical Microbiology*, **38**: 1113–20.

Kahn, J. O. & Walker, B. D. (1998). Acute human immunodeficiency virus type 1 infection. *New England Journal of Medicine*, **339**: 33–9.

Kessler, H. A., Blaauw, B., Spear, J., Paul, D. A., Falk, L. A. & Landay, A. (1987). Diagnosis of human immunodeficiency virus infection in seronegative homosexuals presenting with an acute viral syndrome. *Journal of the American Medical Association*, **258**: 1196–9.

Kleinman, S., Busch, M. P., Hall, L. *et al.* (1998). False-positive HIV-1 test results in a low risk screening setting of voluntary blood donation. *Journal of the American Medical Association*, **280**: 1080–5.

Kourtis, A. P., Bulterys, M., Nesheim, S. R. & Lee, F. K. (2001). Understanding the timing of HIV transmission from mother to infant. *Journal of the American Medical Association*, **285**: 709–12.

Ledergerber, B., Egger, M., Erard, V. *et al.* (1999). AIDS-related opportunistic illnesses occurring after initiation of potent antiretroviral therapy: the Swiss HIV cohort study. *Journal of the American Medical Association*, **282**: 2220–6.

Lindegren, M. L., Byers, R. H., Thomas, P. *et al.* (1999). Trends in perinatal transmission of HIV/AIDS in the United States. *Journal of the American Medical Association*, **282**: 531–8.

Lipman, M. C. I., Gluck, T. A. & Johnson, M. A. (1994). *An Atlas of Differential Diagnosis in HIV Disease*. New York: Parthenon Publishing Group NY.

Mellors, J. W., Kingsley, L. A., Rinaldo, C. R. *et al.* (1995). Quantitiation of HIV-1 RNA in plasma predicts outcome after seroconversion. *Annals of Internal Medicine*, **122**: 573–9.

Murphy, D. G., Cote, L., Fauvel, M., Rene, P. & Vincelette, J. (2000). Multicenter comparison of Roche COBAS Amplicore Monitor Version 1.5, Organon Teknika Nucleosens QT with extractor, and Bayer quantiplex version 3.0 for quantitation of human immunodeficiency virus type 1 RNA in plasma. *Journal of Clinical Microbiology*, **38**: 4034–41.

Quinn, T. C., Wawer, M. J., Sewankambo, N. *et al.* (2001). Viral load and heterosexual transmission of Human Immunodeficiency Virus Type 1. *New England Journal of Medicine*, **34**: 921–9.

Saag, M. S., Holodniy, M. & Kuritzkes, D. R. (1996). HIV viral load markers in clinical practice. *Nature Medicine*, **2**: 625–9.

Sepkowitz, K. A. (2001). AIDS-the first 20 years. *New England Journal of Medicine*, **344**: 1764–72.

Stramer, S. L., Heller, J. S., Coombs, R. W., Ho, D. D. & Allain, J. P. (1988) Transmission of HIV by blood transfusion. *New England Journal of Medicine*, **319**: 513.

Tural, C., Ruiz, L., Holtzer, C. *et al.* and the Havana Study Group (2002) Clinical utility of HIV-1 genotyping and expert advice: the Havana trial. *AIDS*, **16**: 209–18.

Vlahov, D., Graham, N., Hoover, D. *et al.* (1998). Prognostic indicators for AIDS and infectious disease death in HIV-infected injection drug users: plasma viral load and CD4 cell count. *Journal of the American Medical Association*, **279**: 35–40.

Von Sydow, M., Gaines, H., Sonnerborg, A., Forsgren, M., Pehrson, P. O. & Strannegard, O. (1988). Antigen detection in primary HIV infection. *British Medical Journal*, **296**: 238–40.

Zhang, L., Ramratnam, B., Tenner-Racz, K. *et al.* (1999). Quantifying residual HIV-1 replication in patients receiving combination antiretroviral therapy. *New England Journal of Medicine*, **340**: 1605–13.

HUMAN T-LYMPHOTROPHIC VIRUSES

Bazarbachi, A. & Hermine, O. (1996). Treatment with a combined zidovudine and alpha-interferon in naïve and pretreated adult T-cell leukemia/lymphoma patients. *AIDS Human Retrovirology*, **13**(Suppl.1): S186–90.

Brick, W. G., Nalamolu, Y., Jillella, A. P., Burgess, R. E. & Kallab, A. M. (2002). Adult T-cell leukaemia/lymphoma: a rare case in the USA and review of the literature. *Leukemia Lymphoma*, **34**: 127–32.

Centers for Disease Control and Prevention (1993). Recommendations for counselling persons infected with human T-lymphotrophic virus, Types I and II. *Morbidity and Mortality Weekly Report*, **42**(No. RR-9): 1–13.

De The, G. & Kazanji, M. (1996). An HTLV-I/II Vaccine: from animal models to clinical trials? *AIDS*, **13**(Suppl.1): S191–8.

Ferreira, O. C., Planelles, V. & Rosenblatt, J. D. (1997). Human T-cell leukemia viruses: epidemiology, biology and pathogenicity. *Blood Reviews*, **11**: 91–104.

Hall, W. W., Ishak, R., Zhu, S. W. *et al.* (1996). Human T lymphotropic virus type II (HTLV-II): epidemiology, molecular properties, and clinical features of infection. *AIDS Human Retrovirology*, **13**(Suppl.1): S204–14.

Lowis, G. W., Sheremata, W. A. & Minagar, A. (2002). Epidemiologic features of HTLV-II: serologic and molecular evidence. *Annals of Epidemiology*, **12**: 46–66.

Murphy, E. L. (1996). The clinical epidemiology of human T-lymphotropic virus type II (HTLV-II). *AIDS Human Retrovirology*, **13**(Suppl.1): S215–19.

Salemi, M., Vandamme, A. M., Desyter, J., Casoli, C. & Berrazzoni, U. (1999). The origin and evolution of human T-cell lymphotropic virus Type II (HTLV-II) and the relationship with its replication strategy. *Gene*, **234**: 11–21.

Takatsuki, K., Matsuoka, M. & Yamaguchi, Y. (1996). Adult T-Cell leukemia in Japan. *AIDS Human Retrovirology*, **13**(Suppl. 1): S15–19.

Thorstensson, R., Albert, J. & Andersson, S. (2002). Strategies for diagnosis of HTLV-I and –II. *Transfusion*, **42**: 780–91.

Uchiyama, T. (1997). Human T cell leukaemia virus type I (HTLV-I) and human diseases. *Annual Review of Immunology*, **15**: 15–37.

Yamashita, M., Ido, E., Miura, T. & Hayami, M. (1996). Molecular epidemiology of HTLV-I in the world. *AIDS Human Virology*, **13**(Suppl.1): S124–31.

Appendix to Part II. Specimen culture by body site

Specimen	Direct smear	Primary plating	By special request	Comments
Urine Clean-voided midstream; straight catheter; indwelling catheter	Gram stain (unspun urine only) Wet prep-unstained from pellet	BA, Mac or EMB, CNA For suprapubic specimen, 0.1 ml on Ana, add Thio		Clean voided urine: Plate quantitatively at 1:1000; 1:100 if patient is female of reproductive age with leukocytes in specimen and possible acute urethral syndrome
Stool	Methylene blue to detect leukocytes	BA, Mac, HE (or XLD), GN, Campy (incubated @ 42 °C) Mac Sorbitol for *E. coli* O157:H7 Selenite broth for *Salmonella* and *Shigella*	CIN for *Yersinia* TM for *Neisseria gonorrhoeae* acid-fast stain for mycobacteria	Consider: testing for ova and parasites
Gastric aspirate or lavage	Gram stain or AO	BA, C, M, CNA	AFB	May substitute for sputum in child for AFB detection
Gastric biopsy		Skirrow's, BA, CA	Rapid urease test or breath test for *Helicobacter pylori*	
Blood	Giemsa stain or AO	Blood culture bottles	Brucellosis, tularemia, leptospirosis, mycobacteria, cell-wall deficient organisms	Consider: Brucellosis Tularemia Leptospirosis Cell wall-deficient organisms
CSF Do not store for more than 6 h/37 °C unless for viral culture; for viral culture, specimen may be kept at 4 °C for up to 3 days	Gram stain	BA, CA, Thio CNA, Mac, Ana as indicated by smear	Consider cryptococcal antigen	Centrifuge 15 min @ 2500 rpm; use sediment for smear/culture (cytocentrifugation recommended) *Haemophilus influenzae* may require 10 000 g for 10 min Consider rapid testing (e.g. for *Cryptococcus*)
Body fluids: Amniotic, abdominal, ascites (peritoneal), bile, synovial, pericardial, pleural, empyema	Gram stain	BA, CA, Mac, Ana, Thio		Centrifuge non-purulent samples for 15 min at 2500 rpm
Abscess/wound	Gram stain	BA, CA, Mac; add Ana, and Thio for deep abscess; add CNA if smear indicates		Wash granules; emulsify in saline

(cont.)

Appendix to Part II. (*cont.*)

Specimen	Direct smear	Primary plating	By special request	Comments
Ear	Gram stain	BA, CA, Mac. Add thio for inner ear specimens		
Eye Media should be inoculated directly by practitioner	Gram stain, AO; histological stains (Giemsa) for conjunctiva	BA, CA, Mac, CNA, add Ana for specimens other than conjunctiva		Consider *Chlamydia trachomatis* Viruses and fungi For corneal scrapings also consider *Acanthamoeba* spp.
Female genital tract				
Cervix	Gram stain	BA, CA, TM, Ana, Thio		
Cul-de-sac	Gram stain	BA, CA, Mac,TM, Ana, Thio		
Follicular fluid	Gram stain	BA, CA, Mac, TM, Ana, Thio	*Chlamydia, Mycoplasma*	Testing for viruses recommended
Uterine material (include anaerobic transporter)	Gram stain	BA, CA, Mac, TM, Ana,Thio		
IUCD	Gram stain	BA, CA, Mac, HBT, TM	Thio may be added if actinomycosis is considered	
Urethra (Practitioner may plate directly on JEMBEC system)	Gram stain	B, M, TM, Ana, Thio		Consider: *Chlamydia trachomatis Mycoplasma*
Vagina (Practitioner may plate directly on JEMBEC system)	Gram stain or wet prep for diagnosis of bacterial vaginosis		Selective media for Group B strep in pregnancy	Gram stain for bacterial vaginosis, pH and whiff test also performed for this diagnosis
Male genital tract				
Semen	Gram stain	BA, CA, Mac, TM, CNA	*Chlamydia, Mycoplasma* Sabaroud medium for fungi	Testing for viruses and fungi recommended
Prostatic fluid	Gram stain	BA, CA, Mac, TM, CNA, Thio		
Testis/epididymis	Gram stain	BA, CA, Mac, TM, CNA,		
Urethra	Gram stain	BA, CA, TM		Consider: *Chlamydia Mycoplasma*

Upper respiratory tract

Specimen	Stains	Media	Other	Consider
Throat/pharynx		BA		Consider: *Vincent's angina* *Neisseria gonorrhoea* *Neisseria meningitidis* *Corynebacterium diphtheriae* *Arcanobacterium haemolyticum*
Nasopharynx		BA, CA		Consider: *Bordetella pertussis* *Corynebacterium diphtheriae* *Chlamydia* *Mycoplasma*

Lower respiratory tract

Specimen	Stains	Media	Other	Consider
Sputum, Bronchial secretions, Tracheal aspirate	Gram stain and other stains as indicated	BA, CA, Mac	*Mycoplasma*, mycobacteria	Consider: AFB *Nocardia*
BAL, Bronchial washings	Gram stain and other special stains as requested	BA, CA, Mac,	*Bordetella pertussis*	Consider: AFB CMV *Nocardia* *Mycoplasma* *Pneumocystis carinii*
Epiglottis		BA, CA, CNA		

AFB, acid-fast bacillus; Ana, anaerobic agars; AO, acridine orange; BA, blood agar; BAL, bronchial alveolar lavage; Campy, Campylobacter agar; CA, chocolate agar; CIN, cefsulodin-irgasan-novobiocin; CMV, cytomegalovirus; CNA, Columbia agar with colistin and nalidixic acid; EMB, eosin methylene blue agar; GN, gram-negative broth; HBT, human blood-bilayer Tween agar; HE, Hektoen agar; JEMBEC, self-contained CO_2 system with modified Thayer–Martin agar for cultivation of *Neisseria gonorrhoeae*; Mac, MacConkey agar; TCBS, thiosulfate citrate-bile salts; Thio, Thioglycollate broth; TM, Thayer–Martin agar; XLD, xylose lysine desoxycholate.

Table modified from *Bailey & Scott's Diagnostic Microbiology*, 11th edition, Mosby Publishers, St Louis, MO 2002.

Part III

Infection and the assisted reproductive laboratory

Life is short, art (ART) is so long to learn;
opportunity is elusive,
experience is perilous,
judgment is difficult . . .

Hippocrates, Father of Medicine, *c.* 460–377 BC

Infection and contamination control in the ART laboratory

Infection occurs when a susceptible part of the human body is exposed to a microorganism; this exposure may, or may not, lead to disease. Only the body, never the environment, is infected. Contamination may refer to the body (e.g. a wound can be contaminated), or to the working environment. Contamination occurs in the laboratory setting when a microorganism comes into contact with aseptic or sterile materials or supplies being handled or manipulated: contamination with environmental organisms has a negative impact on embryo culture. Gametes or embryos may be contaminated by exposure to organisms in the environment, exposure to pathogens found in body fluids of patients undergoing treatment, or from microorganisms carried by ART staff. When gametes or embryos are exposed to pathogenic organisms, there is the potential to transmit disease to several targets, including the developing embryo, the couple undergoing ART treatment, neighbouring gametes and embryos and subsequently other couples undergoing ART treatment, as well as ART health-care personnel. This unique situation, with multiple targets for contamination and infection, make infection and contamination control crucial in the ART laboratory.

Tissue culture systems used in the ART laboratory are designed to provide a physiological environment that can support and sustain cell metabolism and division, making them an ideal medium for the replication of a variety of microorganisms. These microorganisms can not only thrive and destroy the survival potential of gametes and embryos, but also act as a potential source for transfer of 'foreign' genetic material to the gametes and embryos (Chan *et al.*, 2000). An awareness of the potential sources of infection can help to avoid and eliminate contamination.

Sources of infection

Contaminants can be introduced into a tissue culture system from a variety of different sources:
- patients;
- specimens: blood, serum (e.g. maternal serum used for culture) follicular aspirates, oocytes, semen, embryos, testicular tissue, ovarian tissue;
- staff;
- supplies: water, media, oil, serum, disposables;
- environment: air, gas mixtures, air conditioning/heating systems, walls, floor, instruments, equipment, storage tanks.

The types of contaminants can include a wide range of microbes, described in the first two sections of this book. Those of major concern are summarized in Table 13.1.

Tables 13.2a, 13.2b, 13.2c and 13.2d outline potential sources of infection in an assisted reproduction practice.

Asepsis in all aspects of clinical and laboratory work is extremely important, with the primary objective of excluding all possible pathogens from every potential source as well as preventing the transmission of any that might be introduced. All human tissue should be considered as potentially infectious:

Table 13.1. Medically important organisms in reproduction

Organism	Infection/symptoms	Modes of transmission	Preferred diagnostic testing	Prophylaxis /treatment
HIV	Acute HIV infection often progressing to AIDS	STD Blood transfusion Needle stick exposures Shared needles in IVDA Vertical transmission to fetus in the perinatal period Breast milk	EIA to screen for serum antibodies Western blot to confirm all positives HIV viral load to evaluate response to therapy HIV genotype to evaluate drug resistance	Multi-drug HAART therapy (highly active antiretroviral therapy)
HCV	Chronic hepatitis leading to cirrhosis and occasionally hepatocellular carcinoma	Shared needles in IVDA Blood transfusions Possibly an STD Needle stick exposure Large proportion unknown transmission	EIA to screen for serum antibodies PCR to confirm persistence of infection in all EIA positive patients	Pegylated interferon has been shown to provide sustained viral suppression
HBV	Acute hepatitis with recovery Carrier state Chronic hepatitis with progressive liver damage leading to cirrhosis and possibly hepatocellular carcinoma Highest rate of chronic infection seen following infections acquired at birth or in early childhood	STD Blood transfusion Needle stick exposures Shared needles in IVDA Vertical transmission to child at birth	Screening for HbsAg and antibodies to HBcAg and HBsAg	Vaccination for prevention Alpha-interferon or lamivudine may be used to treat chronic infections Hepatitis B immune globulin and vaccine may be administered for post-exposure prophylaxis
CMV	Majority of infections are asymptomatic, especially in childhood Mononucleosis-like syndrome Opportunistic infections in immunocompromised (pneumonitis, hepatitis, cerebritis, keratitis, etc.) Congenital infections leading to fetal death, eye and brain defects most common	Transmitted in contaminated: oral secretions urine genital secretions Vertical transmission to fetus transplacentally, usually when mother has an acute infection	EIA to screen for serum antibodies PCR or Antigenaemia assay to detect current viremia Culture of semen to detect genital shedding	Gangcyclovir to treat reactivation disease or acute infection in the immunocompromised host

	Clinical features	Transmission	Diagnosis	Treatment
HSV	Asymptomatic infection or shedding Primary or recurrent Vesicular lesions rupture to form shallow painful ulcers HSV-2 most often associated with genital ulcer disease HSV-1 most often seen in non-genital locations (mouth, hands, face etc.) Neonatal HSV infection Hepatitis and pneumonitis seen in immunocompromised hosts	HSV-1 is usually transmitted during childhood via contaminated oral secretions May be fomite transmitted HSV-1 and HSV-2 may be transmitted as STDs in infected genital secretions including semen Vertical transmission occurs at the time of birth when the baby is exposed to infected genital secretions	EIA or RIBA to detect HSV-2 antibodies Viral culture on fibroblast cells to detect virus in genital lesions	Suppressive oral acyclovir, famciclovir or valacyclovir may diminish the frequency, severity and duration of reactivations
HTLV-I and II	Asymptomatic (most cases) May cause T-cell leukemia/lymphomas in humans HTLV-associated myelopathy/tropical spastic paraparesis (HAM/TSP) HTLV-associated uveitis HTLV-associated infective dermatitis HTLV-associated arthropathy	Sexual contact Vertical transmission Blood transfusion Transmission through shared needles in IVDA	EIA to screen for serum antibodies Western blot to confirm all positives	None
HGV	No identified syndrome with this virus	Possibly an STD, high seroprevalence rates seen in prostitutes	EIA to screen for antibodies is available experimentally	None
HPV	Warts (genital and non-genital) High risk HPV serovars may lead to the development of cervical, vaginal, labial, and penile squamous cell carcinomas HPV 6,11 are associated with the development of laryngeal polyps	Direct contact STD (genital HPV serovars) Via fomites Vertical transmission to baby at birth	PAP smears to detect cellular atypia Molecular testing to detect high-risk (cancer-associated) HPV serovars	Cryotherapy to remove exophytic warts TCA or BCA 80–90% applied weekly to vaginal, cervical, or anal warts Podophyllin 10–25% in tincture of benzoin applied to urethral meatus warts Surgical removal may be required
Treponema pallidum	Primary syphilis – chancre (ulcer) Secondary syphilis – generalized rash characteristic of disseminated disease Tertiary syphilis – gummatous lesions form in any organs Lesions in the CNS lead to neurologic manifestations	STD Transplacental Direct contact with infected lesions Blood transfusion (non-refrigerated components only)	RPR to screen for antibodies Treponemal assay (FTA or TPPA) to confirm all positives Dark-field exam of ulcerative lesions or Steiner stained tissue to detect organisms during primary infection	Benzathine Penicillin G 2.4 million units IM in a single dose (Dosage and duration of treatment may depend upon the stage of illness)

(cont.)

Table 13.1. (*cont.*)

Organism	Infection/symptoms	Modes of transmission	Preferred diagnostic testing	Prophylaxis/treatment
Neisseria gonorrhoeae	Urethritis Cervicitis PID Eye infections (in the neonate) Disseminated disease associated with rash and joint infections	STD Vertical transmission to neonate at birth Human is the only reservoir	Urethral or cervical swabs or first void urine amplified molecular diagnosis (PCR and other amplified assays) Culture is not recommended at this time due to low sensitivity	Treatment for uncomplicated genital infection: Cefixime 400 mg orally in a single dose or Ceftriaxone 125 mg IM in a single dose or Ciprofloxacin 500 mg orally in a single dose or Ofloxacin 400 mg orally in a single dose or Levofloxacin 250 mg orally in a single dose **Note: if treating empirically, patients should be treated for both CT and GC** Treatment during pregnancy or for non-genital infections require special treatment regimens
Chlamydia trachomatis	Cervicits Urethritis PID Neonatal infections Associated with involuntary infertility	STD Vertical transmission to neonate at birth	Urethral or cervical swabs or first void urine amplified molecular diagnosis (PCR, LCX, and other amplified assays) Culture and serology are not recommended at this time due to low sensitivity	Treatment for uncomplicated genital infection: Azithromycin 1 gram orally in a single dose or Doxycycline 100 mg orally twice a day for 7 days **Note: if treating empirically, patients should be treated for both CT and GC** Treatment during pregnancy or for non-genital infections require special treatment regimens

Organism	Clinical features / epidemiology	Transmission / source	Laboratory diagnosis	Treatment
Mycoplasma hominis	Normal flora of the vagina; Bacterial vaginosis; Rarely implicated in PID; Causes post-partum sepsis; Vertical intrauterine transmission to the fetus may result in early abortions or still born infants; Infections in pregnancy are associated with premature rupture of the membranes; Infection in the newborn (pneumonia, sepsis, CNS infections)	Normal flora; ?STD; Vertical transmission to fetus and neonate	Culture in SP-4 broth with arginine; Growth on solid medium A7 or A8 under anaerobic conditions produces colonies with a 'fried egg' morphology	Since the genital mycoplasmas are often found in association with CT and GC and anaerobes, empiric treatments should cover these organisms. Cefoxitin and doxycycline or clindamycin and gentamycin are often used in treatments. *M. hominis* is also susceptible to tetracycline
Ureaplasma urea-lyticum	Normal flora of the vagina; Urethritis in males; Causes post-partum sepsis; Vertical intrauterine transmission to the fetus may result in early abortions or still-born infants; Infections in pregnancy are associated with premature rupture of the membranes; Infection in the newborn (pneumonia, sepsis, CNS infections)	?STD; Vertical transmission to fetus and neonate	Culture in A7 broth with urea; Growth on solid medium with Mg^{2+} salts produce small pigmented colonies	See comment for *M. hominis*. Of *U. urealyticum* isolates, 10% are resistant to tetracycline and many of these strains are also resistant to erythromycin.
Anaerobes	Normal flora of the vagina and distal urethra; May overgrow in bacterial vaginosis; May cause PID	Normal flora; Ascending infections are of endogenous origin	Usually not cultured from genital sites unless the specimen is invasively obtained, and not collected transvaginally	See comment for *M. hominis*
Candida spp.	Present on the mucous membrane of the vagina, mouth or the intestinal tract as normal flora, and can invade the tissue; Causes vaginal and oral 'thrush' infections, and opportunistic infection in the immunocompromised.	Overgrows in diabetics causing lesions or when the normal vaginal bacterial flora is destroyed by broad spectrum antibiotics. Transmitted to the newborn through the birth canal	Microscopic identification of the hyphae and yeast cells in the vaginal smears or scrapings of the lesions; Diagnosis is confirmed by culture	Polyene antibiotics are effective, as well as local application of antifungals such as nystatin

Table 13.2a. Sources of infection in ART

Source of infection	Mode of transmission	Original Source	Organisms most likely to be encountered	Comments	Precautions
Semen Male partner or donor	Insemination	GU tract flora	Corynebacteria, Anaerobes, Lactobacillus, Non-hemolytic streptococci, Neisseria species	Additional organisms seen on uncircumcised penis: Mycobacterium smegmatis	Correct collection of semen. Process semen to reduce commensal organisms and selected pathogens. Use of antibiotics in media. Patient and donor testing
		Skin / urethral flora	Staphylococcus spp.	Gram-positive organisms	
		Fecal contamination	Enterobacteriaceae – E. coli, Klebsiella, Pseudomonas Enterococci/Grp B streptococci, E. faecalis		
		STDs/genital tract pathogens	HSV, HPV, Chlamydia trachomatis, Mycoplasma spp., Ureaplasma urealyticum, Trichomonas vaginalis, CMV, Neisseria gonorrhoeae; HBV	Homosexual males also may harbour Giardia lamblia, Entamoeba histolytica, Cryptosporidium, Microsporidium, Salmonella, Shigella, Campylobacter spp., Neisseria meningitides, CMV, Hepatitis A, B, C, E, HTLV and HIV	**Note: Although careful screening, washing, cryopreservation and quarantine of semen should prevent or minimize chance of transmitting infection, virtually all microbes will survive cryopreservation**
			Treponema pallidum, Haemophilus ducreyi and Calymmatobacterium granulomatis are rare; lice and scabies are also rare.		
			Rarely, Adenovirus and Coxsackie viruses may be genital tract pathogens		

Transmission of the following organisms by donor semen has been documented:

Neisseria gonorrhoea, Chlamydia trachomatis, Ureaplasma urealyticum, Mycoplasma hominis
Streptococcus species (Group B)
Trichomonas vaginalis
HIV, HSV-2, HBV

The following organisms have been detected in semen, but no cases have been reported from AI-related transmission

HPV
Transfusion transmitted (TT) virus
CMV, HCV, HSV-1

Table 13.2b. Sources of infection in ART

Source of infection	Mode of transmission	Original Source	Organisms most likely to be encountered	Comments	Precautions
Oocytes: Female Partner or Oocyte Donor • GU tract • Blood • Follicular fluid	Transvaginal oocyte retrieval	GU tract flora	Coagulase-negative staphylococci *Corynebacteria* Non-hemolytic streptococci *Neisseria* species *Enterobacteriaceae* species *Staphylococcus* species Anaerobes, including *Lactobacillus* Non-spore-forming anaerobes, *Clostridium* spp., Anaerobic cocci	May have yeast present as transient flora May carry Group B streptococci	Rinse vagina with normal saline Clean oocytes after retrieval in culture medium containing antibiotics to dilute contaminating organisms and minimize contamination. Patient testing
		Fecal contamination	*Enterobacteriaceae* *Enterococci*, Grp B Strep		**Note: Rinsing the vagina with antiseptics is not recommended since disinfectants may be embryotoxic.**
		Blood	HIV, CMV, hepatitis		
		Follicular fluid	Commensals		
		STDs/genital tract pathogens	HSV, HPV, *Chlamydia trachomatis*, *Mycoplasma* spp., *Ureaplasma urealyticum*, *Trichomonas vaginalis*, CMV, *Neisseria gonorrhoeae*; *Gardnerella vaginalis*, *Mobiluncus* species *Treponema pallidum*, *Haemophilus ducreyi* and *Calymmatobacterium granulomatis* are rare; lice and scabies are also rare. Rarely, Adenovirus and Coxsackie viruses may be genital tract pathogens	Females are often asymptomatic for STDs	

Table 13.2c. Sources of infection in ART

Source of infection	Mode of transmission	Original Source	Organisms most likely to be encountered	Comments	Precautions
Embryos: fresh or donated	Insemination Culture Transfer If frozen, from cryo-preservation media	From semen or follicular fluid, or from laboratory/operating room contamination. Contaminated culture media	Potentially any encountered from the following sources: • Semen • Follicular fluid • Environment • Contamination during embryo culture • If stored, contamination from cryo processing and storage	Washing oocytes and processing semen will diminish selected commensals or pathogens in semen or follicular fluid, but embryos may be contaminated during embryo culture and transfer. If stored, contamination can occur during freezing/thawing processes and during storage.	Adhere strictly to aseptic technique Periodic testing of incubators and workstation to minimize contamination of media and environment

Table 13.2d. Sources of infection in ART

Source of infection	Mode of transmission	Original source	Organisms most likely to be encountered	Comments	Precautions
Staff: Operating room and laboratory Skin Nares	General physical contact	Skin Nares	Coagulase-negative or coagulase-positive staphylococci	Some individuals harbour coagulase-positive *Staphylococcus aureus* in the nares	Aseptic technique Proper attire
		Fecal	Corynebacteria Fecal coliforms		
Laboratory: Atmosphere Inside lab Inside/Outside lab	Physical lab (counter tops, floors, ceilings, walls) Lab equipment Air conditioning (AC) Heating	Contamination of physical area Contamination in AC ducts and ventilation systems	Spore-forming bacillus species Fungal spores, esp. *Aspergillus* species, zygomycetes or other saprophytic moulds		Limit of spread may be accomplished by use of: Positive pressure in embryo culture lab Filtration units (carbon, high efficiency particulate art (HEPA) Sterilization (UV) and chemical methods Proper room ventilation Filtration system in each incubator (HEPA, CODA) Appropriate biological safety cabinets for sterile storage and processing Proper attire in the laboratory Restrict entry of the number of personnel into the laboratory
Laboratory: Materials and Supplies	Collection media Insemination media Culture media Transfer media Manipulation of gametes and embryos Freezing and thawing media	Contamination: Water Commercial media In-house prepared media Lab supplies Oil	Bacteria Fungi Prions	Water may contain organics and pyrogens It is possible to cross-contaminate cultures among patients	Add antibiotics to media Use screened/tested serum supplements Use highly purified water QC programme for water made on-site Test for endotoxin

(cont.)

Table 13.2d. (cont.)

Source of infection	Mode of transmission	Original source	Organisms most likely to be encountered	Comments	Precautions
					Properly sterilize all containers and solutions Use disposable equipment when possible Heat sterilize glassware and plastic pipette tips, etc. Refrigerate media at 4 °C Use sterile technique Exercise Standard Precautions
Operating room: • **Atmosphere**	Air conditioning Heating Physical facility (floors, ceiling, walls, cabinets) OR equipment	Contamination of physical area	Spore-forming bacteria Fungi Fungal spores		Positive pressure to the rest of the institution will minimize contamination.
Operating room: • **Materials and supplies**	Oocyte retrieval Embryo transfer Sperm retrieval (testicular specimens)	Surgical instruments Surgical materials (bandages) Saline Flushing media	Fungi Fungal spores Spore-forming bacteria	Bandages containing spores are common sites of nosocomial infections	Quality control program Use of disposables
Cryostorage tanks and equipment	Transfer of frozen gametes or embryos to patients	Contaminated liquid nitrogen Contaminated or leaking straws/containers, Mixing of specimens in tanks	HBV, possibly HIV and HCV; cases of HBV transmitted via cryo tanks for bone marrow transplants have been reported. The risk is decreased if the cells are in the vapour phase and not in liquid nitrogen	Organisms survive in tanks Quarantine tanks for all unscreened samples Possible medico-legal issues	Observe Standard Precautions Exercise aseptic technique Screen all patients, donors and recipients Separate storage vs. cohorting tanks Process specimens to minimize transfer of organisms Improved containers for freezing Test all donors/recipients before treatment Improved use of antibiotics in media? Vapour phase freezing?

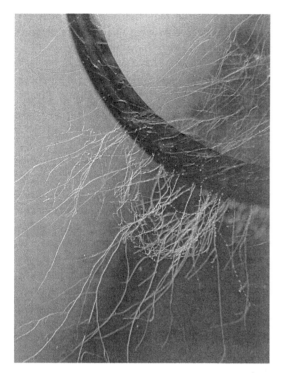

Fig. 13.1. Fungal contamination in an embryo culture dish. Filamentous processes can be seen extending around a drop of culture medium under oil. When viewed by the naked eye, these tufts of hyphae appear as fluffy clumps floating in the culture medium or adhering to the cellular element in culture. The most common fungi causing laboratory contamination are the *Aspergillus* spp., as well as other moulds described in Table 13.3 and Fig. 13.5.

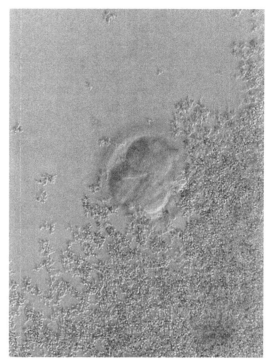

Fig. 13.2. Embryo culture dish with yeast contamination. *Candida* spp. are the most common yeasts to contaminate laboratory cultures. These may present as blastoconidia (budding yeast) as seen in this image, or may form tertiary filamentous structures with pinched off septations, called pseudohyphae. Both forms are often seen in culture simultaneously.

a stringent infection control policy is mandatory in every ART unit, with all staff members suitably trained. A poor standard of hygiene, cleaning and waste disposal results in a much higher risk that infection may be transmitted to patients, staff, gametes, embryos, and contaminate equipment (e.g. incubators), and therefore the policy must clearly specify details including aspects of hygiene, labelling, protective clothing, laundry, safe handling of sharps and specimens, disposal of clinical waste and decontamination procedures. General laboratory rules for safety should also (i) prohibit mouth pipetting, smoking, eating or drinking and application of cosmetics, (ii) mandate that hair, beards and jewellery be worn so as to avoid contamination or tangling into equipment, (iii) require an adequate number of eyewash stations and emergency showers and (iv) include an effective exposure response plan to manage employees who have been exposed to potential blood-borne pathogens. All procedures and manipulations must be carried out with a rigorous discipline of aseptic technique. Figures 13.1, 13.2, and 13.3 illustrate typical examples of IVF laboratory contamination that may result from even minor breaches in sterile technique.

Sterilization refers to the use of physical or chemical agents for the complete and absolute removal of all living organisms: bacteria, viruses, fungi and including spores of either fungi or bacteria.

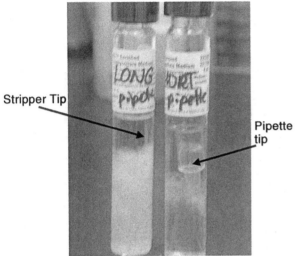

Stripper Tip

Pipette tip

Coagulase negative Staphylococcus

Fig. 13.3. Following an episode of bacterial contamination in an IVF culture, tips of a Pasteur pipette and a 'stripper' were cultured by inoculating them into Enriched Thyoglycollate broth medium. *Staphylococcus* spp., which is what is seen growing in these specimens, are amongst the most common contaminants of liquid culture systems. These organisms are common skin flora and may be introduced into cultures by inadequate sterile technique or poor sterilization of tools, dishes or media. Other bacteria often found to contaminate cell culture systems include *Pseudomonas* spp. and other non-fermentative Gram-negative rods that are found in water supplies such as incubator pans and water baths. Gram-positive rods such as *Bacillus* spp. are also frequently seen.

Disinfection generally refers to the use of chemical agents in order to destroy potential infectivity of a material. The process may reduce the number of pathogenic organisms, but does not destroy them all – spores and some microbes may survive disinfection procedures. The term usually applies to the treatment of fomites (inanimate objects).

Antisepsis refers to the topical application of chemical agents to body surfaces to kill or inhibit pathogenic microbes. An antiseptic is a disinfectant used on living tissue (instruments are disinfected).

Sanitization refers to reduction of the microbial population to a safe level as determined by Public Health agencies, but does not remove all pathogens.

Decontamination refers to the use of any of the above techniques to eliminate microorganisms already present.

Sterilization methods

Sterilizing and disinfecting methods can be physical or chemical, and the methods available must be assessed not only as to their suitability and effectiveness for the material to be treated, but also in terms of potential toxicity to gametes and embryos that may come into contact with the sterilized material. When purchasing sterile supplies, it is prudent to be aware of what method has been used in the sterilization process, and to take precautions such as off-gassing or rinsing to ensure that no residue is left that may be toxic to gametes or embryos.

Sterilization methods can be:

(i) physical: heat (dry and moist), radiation (ionizing – gamma rays and ultraviolet rays);

(ii) mechanical: filtration, ultrasonic and sonic waves;

(iii) chemical agents: alcohols, aldehyes, phenols, ethylene oxide, cationic detergents, chlorinated compounds and oxidants.

Physical methods of sterilization

Heat

Heat is the most effective method of sterilization and is the preferred method for all heat-stable material. Disposable supplies used in the IVF laboratory and media that contain protein (serum or albumin) or other labile factors cannot be heat sterilized. All microorganisms are susceptible to heat; the sensitivity of an organism to destruction by heat is expressed as the 'thermal death point', the lowest temperature at which an exposure of 10 minutes results in destruction of a given culture of microbes: *E. coli* is destroyed at 55 °C, tubercle bacilli at 60 °C and highly resistant fungal and bacterial spores at 120 °C. Steam (moist heat) can reach and penetrate clumps, which cannot always be reached by other methods of sterilization such as chemical agents. However, for effective heat sterilization, it is important that appropriate conditions are applied: the material to be sterilized should be exposed at the appropriate temperature and for an appropriate duration of time. For example, reliable sterilization of spores requires dry heat of 160 °C for 1 to 2 hours. Higher temperatures are required when the material used is thoroughly dried or, in the case of liquids, when the boiling point of the medium is reduced by the presence of high concentrations of glycerol or glucose.

Heat sterilization can be achieved by dry heat or moist heat (steam under pressure). Moist heat has a superior penetration power and requires a shorter duration of time than dry heat for sterilization; for example, the centre of a large package of surgical dressings may not reach 100 °C after an hour in the oven at 160 °C, whereas steam can rapidly penetrate the package. The rapid action of steam is due to the large latent heat of water, so that even cold surfaces are rapidly heated because of surface condensation. Because moist heat requires a lower temperature than is necessary for dry heat, moist heat has the additional advantage of causing less potential damage to material being sterilized.

Different techniques for heat sterilization include:

Incineration

Hazardous material is burned at temperatures of 870 °C to 980 °C. This method is used only for the elimination of hazardous waste, and its use is limited in some urban areas because toxic gases are emitted and the ash may contain heavy metals.

Autoclave

Moist heat sterilization under pressure. Saturated steam under a pressure of 1 atmosphere or 15 psi (pounds per square inch) causes denaturation of structural proteins and enzymes, and spores are also killed. This is the fastest and simplest sterilization method, used to sterilize biohazardous waste and heat-stable supplies. When used to sterilize supplies for an IVF programme, the quality of water used in the autoclave is crucial. Steam penetrates to the inner surface of glassware, pipettes, etc., and substances in the water can leave a residue on drying. Any liquid added to this sterilized container or pipette will dissolve the residue, adding potential toxins to the medium. Some hospital Central Sterile Supplies Departments may add wetting agents to the water used for autoclaving, and this will also leave a potentially toxic residue on glassware, etc.

Media, liquids and instruments: autoclave for 15 min at 121 °C

Infectious waste: autoclave for 60 min at 132 °C

A steam pressure of 15 psi at sea level correlates with a temperature of 121 °C. Higher pressures (3 psi higher) are required at high altitudes (5000 feet or more above sea level).

Dry heat

Oven sterilization, 160–180 °C for 1.5 to 3 hours oxidizes large molecules and kills spores. Dry heat at 180 °C for 3 hours also destroys endotoxins. This is used mainly for glassware, and any other items stable at this temperature.

Boiling at 100 °C

Boiling items that are completely submerged in water for 15 min kills vegetative bacteria. Spores can survive boiling for several hours, and this is therefore not a reliable method for sterilization.

Pasteurization

This is *not* a sterilizing process: it involves very rapid heating to 72 °C for 15 seconds or to 63 °C for 30 minutes. Pasteurization lowers the level of microorganisms, killing food pathogens, but does not kill spores or thermoresistant bacteria. This method has been used primarily for milk as most milk-borne pathogens are destroyed without affecting milk proteins. (UHT, 'ultra-high tempera-ture' milk is sterilized by heating at 150 °C for about 2.5 seconds, then storing in sterile containers.)

Radiation

Ionizing radiation

Short wavelength high energy gamma rays form free radicals that destroy proteins and cause single-stranded breaks and mutations in DNA. Spores are generally resistant to destruction by ionizing radia-tion. This method is commonly used for plastics, e.g. embryo culture dishes, disposable pipette tips and other laboratory disposables.

Non-ionizing radiation

Non-ionizing radiation such as ultraviolet (UV) light causes thymidine in DNA to form dimers, affecting DNA replication and transcription. Since microbes can repair the DNA damage caused by UV light, it is not considered to be an effective means of steriliza-tion. UV light is used to disinfect working surfaces in a biological safety cabinet. Ultraviolet rays are of long wavelength and low energy, and therefore the surface must be directly exposed – items in their path (e.g. microscopes, supplies) will create 'shadows' and reduce effectiveness of the process.

Filtration

A cellulose acetate or cellulose nitrate membrane of pore size 0.10–0.45 μm will remove most bacteria, but not viruses or prions. Filtration is used for heat-sensitive materials including media and other salt solutions, antibiotic solutions, carbohydrates, vac-cines, toxic chemicals and radioisotopes. A vacuum line may be used to pull large volumes of liquid through the filter – however, if the solution contains bicarbonate, the use of a vacuum line may cause the bicarbonate to dissociate. Filters typically contain a wetting agent that may be toxic to gametes/embryos: it is therefore important to discard the first portion of the filtrate.

Air is filtered using a high-efficiency-particulate-air (HEPA) filter designed to remove organisms larger than 0.3 μm from biological safety cabinets, operat-ing rooms, isolation rooms and embryology labora-tories.

Ultrasound

High frequency vibrations coagulate cellular pro-teins and disintegrate their components. This is use-ful for cleaning small objects such as needles, Pasteur pipettes, bulbs, etc., but should not be used as a ster-ilizing process.

Chemical methods of sterilization

Chemical methods of sterilization include gases, fumes and vapours, all of which are toxic, are skin irritants, and also may be carcinogenic.

Ethylene oxide (EtO) gas

This is the most common method of chemical steril-ization, used to sterilize heat-sensitive objects such as syringes and catheters used for embryo transfer or intra-uterine insemination. EtO has a lower pen-etration power than steam, and therefore prolonged exposure to this gas is required for effective steril-ization. It is a highly water soluble gas with strong mutagenic properties and toxic residues can remain after the sterilization process. Complete removal of the gas is absolutely essential before the material is brought into contact with tissue culture media or any biological material; off-gassing and rinsing with cul-ture media before use is advisable. Some patients may be allergic to EtO even at very low concentra-tions.

Alcohols

Ethyl and isopropyl alcohols denature proteins and are effective against lipid-containing viruses. They have a very rapid action, evaporate quickly and are used to disinfect skin, thermometers, exterior of bottles and containers, injection vial rubber septa, etc. They are also useful for wiping down laboratory surfaces and equipment, which should be first wiped with water and in some cases an appropriate detergent to remove organic material. A 70% ethanol solution is more effective as a disinfectant than is 95% or absolute alcohol: anthrax spores can survive in 100% alcohol for up to 50 days! Isopropyl alcohol is slightly more potent than ethanol. If it is used as a sterilizing agent, total immersion for at least 20 minutes is required. Alcohol can also be useful as a final wipe to remove residues after a decontamination procedure using a more toxic agent such as hypochlorite. Ethanol is highly flammable and should not be used near an exposed flame.

> Alcohol is known to cause oocyte activation, and sufficient time (ideally overnight) should be allowed for complete evaporation to avoid exposing gametes/embryos to adverse effects.

Aldehydes

Formaldehyde and glutaraldehyde both produce irritant fumes, and are not used as surface disinfectants; they are commonly used to sterilize surgical supplies. These agents act by replacing the labile H atoms on hydroxyl and amide groups that are present in proteins and nucleic acids. The actions of aldehydes are partly reversible, but since they act on nucleic acids it is not advisable to use them in culture rooms where gametes and embryos are to be handled, unless the complete removal of formaldehyde fumes is ensured. Although aldehydes are not inactivated by organic material, instruments and supplies should be cleaned before immersion in a closed container, kept in a well-ventilated area.

Formaldehyde vapour

Formalin (37% formaldehyde gas dissolved in water) is used to sterilize HEPA filters in biological safety cabinets. It is effective, but produces highly irritant fumes, and reacts with chlorine to form an unstable carcinogenic compound.

Glutaraldehyde

Cidex (2% aqueous glutaraldehyde solution) is less of an irritant than formaldehyde, does not corrode lenses, metal, or rubber, and is used to sterilize medical equipment such as endoscopes and anesthetic equipment. It kills bacteria, fungi, spores and some viruses in 3–10 hours. This method is referred to as cold sterilization. It is also a powerful disinfectant in vapour form.

Halogens

Chlorine and iodine rapidly combine with proteins, disrupting disulfide and other peptide bonds. Halogens are effective sporicidal agents.

Chlorine

Chlorine is used in the form of household bleach, sodium hypochlorite (NaOCl) and is also available as tablets of sodium dichloroisocyanourate. A 10% sodium hypochlorite solution can be used for decontaminating bench-tops, and this is recommended for viral decontamination and for decontamination of spills containing blood or human pathogens. However, it is corrosive to stainless steel surfaces and toxic to gametes and embryos. The *WHO Laboratory Manual for Semen Analysis* (1999) recommends that work surfaces in a semen analysis laboratory should be decontaminated with sodium hypochlorite solution on completing analyses each day, as well as after any spillage. If the exterior of the container in which the semen sample is collected is contaminated, it should also be wiped with the sodium hypochlorite solution.

Iodine

Iodine is prepared either as a tincture with alcohol, or as an iodophore coupled to a neutral polymer (i.e. povidone-iodine). Two percent iodine solutions in alcohol (Betadine, Wescodyne) are effective against all microorganisms, and are commonly used to disinfect skin. They are more effective than bleach against bacteria and spores, but do cause staining, are corrosive to instruments and can be highly irritant to some individuals. Their residual activity is approximately 4 hours.

Phenols

Derivatives of carbolic acid (phenol) precipitate nucleic acids, denature proteins and also cause cell lysis. They have a wide spectrum of activity, are not inactivated by organic material, but are corrosive and toxic with a residual activity of around 6 hours. Products containing added detergent clean and disinfect at the same time.

- Cresols: Lysol, Staphen
- Hexachlorophene (PhisoHex)
- Chlorhexidine (Hibitane, Hibiclens) – is commonly used as an antiseptic in the operating room and other clinical areas because of its low toxicity.
- Phenol-containing soaps or disinfectant solutions such as PhisoHex or Hibiclens are often used to wash hands prior to starting work in a culture laboratory.

Hydrogen peroxide and peroxyacetic acid (peracetic acid)

Oxidizing agents that are widely used as general disinfectants because of their reactive properties. Bacteria vary in their susceptibility, since some (e.g. staphylococci, bacilli) organisms possess catalase, which can denature hydrogen peroxide. Solutions of 3 to 10% hydrogen peroxide may be used for initial soaking of instruments with an internal channel and for cleaning incubators. Peracetic acid is toxic.

Disinfection and decontamination

Quaternary ammonium compounds are cationic detergents with powerful surface-active properties, used for cleaning laboratory surfaces (bench-tops). They are inexpensive, non-corrosive and non-staining, but may be inactivated by organic materials such as blood and anionic detergents and are not recommended as general disinfectants. Blood and spills of other biological material on the

work surface should first be wiped with water before using these detergents as cleaning agents.

Detergents such as trisodium phosphate (TSP) and '7X' (Sigma, ICN) are useful laboratory detergents: they are non-toxic, effective and useful for general cleaning in an ART laboratory. A number of different quaternary ammonium and phosphate preparations are available commercially under different trade names (Roccal, Detergem, Deconex, Labolene, Barricidal, Germekil, etc.), each with a different spectrum of activity and residual activity. It is advisable to obtain specific information from the manufacturer before using any chemical agent in the IVF laboratory.

The same chemical agent may be used to sterilize or to disinfect, depending on the concentration used and duration of exposure time. When all life is destroyed, the agent is referred to as a *biocide*; a disinfectant used on living tissue is an *antiseptic*. Several factors influence the activity of disinfectants, including:

- type of organisms present: spores are the most resistant and lipid enveloped viruses (e.g. *Herpes simplex*) are most susceptible;
- temperature and pH of the process;
- microbial load (number of organisms present);
- concentration of disinfectant;
- amount of organic material present, i.e. blood, mucus, semen, follicular fluid;
- nature of surface to be disinfected: porous or nonporous, potential for corrosion;
- length of contact time;
- water quality: hard water may reduce the rate of microbial killing.

When selecting disinfectants for a particular purpose, consideration should ideally include a number of parameters such as:

- spectrum of activity;
- rapid and irreversible effect;
- stability against certain physical agents;
- no deleterious effect on equipment;
- ease of use;
- lack of toxicity to humans;
- lack of residual irritant odour;
- biodegradability;

- how long a residue may remain in the environment, since most chemical disinfectants have a toxic effect on gametes and embryos.

For virus decontamination

- Formaldehyde alters the genome structure and inactivates virus.
- Phenol reacts with protein capsids, inactivating the virus.
- Lipid solvents and detergents react with viral envelopes (if present).

10% sodium hypochlorite is recommended for decontamination of biological wastes and laboratory surfaces. It is effective against viruses.

Prions

Prions are not affected by agents that destroy nucleic acids or by lipid solvents; the prion protein is extremely heat resistant and autoclaving at 134–138 °C for 60 minutes does not inactivate it completely. The prion protein also remains infective after sterilizing levels of radiation, exposure to strong acids, non-polar organic solvents, incineration at 343–360 °C and passage through 0.1 μm filters. The WHO recommends a combination of strategies aimed towards protein destruction for prion decontamination:

1. Soak in 1N NaOH, 1 hr, 20 °C
2. Soak in 12.5% bleach, 1 hr, 20 °C
3. Steam sterilization, 134–138°C, 18 mins.

Resistant surfaces, such as bench-tops and floors, should be flooded with a 2N NaOH solution or with undiluted sodium hypochlorite. The liquid should remain for 1 hour or longer before mopping and rinsing, and the NaOH or bleach should be disposed of as hazardous waste. The possible sources of prion contamination are discussed in Chapter 5; although the chances of high-risk material entering a routine human IVF laboratory are apparently very low, there is always a potential risk when medical devices are re-used. Universal precautions of asepsis and hygiene are essential in all animal research facilities, as well as in anatomy or pathology laboratories.

Air quality, classification of cleanrooms and biological safety cabinets

The requirements for a clean environment depend upon the nature of the work being carried out, and differ in different industries such as aerospace, food, pharmaceuticals, medical devices, research and healthcare. Air cleanliness is classified according to the number and size of particles within a sample of air, measured in particles per cubic foot or cubic metre of air. The United States Federal Standard 20E and the British Standard 5295 both define terms, identify procedures for collecting and testing the air, and provide statistical analysis required to interpret the data. The British Standard has been superseded by an international standard, BS EN ISO 14644-1 from the International Standards Organization in Switzerland.

The environment in a cleanroom is produced by incorporating parallel streams of HEPA filtered air (laminar flow) that blow across the room, moving at a uniform velocity of 0.3 to 0.45 metres per second, to expel any dust and particles in the airflow by the shortest route. The air velocity must be at a sufficiently high level to ensure that particles do not thermally migrate from the laminar flow. The airflow can be either vertical downflow (entering via filters in the roof, exiting through vents in the floor) or horizontal crossflow (entering through filters in one sidewall and exhausted above the floor in the sidewall opposite and/or recirculated via a bank of filters). The US Federal Standard 209E defines air quality based upon the maximum allowable number of particles 0.5 microns and larger per cubic foot of air: Class 1, 100, 1000, 10 000 and 100 000. The lower the number, the cleaner the air. The ISO classifications are defined as ISO Class 1, 2, 3, 4, etc. through to Class 9. The cleanest, ultra-pure air is Class 1. ISO Class 2 correlates most closely to Federal Standard Class 100 (a summary of detailed technical specifications for both sets of standards can be found at: www.moorfield.co.uk). Class 1/Class 10 are used for semiconductor production in the electronics industry, and Class 2/Class 100 for pharmaceutical production and biological safety cabinets. Drug preparation areas and hospital operating room facilities have Class 5/100 000 or below. New cell culture CO_2 incubators are now available that are equipped with a HEPA filter airflow system that continuously filters the entire chamber volume every 60 seconds, providing Class 100 air quality within 5 minutes of closing the incubator door (www.thermoforma.com, www.shellab.com). These incubators also incorporate a sterilization cycle (Steri-Cycle™), and can be supplied with an additional ceramic filter that excludes volatile low molecular weight organic and inorganic molecules, volatile organic carbon (VOCs). VOCs can arise from a variety of sources both within and outside the laboratory; they are not excluded by HEPA filtration, and can be a potential source of toxicity to gametes and embryos. A number of active filtration units with activated carbon filters and oxidizing material have now been developed specifically for IVF laboratories, to be placed either inside cell culture incubators, or free-standing in the laboratory space itself (Cohen *et al.*, 1997; Boone *et al.*, 1999, www.conception.technologies.com).

Biological safety cabinets (BSCs)

A biological safety cabinet or BSC is an enclosed workspace that provides protection either to workers, the products being handled, or both. BSCs provide protection from infectious disease agents, by sterilizing the air that is exposed to infectious agents. The air may be sterilized by ultraviolet light, heat or passage through a HEPA filter that removes particles larger than 0.3 μm in diameter. BSCs are designated by class based on the degree of hazard containment (see Table 14.1), and the type of protection that they provide. In order to ensure maximum effectiveness, certain specifications must be met.

(i) Whenever possible, a 12-inch clearance should be provided behind, and on each side of, the cabinet, to ensure effective air return to the laboratory. This also allows easy acess for maintenance

(ii) The cabinet should have a 12- to 14-inch clearance above it, for exhaust filter changes.

(iii) The operational integrity of a new BSC should be validated by certification before it is put into service, after it has been repaired or relocated, and annually thereafter.

(iv) All containers and equipment should be surface decontaminated and removed from the cabinet when the work is completed. The work surface, cabinet sides and back, and interior of the glass should be wiped down (70% ethanol is an effective disinfectant) at the end of each day.

(v) The cabinet should be allowed to run for 5 minutes after materials are brought in or removed.

BSC classes

Class I

Class I provides personnel and environmental protection, but no product protection. Cabinets have open front, negative pressure and are ventilated. Non-sterile room air enters and circulates through the cabinet, and the environment is protected by filtering exhaust air through a 0.3 μm HEPA filter (Fig. 13.4(*a*)). The inward air flow protects personnel as long as a minimum velocity of 75 linear feet per minute (l fpm) is maintained through the front opening. This type of cabinet is useful to enclose equipment or procedures that have a potential to generate aerosols (centrifuges, homogenizing tissues, cage dumping), and can be used for work involving Level 2 and Level 3 agents or those that are moderate to high risk.

Class II

Class II provides product, personnel and environment protection, using a stream of unidirectional air moving at a steady velocity along parallel lines ('laminar flow'). The laminar flow, together with HEPA filtration captures and removes airborne contaminants and provides a particulate-free work environment. Airflow is drawn around the operator into the front grille of the cabinet, providing personnel protection, and a downward flow of HEPA filtered air minimizes the chance of cross-contamination along the work surface. Exhaust air is HEPA filtered

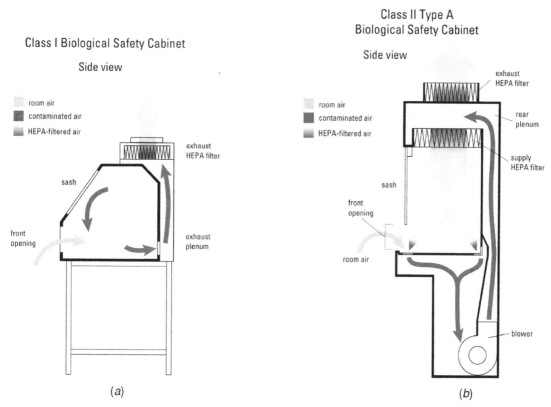

Fig. 13.4(a). Class I biological safety cabinet. Unsterilized room air passes into the cabinet and around the material within the cabinet. Air to be exhausted is passed through a HEPA filter that removes particles larger than 0.3 μm in diameter. Only the air to be exhausted is sterilized. (b). Class II biological safety cabinet. Air flows in sheets (*laminar flow*), acting as a barrier to particles outside the cabinet area and directing the flow of contaminated air into the HEPA filters. Air that enters the cabinet and flows over the infectious material, as well as the air to be exhausted is sterilized. A class II A cabinet is self-contained with ∼ 70% of the air recirculated. The exhaust air in class IIB cabinets is discharged outside the building.

to protect the environment, and may be recirculated back into the laboratory (Type A) or ducted out of the building (Type B). Class II cabinets provide a microbe-free environment for cell culture propagation, and are designed for work involving microorganisms in biosafety levels 2 and 3 or those that are moderate to high risk (Fig. 13.4(b)). They can be modified to accommodate microscopes, centrifuges or other equipment, but the modification should be tested and certified to ensure that the basic systems operate properly after modification. No material should be placed on front or rear grille openings, and laboratory doors should be kept closed during use to ensure adequate airflow within the cabinet.

Class II Type A cabinet is self-contained with a fixed opening. An internal blower draws room air through a HEPA filter in the front grille. The laminar flow air 'splits' as it approaches the work surface, so that approximately 70% of the air is recirculated through the supply HEPA filter back into the work zone, and 30% passes through the exhaust HEPA filter. This type of BSC is recommended for embryo culture procedures.

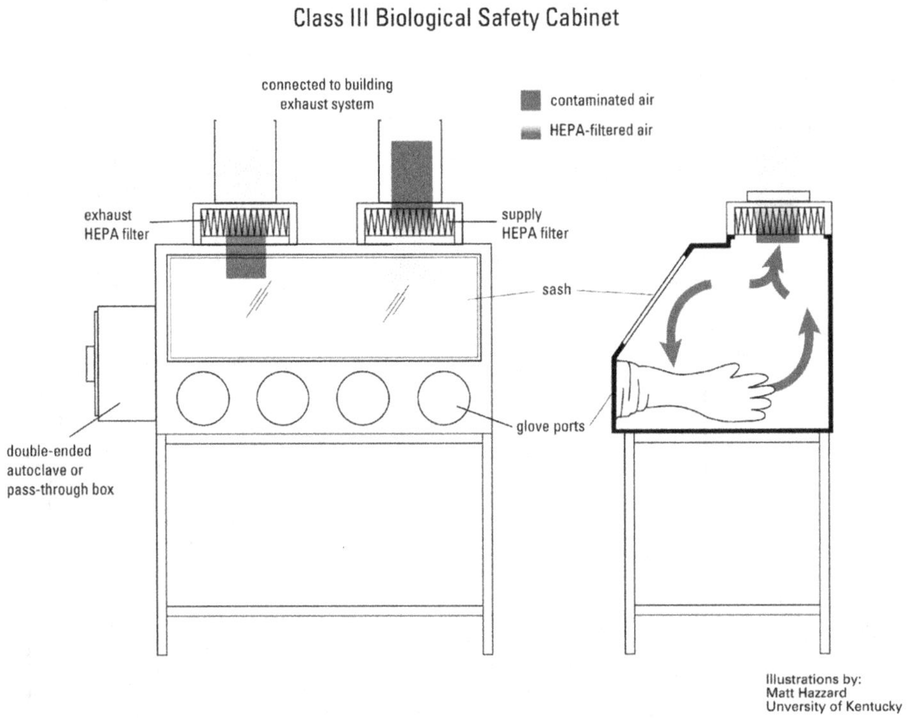

Class III Biological Safety Cabinet

(c)

Fig. 13.4(c). Class III biological safety cabinet. Cabinets are completely enclosed with negative pressure ventilation. Air entering and leaving the cabinet is filter sterilized; infectious material inside the cabinet is handled with rubber gloves attached and sealed to the cabinet. A Class III cabinet affords the greatest degree of protection to the person handling the infectious agents.

Class II Type B cabinet has variable sash opening, and is designed for handling of toxic chemicals and carcinogens or radioisotopes. Approximately 70% of the downflow air exits through the exhaust filter, and 30% is recirculated. These cabinets must be hard-ducted, preferably to their own dedicated exhaust system, or to an appropriate laboratory building exhaust so that air is discharged outside the building.

Class II Type B2 is a total-exhaust cabinet. No air is recirculated within it, providing primary biological and chemical containment.

Class III

Class III is used for routine anaerobe work, and is designed for work with Level 4 organisms in maximum containment facilities. This cabinet provides

maximum protection to the environment and the worker. It is completely enclosed with negative pressure, with access for passage of materials through a dunk tank or double-door pass-through box that can be decontaminated between uses. Air coming into, and going out of, the cabinet is HEPA filtered, and exhaust air passes through two HEPA filters, or a HEPA filter and an air incinerator before discharge to the outdoors. Infectious material within the cabinet is handled with rubber gloves that are attached and sealed to ports in the cabinet (Fig. 13.4(*c*)).

Horizontal laminar flow 'clean bench'

Horizontal laminar flow 'clean bench' – provides only product protection, and is **not** a BSC. HEPA-filtered air is discharged across the work surface towards the user. These can be used for clean activities, but should never be used when handling cell cultures or infectious materials.

Vertical laminar flow 'clean bench'

Vertical laminar flow 'clean bench' – is also **not** a BSC, but is useful in hospital pharmacies for preparation of intravenous drugs. Although they generally have a sash, the air is usually discharged into the room under the sash.

Microbiological testing and contamination

Effective handling, cleaning and maintenance schedules, together with strict adherence to aseptic technique should make routine microbiological testing unnecessary, but may be required in order to identify a source of contamination in a culture system. It is required as part of some of the ISO 9000 series quality management protocols and is recommended by the UK Department of Health for laboratories that offer tissue banking facilities, including ovarian and testicular tissue. Methods used for microbiological testing of the environment include air sampling, settle plates, contact plates and glove print tests. Air sampling by either settle plates or Anderson Air Filtration systems are rarely indicated in an ART laboratory, except in evaluating an episode of contamination or outbreak. Routine culture of bacteria or fungal spores is expected in most environments, and does not reflect the environment in the sterile hood where procedures are performed. Settle plates are non-inhibitory culture media plates that are left out on a work surface so that bacteria and mould spores can settle out of the air onto the plate. This method represents an unconcentrated air volume assessment, and the procedure used should specify the length of time of exposure for the plate (1 h vs. 12 or 24 h). Air filters such as the Anderson Air filter apparatus actively collect (suck in) air through a filter. The filter is then placed on a culture medium to allow bacterial and fungal growth. Using this technique, the number of cubic feet of air to be processed must be specified; it is used mainly in clinical transplant areas (e.g. bone marrow transplant). Isolation

of spores is expected and usually does not correlate with patient disease.

Culture systems should be under constant vigilance to detect early signs of possible microbial contamination, in order to avert serious subsequent problems. Any turbidity or drastic colour change in media is a clear reflection of contamination, and an inseminated culture dish that shows all sperm dead or immotile should prompt further investigation for possible microbial contamination. A practical and simple method that can be used for checking bacterial and fungal contamination in the incubator or culture medium is to leave an aliquot of culture medium in the incubator for 5 days. Organisms contaminating the medium or the incubator that are a hazard under IVF culture conditions will multiply in this optimal growth environment of nutrients, temperature, pH and humidity. The aliquot can then be checked for contamination by looking for turbidity and change in colour (if medium with a pH indicator is used), and stained for microscopic observation of bacteria or fungi. This test can be used as an ongoing procedure for sterility testing of the incubator as well as the culture medium.

Fungal contamination in the laboratory

The ability of fungi to form spores that can survive in a wide range of physical extremes makes them a continuous source of potential contamination, and a laboratory that is not kept strictly and rigorously clean at all times provides an ideal environment for them to thrive. Fungal spores may be introduced from the environment, or from central heating/air conditioning systems, and can grow in incubators, water baths, sinks, refrigerators and on walls and surfaces that escape regular thorough cleaning. They thrive in a moist environment where there is a substrate, such as air filters, heat exchangers, humidifiers, water pumps, cooling units, wet carpet, ceiling tiles, condensation on windows – even indoor plants. In most cases, a thorough routine of regular cleaning together with comprehensive visual inspection should eliminate fungal contamination in the laboratory.

Settle plates are used only rarely, and specifically in patient care areas where patients are immunocompromised. In these areas, an air sampling system that filter a specific volume of air can be used – the filter is then cultured to detect fungi. In the laboratory setting, settle plates and air sampling of any kind is invariably futile. Appropriate use of sterile technique in a sterile laminar flow hood should be sufficient to protect cultures.

Contamination in an incubator is usually detected when the same fungus grows in multiple culture dishes. In this case the incubator must be decontaminated according to the manufacturer's instructions: each manufacturer has specifications about safe and appropriate decontamination procedures. The use of quaternary ammonium compounds, chlorine and alcohol solutions must be dictated by the reactivity of these compounds with the components of the incubator. Following decontamination, the incubators must be wiped down with sterile water to remove any residual cleaning solution that might volatize and contaminate the cultures. Full decontamination procedures should be carried out during laboratory 'down' periods, when no embryos are being cultured. Decontamination should include all surfaces, the water pan and the fan blades (which are very efficient at dispersing spores). Occasionally decontamination may fail – some institutions have been forced to replace the incubators. Incubators have recently been introduced that incorporate a sterilizing cycle (Forma, Steri-Cycle™, Binder, www.binder-world.com). Many are now designed for ease of cleaning and decontamination, featuring seamless internal chambers with rounded corners and simple, easily removable shelf and racking systems that can be sterilized by autoclaving (Micro-Galaxy, www.rsbiotech.com, Binder, www.binderworld.com, Shel Lab, www.shellab.com).

Sloppy technique also carries the risk of introducing organisms and spores from skin or hair into the culture system. Clinical specimens from skin commonly include bacteria (e.g. *Staphyloccocus* spp., see Fig. 13.3), yeasts and filamentous fungi such as *Aspergillus* spp. and *Epidermophyton floccosum* or other dermatophytes: the importance of complete aseptic technique cannot be overemphasized. Since fungal elements including spores are often found in association with hair, hair restraints and head coverings are very important in maintaining a clean working environment.

The Zygomycetes occur in soil and decaying vegetation worldwide, and are occasionally seen as contaminants in the laboratory. They have a very rapid growth rate in culture and produce a high 'cotton-candy-like' mycelium. *Rhizopus* spp., *Mucor* spp., and *Absidia* spp. are the zygomycetes most frequently encountered in the hospital environment causing contamination and infections. Colonies range in hue from white to grey, black or brown. The zygomycetes produce spores in sacklike structures called sporangia. The spores are extremely small and therefore settle very slowly; they remain airborne for long periods of time, particularly when there are only small movements of the air.

Aspergillus spp. are probably the most common type of mould found both as an opportunist and as a contaminant in culture systems. Like those of the zygomycetes, the spores are very small and remain airborne for long periods of time. They are ubiquitous in the environment, even in indoor locations, and may 'fall into' cultures or be introduced into cultures via fomites. *Aspergillus* spores have been identified as contaminants in oil used for overlays, although the source of the spores is not necessarily the oil itself, but may have been introduced into the oil via a breach in sterile technique during its use (see Fig. 13.1).

Aspergillus fumigatus is a truly cosmopolitan mould, and has been found almost everywhere on every conceivable type of substrate, especially in soil and decaying organic debris. *A. fumigatus* colonies show typical blue-green surface pigmentation with a suede-like surface consisting of a dense felt of conidiophores. In addition to being one of the most common fungal contaminants seen in the clinical laboratory, *A. fumigatus* is also the leading filamentous fungal pathogen producing human disease.

Aspergillus niger is one of the most common and easily identifiable species of the genus *Aspergillus*, and may also be a common laboratory contaminant. Colonies consist of a compact white or yellow basal felt covered by a dense layer of dark-brown to black conidial head. Once it contaminates a hood or incubator, *A. niger* is very difficult to eradicate and may cause widespread contamination of cultures.

Aspergillus flavus has a worldwide distribution, typically as a saprophyte in soil and on many kinds of decaying organic matter. On Czapek dox agar the colonies are granular, flat, often with radial grooves, and yellow at first but quickly becoming bright to dark yellow-green with age. *A. flavus* stimulates significant allergic reactions in humans, producing high levels of aflatoxin that may cause life-threatening anaphylaxis in exposed individuals.

Aspergillus terreus occurs commonly in soil and is occasionally reported as a pathogen of humans and animals. Colonies are typically suede-like and cinnamon-buff to sand brown in color with a yellow to deep dirty brown reverse.

Aspergillus nidulans is a typical soil fungus with a worldwide distribution.

Colonies are characteristically plain green in colour, with dark red-brown cleistothecia developing within, and upon, the conidial layer. The reverse side may be olive to drab-grey or purple-brown.

Fungi that may be seen most commonly as contaminants in clinical laboratories are summarized in Table 13.3 and illustrated in Fig. 13.5.

Laboratory cleaning schedules

Monitoring of asepsis, sterilization, and sterile technique should be an integral part of the overall quality management programme for every ART laboratory. Autoclaves and dry heat ovens must be properly maintained, and systematically monitored and checked for effectiveness. Intermittent spore sterilization tests should be part of the routine quality assurance programme. Heat cycles should be recorded for permanent documentation to assure adequate maintenance of both temperature and pressure for each autoclave cycle, with pressure sensitive tapes or strips included with every cycle as an indicator of effective autoclaving.

There must be a well-defined protocol for the routine cleaning of the laboratory environment and equipment, with a schedule appropriate to its level of use. Disposable cleaning materials should be used when practical, and any items that are re-used (mops, etc.) must be dedicated to the laboratory area only and not used in any other part of the building. Sprays should be used with caution; chemicals released from aerosols used for cleaning/disinfection remain in the atmosphere and may be incorporated into the incubator environment.

Above all, common-sense and judgement must be applied, after careful risk assessment to balance the need for cleaning/decontamination against the risk of exposing gametes and embryos to potentially toxic or mutagenic agents. Disinfecting chemical agents should always be used cautiously and judiciously, never indiscriminately. Since a variety of agents and schedules can be used for routine cleaning, the laboratory director should decide how to best implement established protocols, according to the laboratory workload, number of staff, laboratory layout, physical location and environmental atmosphere.

In an effort to reach a consensus of effective cleaning routines currently used in IVF laboratories, a simple questionnaire was made available on the Internet (www.ivf.net) at the beginning of 2003. The questionnaire was designed only to ascertain what methods and protocols are in use and believed to be safe and effective; no data was obtained to correlate this to success rates. Within 2 weeks 88 responses were received. A number of agents were used to clean incubators including sterile water, 70% alcohol, hydrogen peroxide, 0.26% peracetic acid, 1% 7×, Barricidal, and Roccal. Some were used in combination, e.g. sterile water, ethanol and hydrogen peroxide. Sterile water and ethanol, or a combination

Table 13.3. Characteristics of fungi commonly seen as contaminants in clinical laboratories

Fungal contaminant	Colony morphology	Vegetative mycelium	Asexual reproductive structure morphology

Aspergillus spp.
  A. fumigatus
  A. niger
	Low growing velvety colonies with a highly pigmented surface	Hyaline, septate	Swollen vesicles bear conidiogenic cells with strings of small, highly pigmented conidia

Zygomycete spp.
  Rhizopus spp.
  Mucor spp.
  Absidia spp.
	Lid lifter colonies, tall, 'cotton candy'-like morphology	Hyaline, non-septate	Sack-like sporangia contain many small sporangiospores

Penicillium spp.	Low growing velvety colonies, green/blue with white bibs	Hyaline, septate	Septate conidiophore with conidiogenic cells arranged in a tight 'broom-like' arrangement (penicillus)
Paecilomyces spp.	Yellow-tan powdery colonies	Hyaline, septate	Septate conidiophore with open penicillus morphology Conidiogenic cells bear chains of oval golden-coloured conidia
Fusarium spp.	White, cream or pink colonies Low and fuzzy, growing woolly with age	Hyaline, septate	Canoe-shaped multicellular macroconidia are borne singly from simple phialides
Cladosporium spp.	Olive green, low growing velvety colonies	Dematiaceous, septate	Conidiophore is septate ending in shield-shaped conidiogenic cells Small dark conidia are borne in long chains from the shield cells
Bipolaris spp. and *Dreschlera* spp.	Grey-brown colonies turning black with age Velvety texture	Dematiaceous, septate	Oval thick-walled poroconidia with cross septations borne singly from the conidiophore by bent-knee conidiation
Curvularia spp.	Green-brown velvety colonies with folded surface	Dematiaceous, septate	Multicellular macroconidia with cross septations are borne singly by bent-knee conidiation. A middle cell of the macroconidia is asymmetric, leading to a 'boomerang' curve in the spore
Alternaria spp.	Grey colonies turn green and then black with age	Dematiaceous, septate	Chains of club-shaped macroconidia that are multicellular with both longitudinal and cross septation
Aureobasidium spp.	Colonies are at first white to cream-coloured and yeast-like, turning black to brown with age	Dematiaceous, septate	Septate mycelium fragments into thick walled arthroconidia Blastoconidia are also produced

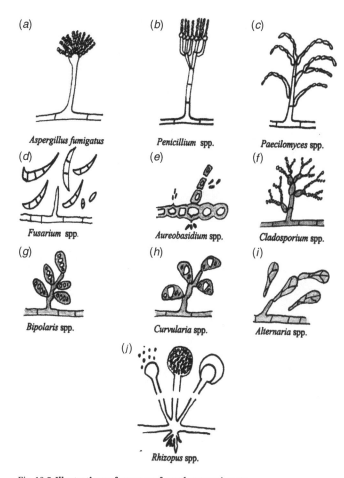

Fig. 13.5. **Illustrations of common fungal contaminants.**

(*a*) *Aspergillus fumigatus* is characterized by a hyaline septate mycelium and conidiophores in a swollen vesicle that bears conidiogenic phialides with a string of small conidia.

(*b*) *Penicillium* spp. have hyaline septate mycelia and septate conidiophores with metula and phillades bearing strings of conidia in a tight or broom-like distribution called a penicillus.

(*c*) *Paecilomyces* spp. are similar to *Penicillium* spp., but the penicillus is more open and the spores are oval in shape.

(*d*) *Fusarium* is a hyaline septate mould that produces canoe-shaped, multicellular macroconidia.

(*e*) *Aureobasidium* spp. grow as a dematiaceous yeast-like mould producing arthroconidia and small blastoconidia.

(*f*) *Cladosporium* spp. are characterized by the production of dematiaceous septate mycelia and conidiogenic cells (shield cells) that bear strings of branching conidia.

(*g*) *Bipolaris* spp. also are septate and dematiaceous. Macroconidia are produced by bent-knee or geniculate conidiation and are thick-walled, containing 3–5 cells.

(*h*) *Curvularia* spp. are morphologically similar to *Bipolaris* spp. with the exception that the macroconidia are 3–4 cells in length and contain an internal cell with a more rapid growth rate that causes the poroconidia to bend or curve.

(*i*) *Alternaria* spp. are characterized by multicelled macroconidia produced in strings from a conidiogenic cell in the septate dematiaceous mycelium. Macroconidia bear both cross and longitudinal septations.

(*j*) *Rhizopus* spp. are hyaline, non-septate moulds that produce long sporangiophores with sacs called sporangia containing small sporangiospores. Rhizoids are found at the bottom of unbranched sporangiophores.

Table 13.4. All routine cleaning schedules are carried out at the end of the working period/day, only distilled water used for cleaning during the working day. Some laboratories use a biologically safe detergent (e.g. 7X, TSP) for daily cleaning, others use only distilled water/EtOh as a daily routine, and detergent during major cleaning routines. Major cleaning should be carried out during a laboratory 'down' period, when no embryos are being cultured. Incubators should be allowed to re-stabilize for at least 2 days after cleaning, or after sterilization in those that incorporate self-sterilizing cycles.

To be cleaned	Cleaning agent/protocol	Time-table for cleaning
Benchtops/Surfaces	(Detergent)/distilled water/70% EtOH	Daily
Microscopes & stages	(Detergent)/distilled water/70% EtOH	Daily
Floors	(Detergent)/distilled water	Daily
Heating blocks	Distilled water/70%EtOH	Weekly
Water baths	70%EtOH/water	Weekly
Incubator water pan	MilliQ water	Weekly
Gas lines – plastic tubing	Distilled water	Monthly
Incubators	Distilled water/70%EtOH or Dist Water/Steri-cycle	Routine cleaning monthly, complete breakdown-clean 2–4 times per year, depending on use/workload
Incubator gas pre-filter		Change 6 monthly
Video monitors	70% EtOH	Weekly
Laminar flow + filters		Prefilter monthly, HEPA filter changed annually
Air filters		Change 6 monthly, or according to manufacturer's instructions
Refrigerators	Detergent/distilled water/70% EtOH	Monthly
Freezers	Detergent/distilled water/70% EtOH	6-monthly
Centrifuges	Detergent/distilled water/70% EtOH	Weekly
Cryotanks	Allow to warm, rinse with distilled water and wipe carefully with 70% EtOH. Allow to dry before re-filling.	not yet defined in the field
Walls, ceilings, and shelves/cupboards	Detergent/distilled water/70% EtOH	6-monthly or annually

using both was the most popular method used, with a schedule of monthly cleaning. Agents for floor and wall cleaning included a number of different proprietary quaternary ammonium detergents, as well as water, alcohol, 7×, chlorhexidine gluconate, bleach and hydrogen peroxide. A schedule for daily cleaning was most popular for floors and annual cleaning for walls. Cleaning and decontaminating cryotanks poses a particular problem, as many chemical agents will damage the tank seals. A number of units use sterile water only, but several confessed that they had no protocol for cleaning cryotanks (see Chapter 15).

Table 13.4 summarizes protocols in most common use according to the survey.

REFERENCES

Boone, W. R., Johnson, J. E., Locke, A. J., Crane, M. M. & Price, T. M. (1999). Control of air quality in an assisted reproductive technology laboratory. *Fertility and Sterility*, **71**: 150–4.

Chan A., Luetjens, C., Dominko, T. *et al.* (2000). Foreign DNA transmission by ICSI injection of spermatozoa bound with exogenous DNA results in embryonic GFP expression and live Rhesus monkey births. *Molecular Human Reproduction*, **6**: 22–33.

Cohen, J., Gilligan, A., Esposito, W., Schimmel, T. & Dale, B. (1997). Ambient air and its potential effects on conception in vitro. *Human Reproduction*, **12**(8): 1742–9.

WHO (1999). *WHO Laboratory Manual for the Examination of Human Semen and Sperm–Cervical Mucus Interaction*, 4th edn. Cambridge, UK: Cambridge University Press.

FURTHER READING

http://www.cap.org/ (home)

http://www.cap.org/html/ftpdirectory/checklistftp.html (all checklists)

ftp://ftp.cap.org/Labchecklist/cklatrlm1102.doc (Repro Checklist)

www.cdc/od.ohs/biosafety/bsc/bsc.htm

www.moorfield.co.uk

www.thermoforma.com

www.IVFonline.com

Baron, E. J., Chang, R. S., Howard, D. H., Miller, J. N. & Turner J. A. (1994). *Medical Microbiology: A Short Course*. New York: Wiley-Liss Inc.

Code of Practice for Tissue Banks: providing tissues of human origin for therapeutic purposes. (2001). UK Department of Health, ISBN 1 84182 329 5. www.doh.gov.uk/humantissuebanking

Cottel, E., McMorrow, J., Lennon, B., Fawsy, M., Cafferkey, M., & Harrison, R. F. (1996). Microbial contamination in an In Vitro Fertilization–embryo transfer system. *Fertility and Sterility*, **66**: 776–80.

Davis, B. D., Dulbecco, R., Eisen, H. N. & Ginsberg, H. S. (1990). *Microbiology*, 4th edn, Philadelphia, PA: Lippincott.

Edwards, R. G. & Brody, S. A. (1995). *Principles and Practice of Assisted Human Reproduction*. Philadelphia, PA: W. B. Saunders.

Elder, K. & Dale, B. (2000). *In Vitro Fertilization*, 2nd edn. Cambridge, UK: Cambridge University Press.

Forbes, B. A., Sahm, D. F. & Weissfeld, A. S. (1998). *Diagnostic Microbiology*, 10th edn. Mosby.

Forbes, B. A., Sahm, D. F. & Weissfeld, A. S. (2002). *Diagnostic Microbiology*. 11th edn. Mosby.

General Services Administration. *Federal Standard FED-STD-209E: Airborne Particulate Cleanliness Classes in Cleanrooms and Cleanzones*. June 15, 1988.

International Organization for Standardization. *ISO 14644-1: Cleanrooms and Associated Controlled Environments – Part 1: Classification of Air Cleanliness*. Geneva, Switzerland, 1999.

Salle, A. (1984). *Fundamental Principles of Bacteriology*. India: Tata-McGraw Hill.

Svalander, PC (1991). Mycocontamination of incubators used for human pre-embryo culture. *Fertility and Sterility*, **56**: 1207–8.

14

Handling infectious agents in the ART laboratory

Rigorous attention to maintaining a clean laboratory environment, a sterile culture microenvironment and aseptic technique at the interface of the two, should minimize exogenous contamination of gamete handling and culture systems in the ART laboratory. All human tissue and samples, regardless of prior testing for infectious agents, must be regarded as a potential hazard and handled accordingly. Samples identified as a biohazard after screening must be handled with extreme caution, according to specified protocols and procedures.

Blood-borne viruses

The **blood-borne viruses (BBV)**, Hepatitis B, C, D and HIV are all potent pathogens capable of causing severe disease and death, with few effective treatments available. Nosocomial transmission of Hepatitis C has been reported (Lesourd *et al.*, 2000, see below), and HBV transmission through contact with environmental surfaces has been demonstrated. The stability of HIV and HBV under different conditions has been determined experimentally.

- HIV in high starting concentrations can remain infectious for 3 weeks or more in dried blood.
- Infectious HIV can be detected for at least 2 months in liquid blood at room temperature.
- HBV in dried plasma can retain infectivity for at least 4 months, and this is likely to be even longer in liquid blood or plasma.

- Infectious HIV has been recovered from bodies up to 16 days after death, and it should be assumed that HBV is at least equally as robust.

In the environment:

- **HBV** is very stable and can persist in the environment for long periods. Risk of infection via contact with contaminated instruments is approximately 30%. It is inactivated by quaternary ammonium compounds, alcohol and hypochlorite solutions.
- **HCV** is more labile and persists in the environment for only a short time. The risk of infection via penetrating injury is approximately 1.8%. It is inactivated by quaternary ammonium compounds, alcohol and hypochlorite solutions.
- **HIV** is labile in the environment; risk of infection is approximately 3/1000 after penetrating injury, and 1/1000 after mucosal exposure. A solution of 10% hypochlorite is recommended for surface decontamination, and steam or ethylene oxide sterilization for instruments.

Transmission of infectious agents to exposed health-care personnel depends upon the type and route of biohazard exposure, the physical containment of the microorganism, frequency of contact and efficacy of transmission and on the operator's protection from biohazardous material during manipulations. The majority of cases (80% approx) of transmission to health care personnel occur via percutaneous exposure (i.e. needlestick) and around 20% via mucocutaneous or conjunctival exposure. Two cases of patient-to-patient transmission of Hepatitis C virus have been reported during assisted conception treatment, and HCV genotyping provided molecular

Table 14.1. Classification of biologic agents based on hazard

Biosafety level	Agents included	Precautions to be taken
Level 1	Agents that have no known potential for infecting healthy people, e.g. *Bacillus subtilis*	Good standard laboratory technique, 'Standard Precautions'
Level 2	All common agents of infectious disease as well as unusual pathogens. Most GU pathogens, including *Chlamydia, Neisseria, Treponema,* HSV, CMV, *Trichomonas*, etc. Hepatitis B/C, HIV	In addition to Level 1 precautions: Limit access to laboratory during working procedures Train laboratory personnel in handling of pathogenic agents Perform aerosol-generating procedures under a BSC Offer Hepatitis B vaccine to all employees at risk of exposure Autoclave for decontamination of all infectious material on the premises
Level 3	Some viruses, *Mycobacterium tuberculosis*, the mould phase of systemic fungi	In addition to Level 2 precautions: Laboratory design and air movement designed to contain potentially dangerous material Protective clothing and gloves for personnel Baseline sera from employees stored for comparison in the event of unexplained illness
Level 4	Certain viruses of the arbovirus, arenavirus and filovirus groups. HIV amplified in culture, Ebola virus, smallpox	Maximum containment facilities Personnel and all materials must be decontaminated before leaving the facility All procedures performed under maximum containment Special protective clothing Class III BSCs Air is piped in from an outside clean source

evidence for nosocomial transmission. Investigation into the probable route of contamination showed this to be through healthcare workers (Lesourd *et al.*, 2000). This type of situation can be attributed to a failure to adhere to strict measures of standard precautions or to inadequate cleaning/decontamination procedures; strict control in the implementation of both is crucial for safe practice in assisted conception treatment. The fact that patients may also be at risk of infection transmitted by healthcare personnel carriers of infectious agents should always be borne in mind.

Biosafety levels

The Advisory Committee on Dangerous Pathogens in the UK and the US Dept of Health categorize organisms into groups according to their risk of transmitting disease and have published recommendations for biosafety in biomedical laboratories (see Table 14.1: Standard Precautions for Good Laboratory Practice (Richmond, 1998)).

- Do not eat, drink smoke or apply cosmetics, including lip balm.
- Do not insert or remove contact lenses.
- Do not bite nails or chew on pens.
- Do not mouth-pipette.
- Limit laboratory access to trained personnel only.
- Assume all patients are positive for HIV and other pathogens that are blood-borne.
- Use appropriate barrier precautions to prevent skin and mucous membrane exposure (wear gloves at all times; wear masks, goggles, gowns and/or aprons if there is risk of droplet formation).

- Thoroughly wash hands and other skin surfaces after any contamination and after gloves are removed.
- Take care to avoid injuries with sharps (needles and scalpels).

A common high standard of handling must be applied in all contact with patient blood, body fluids and tissues. If patients are not screened before treatment, all samples should be handled as potentially hazardous, with Level 2 containment measures. In the setting of assisted conception treatment, this includes semen, vaginal secretions, cervical mucus, follicular fluid, peritoneal fluid and any other body fluid containing visible blood. Current guidelines in the UK recommend Containment Level 2+ for the handling of known infectious samples, with dedicated equipment and facilities physically separated from those used for handling non-infectious routine cases (Gilling-Smith & Almeida, 2003). Infectious cases should also be handled with 'temporal' separation, i.e.

1. As the last case in the day, followed by complete decontamination of the environment, or
2. In a 'series' dedicated to the handling of only seropositive cases of a particular virus, with complete and rigorous decontamination at the end of the series. Throughout all phases of treatment, all samples should be handled as if contaminated, with appropriate containment measures. Detailed protocols and strict safety guidelines must be available to all members of medical, nursing and laboratory staff, who should be vaccinated against HBV and undergo regular training in safety and handling of contaminated body fluids. Vaginal ultrasound probes should be covered with a protective sheath and wiped with a germicidal impregnated tissue after use on each patient. Whenever possible, instruments should be disposable.

Biosafety for ART: level 2

In addition to precautions listed for any Level 2 laboratory, the following are good laboratory practices for ART.

(i) Laboratory personnel should change into clean operating theatre dress, hats and shoes worn by all personnel who enter.

(ii) Hand-washing sink, preferably near the door (in tropical regions of the world with high temperatures and humidity, sinks can be a source of microbial contamination and ideally should be located in an anteroom adjacent to the laboratory).

(iii) Laboratory must be easily cleaned and decontaminated, all work surfaces and floors must be cleaned daily and kept clear of unnecessary equipment, supplies, boxes etc.

(iv) Benchtops should be impervious to acid; plastic-backed absorbent pads available to collect splatters or droplets.

(v) Appropriate chemical decontamination tray available for collecting contaminated implements.

(vi) Waste materials separated according to hazard type, with secure and safe disposal procedure at the end of each day. Use of specified containers for sharp tools.

(vii) Regular hand-washing: liquid soap, 20 seconds of vigorous washing, use towel to turn off taps. Wash hands, change gloves and clean the workstation before working with a new sample from a different patient.

(viii) Supervisor responsible for establishing general laboratory safety procedures and ensuring that personnel are educated.

(ix) Laboratory personnel must accept training and follow proscribed protocols.

(x) Emphasis on avoiding sharps whenever possible and using extreme caution when handling sharps including careful disposal into leakproof and puncture proof containers, readily available in all areas where sharps are used.

Specific policies and procedures must be developed and posted in clear view. There should be a Code of Practice that details procedures and control measures specifically, and full consultation with all staff with respect to containment measures is necessary. The Code of Practice should show clearly who is managerially responsible for the safe conduct of the work.

Documentation is essential! There must be a written protocol for dealing with spills and accidents (see Appendix at end of chapter for control plans) and these must be reported in an incident log book, for future reference and instigation of preventive measures.

Containment Level 2+ (Level 2 with Level 3 precautions): additional precautions for handling HBV/HCV and HIV-positive samples in the ART laboratory

- Dedicated facilities and equipment/instruments are recommended, with separate facilities for semen handling, oocyte/embryo handling and cryostorage procedures
- Train staff rigorously in safe handling procedures.
- Handle only one sample at a time.
- Use only disposable or sterilizable materials.
  - (i) Clearly label all samples and accompanying paperwork as biohazardous, and identify the biohazard.
  - (ii) Seal specimens inside individual plastic bags that can be opened without the use of sharp instruments.
  - (iii) Carry samples in leakproof boxes or deep-sided trays designed to prevent contamination.
  - (iv) Ensure restricted access, established by supervisor.
  - (v) Prevent access of unauthorized persons.
  - (vi) Keep the door closed – do not allow entry by other personnel when material is being handled.
  - (vii) Conduct work in a designated area of the lab with sufficient space to work safely.
  - (viii) Clear workstation of unnecessary equipment; cover ancillary equipment with disposable drapes or cling film.
  - (ix) Use disposable plastic tips (Flexipets, etc.) for manipulations, avoid the use of needles and glass whenever possible.
  - (x) Incubate cultures in a dedicated incubator, or contained within a modular incubator chamber or desiccator.
  - (xi) Use laboratory clothing + fluid impervious laboratory coats or aprons, hats, masks, goggles or visors, and gloves. Used gloves are potentially contaminated and must be removed before touching other laboratory equipment (e.g. refrigerator, incubator, telephone).
  - (xii) Protect breaks in skin with waterproof dressings.
  - (xiii) Use disposable plasticware, preferably screw-top if capped.
  - (xiv) Use disposable counting chambers for semen assessment.
  - (xv) Avoid the use of water baths, gas lines or any procedures that may cause aerosols.
  - (xvi) Carry out any work that can produce aerosols or splatter in BSC Class II.
  - (xvii) Decontaminate infectious waste by steam autoclave or chemical sterilization by immersing in sodium hypochlorite solution – place disposable materials (and any fluid they contain) immediately in a hypochlorite solution and soak for at least 30 minutes before packing it for disposal.
  - (xviii) Decontaminate all surfaces at the end of each procedure.
  - (xix) Treat all linen that has been in contact with patients as potentially infected.
  - (xx) Ensure the laboratory supervisor is a competent scientist who has a technical understanding of the risks and is responsible for restricting access, establishing the protective standards and developing the safety manual.
  - (xxi) Make sure personnel are educated, trained and proficient in the procedures.
  - (xxii) Ensure personnel carrying out the procedures receive hepatitis B vaccination and have a baseline serum sample tested, with written consent.

(A similar set of guidelines must also be in place as applicable for patient and sample handling during surgical procedures in the Operating Room.)

Centrifugation

- Use sealed buckets or rotors.
- In the event of breakage or leakage:
  open the rotor or bucket in a BSC,
  remove centrifuge from use until decontaminated,
  decontaminate surfaces by flooding with fresh
  solution of 10% bleach, left in contact for at least
  30 minutes.

Micromanipulation

- Procedures can be visualized via computer or
  video screen instead of using eyepieces.
- Wear gloves to remove used holding pipettes and
  injection needles
- Avoid the use of sharps as much as possible

Infectious samples for cryostorage must have
a dedicated storage tank (the risks of cross-
contamination associated with cryostorage are discussed in Chapter 15).

Treatment of HBV seropositive couples

If the female partner is positive for HepBs antigen
and the male negative, his immune status should
be checked, and vaccine administered if necessary.
The woman must be further tested for HBeAg and
HBV DNA. If negative after re-testing for confirmation after a further period of at least 1 month, she can
proceed to ART treatment, with vaccination and IgG
therapy for the infant at birth. The risk of transmission to the newborn is around 2–15% and chronic
carrier status is avoided in 85–95% of cases. If further
tests for HbeAg or HBV DNA are positive, the patient
must be referred to a virology specialist for investigation, evaluation and counselling before proceeding
to ART treatment, since risk of transmission to the
baby is 80–90%. Vaccine and immunoglobulin therapy considerably reduce the risk of chronic carrier
status.

If the male partner is positive for HBsag antigen and the female is negative, she must be vaccinated, and antibody status confirmed to be at

protective titres (>10 miU/ml) before ART treatment
is offered. As she is then theoretically protected from
infection, sperm washing is not necessary; samples
should be handled as infectious and handled as high
risk. Although sperm washing techniques have been
shown to reduce the viral load, viral sequences have
been detected integrated into sperm chromosomes,
particularly during acute infection (Hadchouel *et al.*,
1995; Huang *et al.*, 2002). There is therefore a potential risk of vertical HBV transmission via integration
into the germline, and careful follow-up studies are
needed in order to study and quantify this risk. Again,
patients must be carefully counselled before proceeding with treatment.

Treatment of HCV seropositive couples

If either partner is positive for HCV antibodies, they
must be tested for the presence of HCV RNA; if this
is negative for both partners, they may proceed to
ART treatment. If HCV RNA is detected, indicating
active infection, the patient(s) must be referred to
a virology specialist for evaluation and counselling
before proceeding with ART treatment. The actual
risk of vertical transmission is currently unknown,
with published estimates varying widely according
to the study population and the assay methods used;
the factors involved in determining the risk have not
been defined. Published reports vary widely, due to
differences in prevalence of the disease and to differences in detection methodology for diagnosis.

If the female partner is antibody positive but HCV
RNA negative, she can proceed to ART treatment
after repeat testing to confirm the result. In this case,
the risk of transmission to the neonate is very low,
estimated as less than 1%. If the female is RNA positive, the risk of transmission could be as high as
11%, depending on viral load. Concomitant infection with HIV significantly increases the risk of both
sexual transmission and vertical transmission to the
fetus, with reports varying from 16 to 36% (Semprini *et al.* 2001, Guaschino *et al.*, 2003). Women
who are HCV RNA positive and suitable for fertility treatment should first be referred for antiviral

treatment to reduce the viral load, in order to minimize the risk of both vertical transmission and nosocomial transmission during assisted reproduction procedures. Anti-viral treatment is contraindicated in pregnancy, and should be stopped preconceptually.

There is a discrepancy in published results regarding the presence of HCV RNA in semen, probably related to differences in collection and storage of the samples, as well as the wide range of protocols used for RNA extraction and the molecular techniques used to detect HCV RNA. Seminal plasma has been reported to contain inhibitors of the PCR reaction, so that misleading false-negative results can be obtained unless appropriate internal controls are included in the assay (Levy et al., 2002). The presence of RNAses and lipoperoxidases in semen can also interfere with nucleic acid amplification.

If the male partner is HCV RNA seropositive, it must be assumed that his semen will also contain viral RNA, although viral loads may vary through time and different ejaculates may yield a different result. Each semen sample should be tested for viral load prior to use. Viral RNA has also been found in some of the fractions of motile sperm after gradient selection and washing, possibly due to passive adsorption (Levy et al., 2002). These authors recommend that semen samples and corresponding motile sperm fractions should be tested and cryopreserved in highly secure straws in liquid nitrogen prior to use for ART. Only sperm fractions that test negative for HCV RNA can be considered for ART. Men positive for HCV RNA should also be referred for antiviral treatment to reduce the viral load during assisted reproduction procedures.

Treatment of HIV seropositive couples

HIV primarily affects people of active reproductive age (86% are between ages 15 and 44), and the risk of viral transmission to sexual partners and offspring is considerable. For HIV serodiscordant couples, where one partner is seropositive for the virus, the greatest risk is transmission of the virus to the seronegative partner during unprotected sexual intercourse. The transmission rate to an uninfected partner is estimated to be approximately 1 in 500 to 1 in 1000 episodes of unprotected intercourse, but this increases if the viral load is high, and in the presence of concomitant genital infection, inflammation or abrasions. Therefore, these couples may now seek assisted reproduction in starting their families. Concerns regarding offering assisted reproductive treatment to patients with HIV have been repeatedly expressed and debated, including potential transmission of the virus to offspring, as well as the welfare of the child with one or both parents having a potentially shortened lifespan. Complex ethical issues are involved, all of which are beyond the scope of this text. The recent introduction of more effective treatment regimens has altered the perspective and prognosis for HIV patients from that of a serious life-threatening disease to a chronic illness. In 1998, the United States Supreme Court ruled that a person with HIV is considered 'disabled' and therefore is protected under the Americans with Disabilities Act (Annas, 1998; Bragdon vs. Abbott, 1998). The Court determined that having HIV was a disability because it interfered with the 'major life activity' of reproduction due to the risk of transmitting HIV to offspring. According to that decision, persons with HIV are entitled to medical services unless it can be demonstrated 'by objective scientific evidence' that treatment would pose a significant risk of infection. Unless healthcare workers can show that they lack the skill and facilities to treat HIV-positive patients safely, they may be legally obliged to provide them with any requested reproductive treatment. When a clinic lacks the skills and facilities to manage HIV-positive patients, they should be referred to a clinic that has these resources.

However, the availability of adequate facilities for handling infected material in fertility centres worldwide is currently limited, due to health concerns both for patients and for the healthcare practitioners who may be exposed during treatment procedures. The decision to set up a treatment programme for these patients is a complex one, and should be preceded by careful consideration of all the issues involved, including legal concerns. There should be a multidisciplinary team available with expertise in appropriate patient selection, the risks involved for different categories of patients, prognosis and the type of treatment to offer. Specialist HIV evaluation, treatment, monitoring, counselling and follow-up facilities are essential. Particular attention must be paid to correct training of medical, nursing and laboratory personnel in the handling of infected material, and emphasis placed on provision of adequate facilities and environmental conditions to minimize the possibility of accidents that may lead to contamination with infected material.

If a woman is HIV positive and her partner HIV negative, transmission of infection to her partner can be avoided by homologous insemination with the partner's sperm, using quills. If the woman is <35 years of age, with no overt signs or symptoms of infertility, this can be advised for a period of 6–12 months before considering intensive fertility investigations. If assisted conception treatment is indicated, this should be planned carefully to minimize the risk of multiple pregnancy; HIV-infected women are more prone to ill health, and a multiple pregnancy represents a severe risk from several different perspectives during pregnancy, birth, and in terms of caring for the children. The resulting pregnancy poses risks to both mother and child, due to opportunistic infections and to medications that may affect the developing fetus. Amniocentesis must be avoided, as it carries the risk of viral transmission into the amniotic sac and to the fetus. If an HIV-positive pregnant woman does not receive active antiretroviral therapy, the risk of transmission to the infant is greater than 20%, regardless of the mother's viral load. Zidovudine treatment during pregnancy and treating the baby for the first 6 weeks of life can reduce the risk of transmission to 5–8%. The risk can be further reduced by Caesarean section delivery and by avoiding breast feeding.

If a man is HIV positive and his partner is HIV negative, the risk of transmitting the virus to his partner is reduced, but not eliminated, by using condoms during intercourse with timed unprotected intercourse during ovulation. This practice is unsafe and is not recommended. Highly active antiretroviral therapy can lower the virus load in serum and semen, and sperm washing techniques can be used to prepare samples with PCR-undetectable levels of virus RNA for insemination or IVF. This technique has been used mainly for insemination procedures, and in studies published to date mothers and children were negative for HIV when tested at 3 months and 1 year (Semprini et al., 1992; Marina et al., 1998; Gilling-Smith & Almeida, 2003). This data is reassuring, but more follow-up studies are needed and couples must be carefully counselled about the potential risk of HIV transmission to the uninfected partner and to their offspring.

If both partners are HIV positive, both may have normal fertility potential, or one or both may have impaired fertility and seek assisted reproduction. There is a chance that male and female partners may be infected with different HIV strains, and may have different treatment regimens. Therefore, the sperm sample should be washed to minimize the risk of transmitting mutated, resistant HIV strains from male to female and offspring. Although aggressive antiretroviral therapy can extend life and improve health, the long-term prognosis is still uncertain. They must be carefully counselled to consider the risk of having a child that may be infected, and to consider the fact that the child may lose one or both parents to AIDS before reaching adult life. To date, insufficient data is available regarding the effects of antiretroviral therapy on spermatogenesis or fetal development, and follow-up studies are necessary to monitor the growth and development of children born to these couples after assisted conception treatment.

It has been suggested that the CD4 receptor may be expressed on spermatozoa (Scofield et al., 1994), and that HIV particles can also penetrate human spermatozoa through an alternative receptor, galactosylalkylacylglycerol (GalAAA). This molecule is distributed in a variety of sites on the surface of the sperm membrane (Piomboni & Bacetti, 2000). It is now generally accepted that virus transport by human spermatozoa is possible and that virus sequences may be integrated into the spermatozoal DNA. HIV-1 sequences were found in spermatogonia, spermatocytes and spermatids from the testes of men who had died of the AIDS syndrome (Nuovo *et al.*, 1994; Shevchuk *et al.*, 1998). Experiments using intra-cytoplasmic sperm injection (ICSI) in mouse and non-human primate systems demonstrate that exogenous DNA bound to sperm can be retained in oocytes and expressed at a high rate in the resulting embryos (Kiessling, 1998; Perry *et al.*, 1999). Chan *et al.* (2000) showed that exogenous DNA tagged with green fluorescent protein (GFP) bound on the sperm surface was retained in non-human primate oocytes after ICSI, but could not be detected after IVF. Although this experiment may suggest that IVF could be a 'safer' procedure than ICSI, if the proviral DNA is already incorporated into the genome of the sperm cell, both techniques share the same risk. Although successful cases of IVF and ICSI without apparent vertical transmission have been reported, the consequences of germ-line integration after assisted reproductive techniques are completely unknown.

In vitro experiments indicate that HIV does not infect oocytes of healthy women that are exposed to inocula of cell-free virus (Bacetti *et al.*, 1999). These experiments demonstrated that cell-free HIV-1 did not bind to or penetrate the human oocyte in vitro, and both virus receptors, CD4 and GalAAG were absent from oocytes and cumulus cells.

The study of HIV has provided new insights into the biology of eukaryotic cells and it is clear that the virus has an extraordinary capacity to exploit the cell's molecular machinery in the course of infection. The most damaging characteristic of the virus is possibly its ability to establish stable post-integration latent forms of infection, ensuring persistence even in the presence of intensive drug therapy and an antiviral immune response. Although the development of potent antiviral drugs has allowed HIV-infected individuals to live longer and to enjoy a higher quality of life, it is clear that these drugs do not cure the infection. Their prolonged use often can be significantly toxic, and does result in the emergence

of drug-resistant viruses. The combination of virus persistence, together with a high rate of mutation, allows HIV to escape from traditional vaccination strategies.

In all cases and situations, couples should always be advised that the absolutely safest courses to consider are adoption, child-free living, or, if only the male is HIV positive, donor sperm.

Semen washing procedures for HBV/HCV/HIV serodiscordant couples

(Semprini *et al.*, 1992; Marina *et al.*, 1998)

Note: tests carried out on semen for the presence of virus must have appropriate internal amplification controls to detect possible inhibitors of the PCR reaction that will yield false-negative results. It has been noted that there may be a dissociation between HIV serum viral load and the amount of virus shed in semen: even if viral load in the serum is undetectable, there may still be HIV in the semen. In order to validate standardized techniques for the detection of HCV in semen, Bourlet *et al.* (2003) carried out a multicentre quality control study and reported on the different aspects of diagnostic methodology that can influence the results.

> *All procedures must be carried out in a Class 2 biosafety cabinet with vertical laminar flow, using disposable sterile supplies and complete aseptic technique. Although preparation protocols can reduce the risk of infection, their efficacy may be variable, dependent on viral loads, and should never be assumed to be absolute. Final preparations must always be re-tested before use.*

- Evaluate the semen sample with respect to count, motility and morphology, using a disposable counting chamber.
- Prepare a two- or three-layer discontinuous buoyant density gradient (e.g. 2 ml of 90% overlaid with 2 ml of 47%, or 90%, 70%, 50%).
- Layer 2–4 ml of the semen sample on top of the gradient
- Centrifuge at 600–800g for 30 minutes.

- Carefully remove the supernatant by pipetting and transfer to a clean test tube.
- Resuspend the pellet in 3 mls of sperm washing medium and transfer to a clean test tube.
- Centrifuge at 600–800g for 10 minutes.
- Remove the supernatant with a clean pipette and carefully layer 1 ml of sperm washing medium over the pellet.
- Cap the tube and incubate the sample at 37 °C for 1 hour.
- Recover approximately 0.5 ml of the superficial swim-up layer and transfer to a clean test tube.
- Evaluate the count, motility and morphology of the swim-up sperm sample.
- Aliquot 100 μl of this sample for virus RNA testing.
- Store the remaining 400 μl at 4 °C.

If the aliquot tested is negative for virus RNA, re-warm the sample at 37 °C for 15 minutes and proceed with the ART procedure. If it is positive, the sample must be discarded. If virology results cannot be obtained on the same day that the sample is processed, samples may be cryopreserved and stored in tanks dedicated to high-risk samples until test results are available.

Virus decontamination

Heat

Heat is the most effective routine means of destroying the infectivity of all microorganisms, including BBV.

(i) Autoclave – pressure steam sterilization, 30 min at 15 psi pressure (high altitude locations require higher pressure, approximately 18 psi at 5000 feet above sea level).
(ii) Full immersion in boiling water for a minimum of 5 minutes, longer for large objects.
(iii) Dry heat ovens.

Chemical disinfection

(i) Clean the item first if it is safe to do so.
(ii) Hypochlorite, alcohol, formaldehyde and glutaraldehyde solutions are effective: these must be used at the correct recommended concentration, and only a freshly prepared dilution should be used on each occasion, as disinfectants lose their activity with time after dilution. Adequate precautions should be taken to avoid exposure of gametes and embryos, as all of these agents are toxic.

- Hypochlorite is corrosive to metals.
- Formalin may be used for fumigation.

(iii) The agents are effective only if sufficient contact time is allowed: at least 30 minutes (one hour for 70% alcohol).
(iv) A solution of 70% acohol can be used to remove residues after chemical disinfection with hypochlorite, formaldehyde or glutaraldehyde.
(v) There must be a protocol for dealing with spills that describes cleaning of spillages, disinfecting equipment and waste disposal. All personnel must be familiar with procedures to follow in case of a contaminated sample spill.

Accidental exposure

There must be a written procedure to be followed in case of accidental exposure of laboratory personnel to a sample known to be a biohazard, with recommendations for post-exposure prophylaxis (PEP).

(i) Prevention is the primary strategy, i.e. use of standard precautions and vaccine availability.
(ii) The system must include written protocols for prompt reporting, evaluation, counselling, treatment and follow-up of occupational exposures.
(iii) There should be 24-hour access to clinicians who can provide post-exposure care immediately.
(iv) All personnel must be familiar with evaluation and treatment protocols for PEP.

Any splashes to skin should be washed immediately with soap and running water; wounds should be rinsed under running water. Mucous membranes should be flushed with water and an eye wash bottle must be available for washing splashes to the eye. For skin exposure, first assess the risk: follow-up is indicated only if there is compromised skin integrity (dermatitis, abrasion, open wound).

The source of contamination should be recorded and an incident report completed to document the circumstances of the exposure. This incident report should document details of:

(i) date and time of the exposure;
(ii) description of procedure, including where and how the exposure occurred;
(iii) type and amount of fluid involved, severity of the exposure;
(iv) exposure source, whether of known or unknown risk;
   • (If the status is unknown, the source should be tested for HBV, HCV, and HIV if possible.)
(v) immune status of the exposed person;
(vi) counselling, management and follow-up.

HBV prophylaxis

If the exposed person is unvaccinated, HepB Immunoglobulin should be administered, at a dose of 0.06 ml/kg, and a vaccine series initiated. If he/she is vaccinated and immune, no further treatment is indicated (Table 14.2).

HCV prophylaxis

No protective antibody response has been identified following HCV infection, and post-exposure immunoglobulin is not relevant or effective. Therefore, post-exposure management is aimed at early detection of disease and referral for evaluation of treatment options: a short course of interferon administered early in disease may be effective. Serum should be tested for anti-HCV and alanine amino transferase (ALT) as a baseline, with follow-up at 4–6 weeks, then 4–6 months. If HCV infection is identified early, the patient must be referred to a specialist for treatment and advice. With the advent of pegylated interferon treatments, early aggressive therapy may be warranted.

Table 14.2. Procedure after accidental exposure to HBV

Status of exposed person	Treatment
Unvaccinated	Administer HepB Immuno-globulin within 1 week, 0.06 ml/kg, multiple doses
	Initiate vaccine series
Vaccinated and immune	No further treatment is indicated
Vaccinated and not immune	HBIgG ×1 and re-vaccinate, or HbIgG × 2

HIV prophylaxis

Theoretically, antiretroviral PEP soon after exposure might prevent or inhibit systemic infection, by limiting the proliferation of virus in the initial target cells or lymph nodes. Personnel exposed to HIV should be evaluated within hours, tested for HIV as baseline, and re-evaluated at 72 hrs. Follow-up should be carried out at 6 weeks, 12 weeks, 6 months and 12 months, whether or not antiretroviral treatment is administered. If any illness compatible with acute retroviral syndrome develops, the patient must be re-tested for HIV. Failure of PEP to prevent HIV infection has been reported in at least 21 cases (USPHS, 2001) with different combinations of drugs; 13 of the source persons had been treated with antiretrovirals before the exposure and it is possible that a resistant strain had developed. Three classes of drugs are currently available:

• nucleoside reverse transcriptase inhibitors (NRTIs);
• non-nucleoside reverse transcriptase inhibitors (NNRTIs);
• protease inhibitors (PIs).

Resistance to HIV infection occurs with all of the available drugs, and cross-resistance within drug classes is frequent. Primary genetic mutations are associated with resistance to NRTI and PI. Occupational transmission of resistant HIV strains, despite PEP with combination drug regimens, has been reported.

The emotional effect of exposure is substantial; there must be a secure management system in place, with written procedures and protocols and ready access to expert advice.

Air transport of biohazardous materials

International regulations for the transport of dangerous goods by any mode of transport are based upon recommendations of the United Nations Committee of Experts on the Transport of Dangerous Goods (UN). Other specialized agencies of the United Nations, including the Universal Postal Union (UPU), the International Civil Aviation Organization (ICAO), and the International Air Transport Association (IATA) have incorporated the UN recommendations into their regulations. The majority of international air carriers belong to IATA and follow the IATA *Dangerous Goods Regulations* for transport of dangerous goods, which is updated and published annually by IATA (800 Place Victoria, Suite 6035-Promenade, Montreal, Quebec, Canada H4Z 1M1).

The IATA (2003) defines dangerous goods as '*articles or substances which are capable of posing a risk to health, safety, property or the environment –*'. Dangerous goods include *Division 6.2-Infectious Substances*, further categorized in the 12th revised edition of the *UN Model Regulations* as infectious substances, biological products, diagnostic specimens, genetically modified microorganisms and organisms, and wastes from medical treatment or bioresearch. Information for identifying, classifying, and documenting the transport of *Division 6.2 – Infectious Substances* is available from a variety of sources; rules governing air transport are the most stringent. International regulations that affect air transport of infectious substances, diagnostic specimens, and biological products will be covered here.

Regulations that cover transport of dangerous goods by surface (land or water) vary according to specific national regulatory agencies, and are generally less restrictive than those governing air transport. In the United States the Department of Transportation (DOT) regulates surface and air transport of dangerous goods and the United States Postal Service (USPS) regulates transport of dangerous goods by mail. DOT regulations are covered in the *49 Code of Federal Regulations* (CFR), parts 171–178. This regulation allows exceptions (listed in *49 CFR*) for transport of some diagnostic specimens by motor vehicle. ICAO Technical Instructions for air transport are referred to in *49 CFR*. New regulations for transport of infectious substances and diagnostic specimens are being proposed by the USPS, so that these are in line with other regulatory agencies. Current USPS regulations can be found in the *Domestic Mail Manual* and proposed USPS regulations can be found in the *Federal Register*.

International and national regulatory agencies require that anyone involved in the shipping and packaging of dangerous goods should receive training and certification in the proper regulations that govern transport, packaging, and labelling of those substances. In order to keep abreast of frequent changes regarding shipping regulations, certification training must be repeated at intervals set by the regulatory agencies or when new regulations take effect. In the United States, select agents have been identified and classified as imported or exported biological materials, and agents that have the potential to pose a severe threat to public health. Special regulations that apply to the transport of select agents within the USA and between the USA and other countries can be found on the Centers for Disease Control (CDC) website.

The 12th revised edition of the UN Model Regulations has the following definitions:

A. *Infectious substances* are those substances known or reasonably expected to contain pathogens, including bacteria, viruses, rickettsiae, parasites, fungi or recombinant microorganisms. Infectious substances are classified into two categories:

- UN 2814, affecting humans and animals,
- UN 2900, affecting animals only.

The World Health Organization (WHO) has defined three risk groups, characterized by criteria that include pathogenicity, mode and ease of transmission, degree of risk to both an individual and community, and availability of effective disease treatment or preventative agents.

- Risk Group 1 includes substances unlikely to cause human or animal disease.
- Risk Group 2, 3, and 4 pathogens include pathogens that have an increasing risk for causing individual or community disease.
- Risk group 4 pathogens have the highest risk of causing disease and effective treatment and preventative measures are not usually available to treat that disease.

In the United States, infectious substances include any agent that causes or may cause severe, disabling or fatal disease, and agents listed in 42 CFR 72.3 of the regulations of the Department of Health and Human Services. Risk group 1 substances are not subject to 'infectious substance' shipping or packaging regulations.

B. A *diagnostic specimen* is any human or animal specimen shipped for purposes of diagnosis. It includes, but is not limited to excreta, secreta, blood, blood components, tissue, and tissue fluids. Diagnostic specimens that do not contain pathogens or may contain risk group 1 pathogens are not subject to international air transport regulations. Diagnostic specimens containing risk group 2 or 3 pathogens are packaged and shipped according to regulations governing 'diagnostic specimens'. Diagnostic specimens that contain or may contain risk group 4 pathogens must be classified and conform to the regulations governing 'infectious substances'.

C. *Biological products* are materials derived from living organisms and manufactured in accordance with the regulations of national governmental authorities. Biological products are used in the prevention, diagnosis or treatment of disease in humans or animals. These include certain viruses, therapeutic serums, toxins, antitoxins, vaccines, blood and blood products. Biological products that have a very low probability to produce disease and those packaged for final distribution for use by medical practitioners in personal health care are not subject to special shipping regulations.

Biologic specimens packed with dry ice or liquid nitrogen must meet special packaging instructions that include types of material used for primary receptacle, and support for secondary packaging. If a sample preservative (e.g. ethanol) is classified as a dangerous good, proper instructions for that substance must also be followed.

Infectious substances and diagnostic specimens are shipped for transport by air using *triple packaging* with minor modifications as illustrated in Fig. 14.1.

UN specification packaging is required for shipping infectious substances.

Primary receptacle

- Holds the biological material.
- Must be leak-proof or sift-proof.
  - leak-proof seal is required.
  - if the container has a threaded edge, it must be secured with adhesive tape.
  - if lyophilized substances are being shipped, flame sealed glass ampoules or rubber stopped glass vials with metal seals are required.
- Label.

Secondary container

- Holds one or more primary containers.
- Must be leak-proof or sift-proof.
- If liquid is being shipped, must include enough absorbent material to absorb total contents of liquid in the primary receptacle(s).
- If multiple primary receptacles are included, each must be cushioned to prevent contact and potential for breakage during transport.

Primary or secondary container must be capable of withstanding internal pressure of 95 kpa at a range from −40 °F to 131 °F (−40 °C to 55 °C).

An itemized list of package contents must be included between the secondary container and outer packaging.

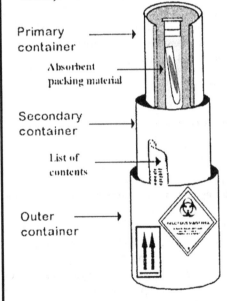

Infectious substances
packaging
(49 CFR 173.196)

- Watertight primary and secondary inner containers
- Primary *or* secondary inner containers capable of withstanding internal pressure of 95 kpa at −40 ° F to 131 ° F
- Outer packaging – smallest external dimension at least 100 mm (3.9 in)
- Capable of passing:
  - 9 m (30 ft) drop test
  - Penetration test
  - Vibration standard

A typical infectious substance packaging configuration (closures not shown):

Primary container

Absorbent packing material

Secondary container

List of contents

Outer container

Fig. 14.1. Instructions for triple packaging of biohazardous materials, UN. From: US Department of Transportation, Research and Special Programs Administration, Hazardous Materials Safety, Washington, DC.

Outer packaging

- Smallest external dimension must be at least 100 mm (3.9 inches) in order for required markings and labels to fit.
- Must be marked to identify hazardous contents.
- If infectious substance is being shipped:
  - Must include proper shipping name, UN number and net quantity for each substance
  - Must include name and telephone number of the individual responsible for the shipment

Labelling and weight limits are based on the type of specimen(s) being shipped as outlined in Table 14.3, and examples of standard labels are illustrated in Fig. 14.2.

Other packaging requirements:

1. Overpacks – used to combine several triple packages into one package.
   - Each triple package inside the overpack must be properly labelled.
   - The outside of the overpack must bear the same markings and labels as the triple packages within.
   - If packed in dry ice, the total net quantity of dry ice must be listed on the outer container.
   - Must be marked with the statement 'inner packages comply with prescribed specifications' (Fig. 14.2(*d*)).
2. Ice and dry ice require special packaging.
   - With ice, all packaging must be leak-proof.
   - With dry ice, outer packaging must allow for the release of carbon dioxide gas and the solid supports must be provided to secure the secondary container as the refrigerant melts.
3. Liquid nitrogen or dry shipper.
   - Special packing regulations apply.

A ***Shipper's Declaration for Dangerous Goods*** must accompany the air bill when shipping infectious substances. A shipper's declaration is not required for diagnostic specimens. A specimen form is illustrated in Fig. 14.3; these are generally provided by each carrier and are also often included with purchased shipping materials.

The Shipper's Declaration for Dangerous Goods includes the following information and warnings:

Table 14.3. Air transport of hazardous materials

Specimen name of shipping	UN	Packing instruction	Labels	Other	Hazard class	Maximum quantity for passenger aircraft	Maximum quantity for cargo aircraft
Infectious substance affecting humans or humans and animals	UN 2814	602	• Class 6 infectious substance Label on outer container	Limit for primary receptacle	6.2	50 ml or 50 g	4 L or 4 kg
Infectious substance affecting animals	UN 2900	602	• If packaged in dry ice, Class 9 diamond label must be placed on one side of outer package – Overpacks containing > 50 ml or 50 g of material, add cargo aircraft label on outer container	500 ml or 500 g	6.2	50 ml or 50 g	4 L or 4 kg

				Ship as infectious substances if reason to suspect that specimen may contain Group 4 pathogens	4 L or 4 kg	4 L or 4 kg
Diagnostic specimen	UN 3373	650	• If shipped by air, include 'diagnostic specimen packed in compliance with IATA packing instruction 650' • If packaged in dry ice, Class 9 diamond label must be placed on one side of outer package • In US, may need international Biohazard symbol on primary or secondary container, if there is the possibility of a blood-borne pathogen	–		
Biological product that meets definition of an infectious material			Treat as infectious material (see above)			
Biological product with low probability to produce disease and those packaged for use by health professionals			Not subject to special shipping regulations: If packaged in dry ice, Class 9 diamond label must be placed on one side of outer package			

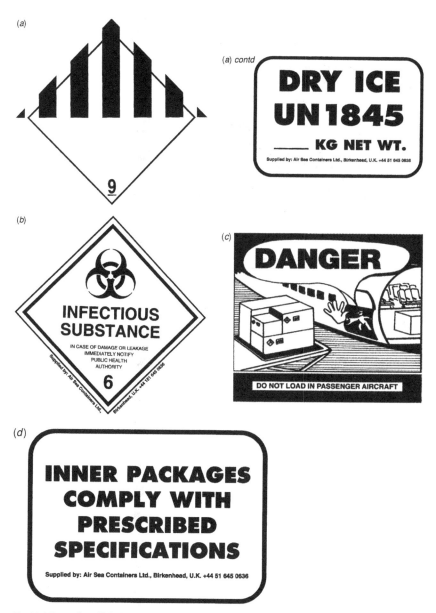

Fig. 14.2. Examples of labels used for mailing of hazardous substances (*a*) dry ice (*b*) infectious substance (*c*) > 50 g or 50 ml of material (*d*) inner package label.

SHIPPERS DECLARATION FOR DANGEROUS GOODS

Shipper	Air Waybill No.
	Page of Pages
	Shipper's Reference Number *(Optional)*

Consignee	
	△ *Air Sea*

Two completed and signed copies of this Declaration must be handed to the operator	**WARNING**
TRANSPORT DETAILS	Failure to comply in all respects with the applicable Dangerous Goods Regulations may be in breach of the applicable law, subject to legal penalties. This Declaration must not, in any circumstances, be completed and/or signed by a consolidator, a forwarder or an IATA cargo agent.
This shipment is within the limitations prescribed for *(delete non applicable)* / Airport of Departure	
PASSENGER AND CARGO AIRCRAFT / CARGO AIRCRAFT ONLY	
Airport of Destination	Shipment type *(delete non-applicable)* NON-RADIOACTIVE RADIOACTIVE

NATURE AND QUANTITY OF DANGEROUS GOODS

Dangerous Goods identification

Proper Shipping Name	Class or Division	UN or ID No.	Packing Group	Subsidiary Risk	Quantity and type of packing	Packing inst.	Authorization

Additional Handling Information

I hereby declare that the contents of this consignment are fully and accurately described above by the proper shipping name, and are classified, packaged, marked and labelled/placarded, and are in all respects in proper condition for transport according to applicable international and national governmental regulations.	Name/Title of Signatory
	Place and Date
	Signature *(see warning above)*

Fig. 14.3. Example of shipper's declaration form: From US Department of Transportation, Research and Special Programs Administration, Hazardous Materials Safety, Washington, DC.

- Shipper:
  - Full name
  - Address
  - Telephone number may be required by contract carriers
- Consignee:
  - Full name and address
  - Name and telephone number of the person responsible for the shipment (this may be shipper, consignee, or another person who should be contacted if there is a delay in shipment).
- Transport details:
  - Include whether or not shipment is restricted to cargo aircraft only (e.g. more than 50 ml or 50 g of infectious substance)
  - Airport of departure – *completed by carrier*
  - Airport of destination – *completed by carrier*
- Nature and quantity of dangerous goods:
  - Mark out "radioactive" to indicate you are shipping non-radioactive materials
- Shipment type:
  - Enter proper shipping name (e.g. infectious substance affecting humans, ***)
  - *** denote the technical name of the substance, e.g. gram-positive rod or *Salmonella* sp.
- Class or division:
  - Enter appropriate hazard class (6.2)
  - UN or ID Number
- Enter appropriate UN number, e.g. UN 2814 for infectious substance affecting humans or animals, UN 2900 for infectious substance affecting animals only.
- Packing group:
  - Dry ice = III (Note: infectious substances are not assigned packing groups)
- Subsidiary risk:
  - Leave blank
- Quantity and type of packaging:
  - Enter net quantity for each material using metric units. At the end of the column, indicate the number and type of packages used (e.g. all packed in one fibreboard box)
- Packaging instructions:
  - Enter appropriate number (e.g. 602 for infectious materials)

- Authorization:
  - Leave blank
- Additional handling instructions:
  - Give emergency contact telephone number
  - Include the statement 'Prior arrangements as required by the IATA Dangerous Goods Regulations 1.3.3.1 have been made'
- Signature and Date

The individual who signs and dates the form declares that the contents of the shipment are fully and accurately described and meet all conditions of transport according to national and international governmental regulations. The form includes the warning that failure to comply with the Dangerous Goods Regulations is subject to legal penalties. The form is completed in triplicate (keep one copy; two for carrier), and regulations require that you keep the copy for 375 days.

Some carriers and other governmental agencies may have additional requirements. Shippers are advised to check with carriers and other agencies that regulate infectious substances and diagnostic specimens (e.g. OSHA in the USA, Department of Health in the UK) to determine additional requirements pertaining to shipment. Instructions must be updated yearly with attention to IATA addendums when the new IATA *Dangerous Goods Regulations* are published.

If shipping by land (e.g. cab, bus, motor vehicle), check with competent regulatory agencies within your governmental jurisdiction for a copy of the regulations that apply to your location.

(With thanks to Patricia L. Payne, Ph.D., JBM Associates, USA, for consultation and editing.)

Useful addresses for air transport of hazardous materials

NIH Infectious Materials Shipping Requirements
National Institutes of Health
Division of Safety
Office of Research Services
Bethesda, MD

Infectious Substances: What You Need to Know
US Department of Transportation
Research and Special Programs Administration
Hazardous Materials Safety
400 Seventh St., SW
DHM-50
Washington, DC 20590

http://www.iata.org/dangerousgoods/
dgr_44edition_changes.htm
http://www.nih.gov/od/ors/ds/shipping/
infectious.html
http://www.nih.gov/od/ors/ds/shipping/
biologic.html
http://www.nih.gov/od/ors/ds/shipping/
documents/infect.pdf
http://www.unece.org/trans/danger/publi/unrec/
12_e.html
http://www.iata.org/NR/ContentConnector/
CS2000/SiteInterface/pdf/
cargo/dg/Consignment_diagnostic_specimens_
2003.pdf
http://www.access.gpo.gov/nara/cfr/waisidx_02/
49cfrv2_02.html
http://www.cdc.gov/od/ohs/biosfty/shipregs.htm

Appendix: general laboratory safety issues

Chemical safety

In the USA this is mandated by OSHA and includes the 'employee right-to-know':
- labelling according to the National Fire Protection Association health risks, including carcinogens and teratogens and hazard class (corrosive, poison, flammable, oxidizing).
- Chemical hygiene plan includes:
  - guidelines of proper labelling of chemicals and materials safety data sheets (MSDS) sheets,
  - personnel safety training,
  - guidelines for annual inventory of hazardous chemicals,
  - information for labelling,

- requirement for fume hoods to prevent inhalation of toxic fumes,
- guidelines for cleaning spills.

Fire safety

- Laboratory must post fire evacuation routes.
- Fire drills must be held quarterly or annually (depends on local laws).
- There must be: fire alarms
  clear exits
  employee training.
- Use of fire extinguishers types A (for trash wood and paper), B (for chemical fires, and C (for electrical fires). Most laboratories use ABC extinguishers, but type C with carbon dioxide are also used because this does not damage equipment.

Electrical safety

- Cords checked regularly
- Plugs 3-prong, grounded
- Sockets checked annually for electrical grounding
- Extension cores

Handling of compressed gases

- Tanks should be chained and stored in well-ventilated area (includes cryotanks).

REFERENCES

Annas, G. (1998). Protecting patients from discrimination: The American with Disabilities Act and HIV infection. *New England Journal Medicine*, **339**: 1255–9.

Baccetti, B., Benedetto, A., Collodel, G. *et al.* (1999). Failure of HIV-1 to infect human oocytes directly. *Journal of Acquired Immune Deficiency Syndrome*, **21**: 355–61.

Bourlet, T., Levy, R., Laporte, S. *et al.* (2003). Multicenter quality control for the detection of hepatitis C virus RNA in seminal plasma specimens. *Journal of Clinical Microbiology*, **41**(2): 789–93.

Bragdon vs. Abbott (1998): 524. US 624.118 S. Ct 2196.

Chan, A. N., Luetjens, C. M., Dominko, T. *et al.* (2000). Transgenic ICSI reviewed: foreign DNA transmission by intracytoplasmic sperm injection in rhesus monkey.

Molecular Human Reproduction and Development, **56** (Suppl.): 325–8.

Dangerous Goods Regulations (2003), 44th edn. Montreal, Quebec, Canada: IATA.

Gilling-Smith, C. & Almeida, P. (2003). HIV, hepatitis B and hepatitis C and infertility: reducing the risk. *Human Fertility*, **6**: 106–12.

Guaschino, S., Ricci, G., De Seta, F., Nucera, G., Pozzobon, C. & Guarnieri, S. (2003). Percorso diagnostico e comportamentale 'counselling' per la coppia infetta a rischio di trasmissibilità. In *Infezioni e Riproduzione*, ed. M. E. Coccia, A. Borinini, A. Massacesi & G. Ragusa, pp. 49–60. Roma: CIC Edizioni Internazionali.

Hadchouel, M., Scotto, J., Huret, J. *et al.* (1995). Presence of HBV DNA in spermatozoa: a possible vertical transmission of HBV via the germ line. *Journal of Medical Virology*, **16**: 61–6.

Huang, J. M., Huang, T. H., Qiu, H. Y., Fang, X. W., Zhuang, T. G. & Qiu, J. W. (2002). Studies on the integration of hepatitis B virus DNA sequence in human sperm chromosomes. *Asian Journal of Andrology*, **4**(3): 209–12.

Kiessling, A. A. (1998). Expression of human immunodeficiency virus long terminal repeat-coupled genes in early cleaving embryos. *Journal of Reproductive Immunology*, **41**: 95–104.

Lesourd, F., Izopet, J., Mervan, C. *et al.* (2000). Transmission of hepatitis C virus during the ancillary procedures for assisted conception. *Human Reproduction*, **15**(5): 1083–5.

Levy, R., Bourlet, T., Maertens, A. *et al.* (2002). Pregnancy after safe IVF with hepatitis C virus RNA-positive sperm. *Human Reproduction*, **17**(10): 2650–3.

Marina, S., Marina, F., Alcolea, R. *et al.* (1998). Human immunodeficiency virus type 1-serodiscordant couples can bear healthy children after undergoing intrauterine insemination. *Fertility and Sterility*, **70**: 35–9.

Nuovo, G. J., Becker, J., Simsir, A., Margiotta, M., Khalife, M. & Shevchuk, M. (1994). HIV-1 nucleic acids localize to the spermatogonia and their progeny: a study by polymerase chain reaction *in situ* hybridization. *American Journal of Pathology*, **144**: 1142–8.

Perry, A. C. F., Wakayama, T., Kishikawa, H. *et al.* (1999). Mammalian transgenesis by intracytoplasmic sperm injection. *Science*, **284**: 1180–3.

Piomboni, P. & Bacetti, B. (2000). Spermatozoa as a vehicle for HIV-1 and other viruses: a review. *Molecular Reproduction and Development*, **56**: 238–42.

Semprini, A., Levi-Setti, P., Bozzo, M., Ravizzi, M. & Pardi G. (1992). Insemination of HIV-negative women with processed semen of HIV-positive partners. *Lancet*, **340**: 1317–19.

Scofield, V. L., Rao, B., Broder, S. *et al.* (1994). HIV interaction with sperm. *AIDS*, **8**(12): 1733–6.

Shevchuk, M. M., Nuovo, G. J. & Khalife, G. (1998). HIV in testis: quantitative histology and HIV localization in germ cells. *Journal of Reproductive Immunology*, **41**: 69–80.

Updated US public health service (USPHS) guidelines for the management of occupational exposure to HBV, HCV, and HIV, and Recommendations for postexposure prophylaxis (2001). http://www.cdc.gov/mmwr

FURTHER READING

US Department of Health and Human Service, CDCP & NIH (1999). *Biosafety in Microbiological and Biomedical Laboratories*, 4th edn. Washington, DC: US Goverment Printing Office.

Health and Safety Executive, UK (2001). *Blood-borne Viruses in the Workplace: Guidance for Employers and Employees*. Sudbury, Suffolk: HSE Books.

Advisory Committee on Dangerous Pathogens (1995, 2000). *Categorisation of Biological Agents According to Hazard and Categories of Containment*, 4th edn (1995), 2nd Suppl. (2000). London: HMSO Publications.

Coccia, M.E., Borini, A., Massacesi, A. & Ragusa, G. (eds.)(2002). *Consensus Conference: Infezione e Riproduzione.* Romai CIC Edizioni Internazionali.

Dimitrakopoulos, A. A. (2003). HIV and gamete interactions. *Human Fertility*, **6**: 81–3

Ethics Committee of the American Society for Reproductive Medicine (2002). Human immunodeficiency virus and infertility treatment. *Fertility and Sterility*, **77**(2): 218–22.

Advisory Committee on Dangerous Pathogens (1996a). *Microbiological Risk Assessment: An Interim Report*. London: HMSO.

(1996b). *Protection Against Blood-borne Infections in the Workplace: HIV and Hepatitis*. London: HMSO.

—2002 Revised advice on laboratory containment measure for work with tissue samples in clinical cytogenetics laboratories, Health & Safety Executive, UK.

Medical Microbiology: A Short Course. Baron E.J., Chang, R.S., Howard, D.H., Miller, J.N. & Turner, J.A. (eds.)(1994). New York: Wiley-Liss.

Alexander, N. J. (1998). HIV and germinal cells: how close an association? *Journal of Reproductive Immunology*, **41**: 17–26.

Baccetti, B., Benedetto, A., Borini, A. *et al.* (1994). HIV-particles in spermatozoa of patients with AIDS and their transfer into the oocyte. *Journal of Cell Biology*, **127**: 903–14.

Baccetti, B., Benedetto, A., Collodel, G., di Caro, A., Garbuglia, A. R. & Piomboni, P. (1998). The debate on the presence of HIV-1 in human gametes. *Journal of Reproductive Immunology*, **41**(1–2): 41–67.

Blank, S., Simonds, R. J. & Weisfuse, L. (1994). Possible nosocomial transmission of HIV. *Lancet*, **334**: 512.

The BLEFCO Federation (1997). The proposed position statement on the preliminary screening of hepatitis B and hepatitis C of tentative intra-couple medically assisted reproduction. *Contraception Fertilité Sexualité*, **25**(4): 313–24.

Bourlet, T., Levy, R., Maertens, A. *et al.* (2002). Detection and characterization of hepatitis C virus RNA in seminal plasma and spermatozoon fractions of semen from patients attempting medically assisted conception. *Journal of Clinical Microbiology*, **40**(9): 3252–5.

Chrystie, I., Mullen, J., Braude, P. *et al.* (1998). Assisted conception in HIV discordant couples: evaluation of processing techniques in reducing HIV viral load. *Journal of Reproductive Immunology*, **41**: 301–6.

Connor, E., Sperling, R. & Gelbert, R. (1994). Reduction of maternal-infant transmission of HIV type 1 with zidovudine treatment. Paediatric AIDS clinical trials group. Protocol 076 study group. *New England Journal of Medicine*, **331**: 1173–80.

Greene, W. C. & Peterlin, B. M. (2002). Review: charting HIV's remarkable voyage through the cell: basic science as a passport to future therapy. *Nature Medicine*, **8**: 673–80.

Levy, R., Tardy, J. C., Bourlet, T. *et al.* (2000). Transmission risk of hepatitis C virus in assisted reproductive techniques. *Human Reproduction*, **15**(4): 810–16.

Marcus, S. F., Avery, S. M., Abusheikha, N., Marcus, N. K. & Brinsden, P. R. (2000) The case for routine HIV screening before IVF treatment: a survey of UK IVF centre policies. *Human Reproduction*, **15**(8): 1657–61.

McKee, T. A., Avery, S., Majid, A. & Brinsden, P. R. (1996). Risks for transmission of hepatitis C virus during artificial insemination. *Fertility and Sterility*, **66**: 161–3.

Muciaccia, B., Filippini, A., Ziparo, E., Colelli, F., Baroni, C. D. & Stefanini, M. (1998). Testicular germ cells of HIV seropositive asymptomatic men are infected by the virus. *Journal of Reproductive Immunology*, **41**: 81–93.

Passos, E. P., Silveira, T. R. & Salazar, C. C. (2002). Hepatitis C virus infection and assisted reproduction. *Human Reproduction*, **17**(8): 2085–8.

Richmond, J. (1998). The 1,2,3's of biosafety levels. Adapted from *Biosafety in Microbiological and Biomedical Laboratories*, 3rd edn. US Department of Health and Human Service, CDCP & NIH. Washington, DC: US Government Printing Office.

Semprini, A. E., Savasi, V., Hollander, L. & Tanzi, E. (2001). Mother-to-child HCV transmission. *Lancet*, **357**(9250): 141.

Steyaert, S. R., Leroux-Roels, G. G. & Dhont, M. (2000). Infections in IVF: review and guidelines. *Human Reproduction Update*, **6**(5): 432–41.

Tesourdi, L., Testart, J., Cerutti, L., Moussu, J. P., Loeuillet, AL. & Courto, A.-M. (2002). Failure to infect embryos after virus injection in mouse zygotes. *Human Reproduction*, **17**(3): 760–4.

15

Prevention: patient screening and the use of donor gametes

Routine screening

Prevalence of BBV: geographic distribution

The risk of introducing infection into the laboratory can be minimized by screening patients for infectious agents where indicated by medical history and physical examination. The risk of infectious agent transmission in ART procedures varies in different populations and geographical regions; a risk assessment should be carried out according to the prevalence of disease in the specific patient population, bearing in mind the possibility of 'silent' infection prior to detectable seroconversion. Figures 15.1–15.4 illustrate the current geographic distribution for infections due to HIV/AIDS, HBV and HCV.

National and international guidelines in many countries now recommend that patients presenting for ART procedures should undergo routine testing for Hepatitis B and C annually; screening for HIV-1 and HIV-2 should be carried out within 3–6 months of starting treatment to allow for the lag time to seroconversion. Human T-cell lymphotrophic virus (HTLV-I and HTLV-II) has a low prevalence in Western countries, with HTLV-I principally endemic in Japan, Central Africa, the Caribbean and Malaysia, and HTLV-II prevalent in Central America and the southern USA. Screening for these viruses prior to blood or organ donation is now mandatory in some countries; guidelines for HTLV-I and HTLV-II patient screening prior to ART procedures should be adapted to local regulations and epidemiology. Routine screening for genital infections, i.e. syphilis,

gonorrhea, chlamydia, herpes simplex, human papilloma virus and vaginal infections should be assessed within the context of patient population, prevalence of disease and full medical history/physical examination of both partners.

The use of donor gametes

Infectious agents in semen can be transmitted by artificial insemination; those associated with oocytes as well as with semen can be transmitted via IVF and ICSI. Infectious agents may produce local or disseminated disease in the inseminated woman as well as possibly affect the outcome of a resulting pregnancy. Complete and rigorous screening is mandatory when donor gametes are used in ART procedures in order to ensure safety and good practice for patients and donors. Although legislation, regulations and practice differ among countries and in different parts of the world, consensus guidelines regarding minimum requirements for testing of semen and oocyte donors have been published both in Europe (Englert, 1998) and in the USA (FDA). Guidelines should be assessed and adapted in the context of local situations, according to geographical region and prevalence of disease in that specific region.

In 1998, a European multidisciplinary group of experts drew up a consensus document of guidelines surrounding both sperm and oocyte donation. These guidelines, based upon several meetings, critical discussion and review by experts are published as

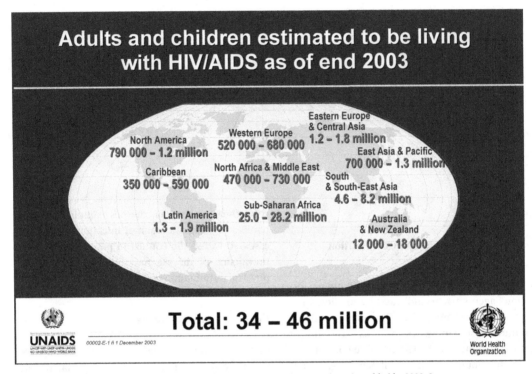

Fig. 15.1. Number of adults and children estimated to be infected with HIV and AIDS worldwide, 2002–3.
Source: Joint United Nations Program on AIDS.

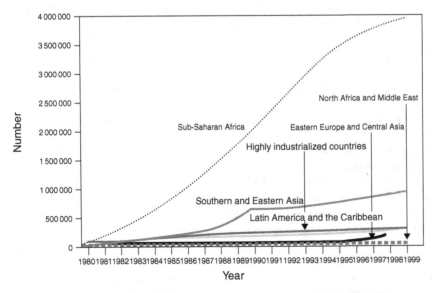

Fig. 15.2. Estimated number of new HIV infections, by region and year – worldwide, 1980–1999.
Source: Joint United Nations Program on AIDS.

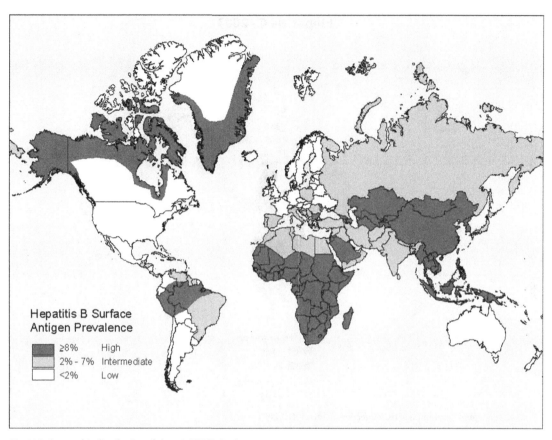

Fig. 15.3. Geographic distribution of chronic HBV infection.
http://www.cdc.gov/ncidod/diseases/hepatitis

The Corsendonk Consensus Document for the European Union (Barrat *et al.*, 1998), and the following is an excerpt from the book published as a supplement to *Human Reproduction* in 1998 (*Gamete Donation: Current Ethics in the European Union*, ed. Y. Englert):

Recruitment of donors

(i) Donors must be informed about the use of their gametes, the maximum number of family units into which children can be born using their gametes, medical risks of the procedures and the legislation and rules of the centre.

(ii) Counselling must be offered.

(iii) Fully informed consent must be obtained; the donors must be allowed to withdraw their consent for further use of their gametes at any time.

(iv) Donors must be at least 18 years of age and a mandatory upper age limit set. The upper limit should be 45 years for semen donation, and it should be <36 years for oocyte donation.

(v) A staff member must not be accepted as a donor in his(her) own centre.

(vi) Anonymous donation should be encouraged.

(vii) Gametes should not be donated in exchange for money. Documented travel costs may be reimbursed. The amount of payment given must be limited so that it is not the primary reason for donation.

Hepatitis C, 2003

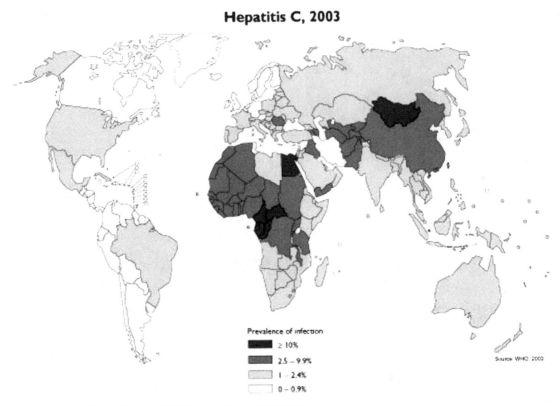

Prevalence of infection

▉	≥ 10%
▉	2.5 – 9.9%
░	1 – 2.4%
☐	0 – 0.9%

Source: WHO 2003

Fig. 15.4. Geographic distribution of HCV infection. *Source*: WHO, 2003.

(viii) When possible, centres should recruit gamete donors who already have children without major hereditary disease.

- A physician must evaluate the health status and the medical history of the donor, in order to avoid any major problems interfering with fertility or transmission of disease.
- Information on donor identification available to the offspring is a matter of debate; this is covered by legislation in some countries.

Screening

Infectious disease

(i) The following tests, carried out with clinically acceptable procedures, must be negative at the initial screening:

- HIV-1 and HIV-2 in serum,
- HTLV in serum according to local prevalence
- syphilis, hepatitis B and hepatitis C,
- *Neisseria gonorrhea* and *Chlamydia trachomatis* in semen or urine.

(ii) The following tests (with the use of reliable techniques) must be negative at the end of the donation period:

- *Neisseria gonorrhea* and *Chlamydia trachomatis* in semen or urine

(iii) The following tests, carried out with clinically acceptable procedures, must be negative after 6 months of quarantine:

- HIV-1 and HIV-2, and HTLV when applicable
- syphilis, hepatitis B and C.

(iv) Donors must be tested for cytomegalovirus (CMV) antibodies, IgG and IgM, initially and after a 6-month period of quarantine. If seroconversion is detected, the donor must be rejected.

Screening for genetic disease

(i) A physician must record the donor family history for genetic diseases.
(ii) Karyotyping should be performed.
(iii) Selective testing for recessive genetic diseases prevalent according to ethnic origin should be performed.
(iv) Donors with major hereditary diseases must be rejected.
(v) If a genetic risk factor is detected in the donor, the decision concerning the use of his/her gametes must be made in collaboration with a geneticist.

Procedures and technical aspects

(i) Centres must ensure that the highest possible standards are maintained in the handling and storage of gametes.
(ii) The regulations and the procedures involved in the handling and storage of gametes must be clearly and specifically defined.
(iii) Gamete donation centres must have well-trained staff who have access to the necessary equipment.
(iv) Gamete donation programmes should be run by multidisciplinary teams. They should have a minimum level of activity as defined according to various geographical situations.
(v) Appropriate quality control and quality assurance in the laboratory and other procedures must be applied.
- Gametes must be collected in the centre, with documented chain of custody.
- Strict measures must be taken in order to respect the confidentiality of donors and recipients.
- The exchange of gametes between centres using comparable standards should be possible. Commercial trading of human gametes should be prohibited.

- Only frozen and thawed samples quarantined for 6 months may be used for semen donation. Appropriate tests to avoid risks of infectious disease transmission must be done initially and at the end of the quarantine period.
- In the absence of an effective technique to freeze oocytes, only frozen embryos should be used in a donor oocyte programme. This practice allows for a quarantine period so that necessary tests can be repeated for the oocyte donors. If fresh embryos are transferred in the donor oocyte programme, the recipient must be clearly informed that there is a risk of infectious disease transmission.
- Spermatozoa or semen from two different men or oocytes from two different women must not be used in the same treatment cycle.
- Accurate medical records of all donors must be kept in separate files by the centre.

Use of gametes for donation

(i) Recipients must receive information regarding the methods of donor recruitment and screening, the medical risks of treatment, the legislation, the procedures and the success rates of the centres.
(ii) Counselling must be offered to the recipients.
(iii) Fully informed signed consent must be obtained from recipients.
(iv) Gamete donation must not be used for eugenic purposes.
(v) Donor and recipient phenotypic characteristics should be matched.
(vi) Recipients seronegative for CMV markers must receive gametes only from seronegative donors.
(vii) Although the risk of consanguinity as a consequence of gamete donation is extremely low, the number of children born from a single donor must be limited and controlled.
(viii) The number of children born from a single donor should be limited to a low number for social and psychological reasons.

(ix) Since several children could be conceived in a single family with gametes of the same donor, it is the number of recipient family units with such children that should be limited in gamete donation.

Treatment evaluation

(i) The outcome of treatment using donated gametes (including pregnancies) must be recorded by the centre.

(ii) Each centre must provide public information on an annual basis regarding treatment and success rates.

(iii) Centralization of statistics and data readily accessible to the public should be an objective.

Summary of donor testing practices and proposals in the USA

Current guidelines/proposed legislation in the United States are summarized in Tables 15.1 and 15.2.

Cryopreservation and transmission of infection

Cryopreservation and liquid nitrogen cryostorage for sperm and embryos has been a routine component of ART laboratories since the early 1980s and is now essential for any ART laboratory that offers the use of donor gametes in patient treatment. The identification of viruses in semen, the lag time to seroconversion and reports of infection transmitted to recipients has made the use of fresh semen absolutely unacceptable. Only cryopreserved semen that has been quarantined and the donors re-tested before clinical use is acceptable for insemination procedures. However, in many cases samples from several donors may share the same liquid nitrogen Dewar during the 'quarantine' period, so that semen from an uninfected donor could be stored with infected semen, with the potential for cross-contamination unless suitable precautions in sample processing and storage are in place. Oocytes and embryos for

donation should also preferably be quarantined and the donors screened before transfer to a recipient. The recent introduction of long-term storage for cryopreserved ovarian and testicular tissue presents a further set of ethical and logistic problems and considerations for the ART laboratory.

Transmission of viruses through assisted reproduction techniques is a major concern in the bovine embryo transfer industry. International Embryo Transfer Society (IETS) guidelines for washing and trypsin treatment of bovine embryos derived in vivo were designed to eliminate a variety of pathogens before embryo transfer, but these procedures appear to be less effective for some viruses when applied to embryos produced in vitro (IVP). It appears that there are differences in the zona pellucida (ZP) of embryos produced in vitro and in vivo, making IVP embryos more difficult to decontaminate following exposure to viruses – some viruses are easier to remove than others. Ultrastructural differences in the ZP from IVP embryos can allow viral particles to become entrapped in 'pores' (Stringfellow *et al.*, 2000). In addition, the ability of trophectoderm projections of these embryos to penetrate the zona could be a means of transit for viral infection around the time of implantation (Gonzales *et al.*, 1996). Experiments that deliberately exposed IVP embryos to bovine viral diarrhea virus (BVDV) or bovine foot and mouth disease virus (FMDV) showed that embryos can retain virus, with an effect on cleavage rates and development. ZP-free embryos are particularly susceptible to infection. As a result of this experimental data, embryos produced in vitro can no longer be moved across state or national boundaries. Risk assessment has become very sophisticated, and risk management is now commonly applied in connection with animal health and import/export of livestock genetic material (for list of references, see www.iets.org, import/export link).

Apart from the hazards of storing potentially infected samples, liquid nitrogen has been clearly identified as a source of potential exogenous contamination, as well as a medium for allowing cross-contamination between samples. In 1995 Tedder *et al.* reported a cluster of hepatitis B infections in

Table 15.1. Summary of donor testing practices and proposals (FDA Proposed Regulation, September 1999)

Test	Sperm donation				Oocyte donation			Embryo donation		
	Male partner	Female recipient	Male donor		Male partner	Female recipient	Female donor	Donors		Recipients
			Initial	6 mo				Initial	6 mo[a]	Initial
HIV-1			×	×			×	×		
HIV-2			×	×			×	×		
Hep B/C			×	×			×	×		
Syphilis			×	×			×	×		
CMV			×	×				× (male)		
HTLV-I/II			×	×				× (male)		
Gonorrhoeae			×	×			×	×		
Chlamydia			×	×			×	×		
Other STD			×					×		

[a] Under discussion.

Table 15.2. Summary of donor testing practices and proposals (ASRM Guidelines, June 2002)

Test	Sperm donation				Oocyte donation			Embryo donation		
	Male partner	Female recipient	Male donor		Male partner	Female recipient	Female donor	Donors		Recipients
			Initial	6 mo				Initial	6 mo	Initial
HIV-1	×-R	×	×	×	×	×-R	×	×		×-R
HIV-2		×	×	×			×			
Hep B/C		×	×	×	×	×-R	×	×		×-R
Syphilis		×	×	×	×	×-R	×	×		×-R
CMV		×	×	×	×	×-R	×			
HTLV-I/II		×	×	×						
Gonorrhoeae		×-R	×	×			×			
Chlamydia		×-R	×	×			×			
Other STD	×-R									

R = recommended.

Note: *Tables for FDA and ASRM testing proposals modified from handout provided by Martha Wells, CBER, FDA* bone marrow/peripheral blood stem cell recipients. The source of infection was definitively traced to a single infected bone marrow sample stored in the same liquid nitrogen tank as non-infected samples. Hepatitis B viral DNA was found in detritus extracted from the storage tank; contamination of the liquid nitrogen apparently occurred via a cracked and leaking cryopreservation bag that allowed infected material to come into contact with liquid nitrogen and then penetrate other specimens. Other viruses have also been shown to survive direct exposure to liquid nitrogen, including vesicular stomatitis virus, herpes simplex virus, adenovirus and papilloma virus. Liquid nitrogen itself may carry exogenous contamination; specifications for purity from suppliers are chemical, not biological. Fountain *et al.* (1997) grew a wide range of bacterial and fungal species after taking swabs from five liquid nitrogen vessels. One liquid nitrogen tank was found to be heavily contaminated with an *Aspergillus* species. Liquid nitrogen may be supplied from a non-sterile source, and/or organisms from the environment can contaminate nitrogen or any of its container vessels during handling procedures.

All of the above data make it imperative that every ART laboratory should be aware of the hazards involved in cryostorage and have clear guidelines and protocols in place regarding patient screening and safe handling of samples and liquid nitrogen. Vapour phase controlled rate freezers spray non-sterile liquid nitrogen directly onto the samples. Any direct contamination may be further compounded by liquid condensate accumulating within ducting between freezing runs, becoming contaminated by microbes and then blown onto samples. Cross-contamination of IVF samples may arise at various steps during cryopreservation, and storage tanks, containers, freezing equipment and water baths must be kept clean, with a schedule for regular decontamination. Pipetting devices and sealing instruments must be similarly cleaned and decontaminated regularly. Samples that have not been screened, and those from known infected patients, should be stored in separate containers, and transfer of liquid nitrogen between vessels must be avoided.

The type of container used for cryostorage, and the techniques used for transferring cells to and from the containers affect the risk for potential cross-contamination. Containers must be filled and sealed very carefully to avoid contamination of the external surface and to minimize the chance of leakage and rupture during freezing/thawing.

(i) Traditional straws used for semen storage can be difficult to fill aseptically, and the end/outside is easily contaminated. Overfilled straws can crack or release their plugs during freezing, and straws that are inadequately sealed can absorb potentially contaminated liquid nitrogen, leading to possible cross-infection. Polyvinyl alcohol (PVA) powder used for sealing straws is not only ineffective in creating an impermeable seal, but can also harbour microorganisms that may be introduced into samples and thence to recipient patients.

(ii) Plastic cryovials with a screw cap do not maintain their seal when placed in liquid nitrogen: Clarke (1999) demonstrated that 45% of cryovials without an O-ring and 85% of those with an O-ring, absorbed up to 1 ml of liquid nitrogen during a 3-hour immersion. There was no evidence of liquid nitrogen condensation inside the vials when they were stored in the vapour phase for 16–24 hours.

(iii) If completely and effectively sealed, glass ampoules should theoretically be safe from cross-contamination; however, this can be difficult to achieve in practice.

Awareness of the above problems has led to the development of new packaging for bone marrow cells, encasing them in a secondary container ('double-bagging') in order to overcome the problem of leakage from cracked bags.

A leak-free system has also been developed for gametes and embryos, the Cryobiosystem (CBS™) 'high security' straw system. These straws are made of highly resistant, non-toxic ionomeric resin (IR) that contains no plastifying agent. This ensures that they will not fracture under normal stress conditions of freezing/thawing. These straws can be filled via a sterile nozzle so that the outside of the straw is free of contamination after filling, and the ends should be heat sealed to ensure that the seal is leakproof. The straws can be identified by using internal rods, providing a tamper-proof printed identification label that is sealed within the straw.

Schnauffer *et al.* (2003) designed an experiment to determine the efficacy of CBS straws in preventing bacterial cross-contamination, by loading them with samples inoculated with *E. coli* and *E. facecalis*. Their results demonstrated that the straws can be contaminated externally even when filled via the nozzle, and that the sealing machine can also become contaminated and transmit infection. The level of contamination was decreased by wiping the exterior of the straws after filling. Letur-Könirsch *et al.* (2003) tested the safety of three different kinds of straws under cryopreservation conditions: polyvinyl chloride (PVC), polyethylene terephthalate glycol (PETG) and high-security ionomeric resin (IR). After filling, sealing, freezing and thawing straws that had been filled with 100 µl of a supernatant containing a high load of HIV-1 (15 000 cpm/50 µl reverse transcriptase activity), the authors were able to identify potential sources of contamination during the process.

- The straw material or cotton plug of PVC straws might be permeable.
- The sealing system for both PVC and PETG straws may be defective, either splashing the straw contents at the time of sealing, or contaminating the outside of the straw from a seal that is not impervious. Decontaminating the straw with bleach after sealing did not completely eliminate this risk.
- The sealing instrument can become contaminated.
- They were not able to demonstrate cross-contamination in their experiments using IR straws, and concluded that these straws appear to be safe for storing HIV positive samples in ART. Wiping straws externally to decontaminate after filling is recommended.

The results of both the above experiments confirm that extreme caution and care must always be exercised when handling material for cryopreservation, even when 'high security' systems are used.

Sterilization of liquid nitrogen Dewars is difficult to achieve; many of the available disinfectants cause severe corrosion problems with aluminium Dewars, which may result in a catastrophic loss of vacuum. Potential contamination can be reduced by allowing them to warm periodically, carefully disposing of any accumulated liquid, then washing with alcohol and drying.

Vapour-phase storage has been recommended as a means of minimizing the chance of cross-contamination and has been shown to be effective for short-term storage of semen samples. However, there are temperature gradients from the nitrogen surface to the top of the vapour column, with the top of the column rapidly warmed each time the vessel is opened, making it difficult to maintain all samples at an adequately low temperature. The long-term reliability of this strategy, especially for embryos, is unknown. Fungal and bacterial contamination has been found in the vapour phase of a freezer used to store hematopoietic cells (Fountain *et al.*, 1997): the risks of environmental contamination therefore still remain.

Tissue banking: ovarian and testicular tissue

Recent research suggests that primordial oocytes and spermatogonia can be cryopreserved by freezing small biopsies of ovarian cortex or testis: this procedure might be used to preserve fertility for oncology patients who are likely to lose ovarian or testicular function after treatment for malignant disease. These procedures are currently experimental and successful restoration of fertility following gonadal cryopreservation and autotransplantation has not so far been reported. The potential for future application of these techniques is therefore yet to be determined. A working party set up by the UK Royal College of Obstetricians and Gynaecologists published a report (RCOG, 2000) that reviewed the scientific background and ethical procedures to be considered, and developed a voluntary code of best practice for the storage of gonadal tissue. Following new guidelines for tissue banking published by the

Department of Health (DoH) in February 2001, the Association of Clinical Embryologists UK (ACE), the British Fertility Society (BFS) and the RCOG issued a joint statement of advice on good clinical practice regarding cryopreservation for fertility preservation. The DoH guidelines apply to laboratory practices required for specimen preparation, handling and cryopreservation of ovarian and pre-pubertal tissue, and also include recommendations on screening, infrastructure and management. Based on these guidelines, the tissues should be stored separately from embryos and sperm and a quarantine period applied in order to allow for complete infection screen. The DoH Guidelines suggest that a total Quality Management System, based upon the ISO 9000 series, should be in place. This quality system must be documented and maintained, including standard operating procedures, specifications and records, and should cover:

- tissue bank, buildings and premises,
- environmental controls,
- managerial responsibilities,
- donor selection and testing,
- written agreements of contracts with third parties,
- testing of tissues to specifications,
- record keeping,
- transport of tissues,
- regular review meetings by key personnel,
- provision of resources.

The facilities should be housed in buildings that are appropriate for the purpose, with efficient cleaning and maintenance, as well as environmental controls designed to avoid contamination. Processing areas should have standard precautions in place and critical work areas where the tissue is manipulated openly must have Level 2 facilities. These must be monitored by microbiological testing according to a documented procedure and defined plan, using measures such as settle plates or glove prints. All tissue must be traceable using documented procedures through all stages.

In the UK, the Department of Health Code of Practice on Tissue Banking has ruled that from 1 April, 2003, ovarian and testicular tissue must be stored in accredited tissue banks only.

In view of the stringent measures that are necessary to maintain strict safety levels, the ethical dilemmas involved and the relatively limited number of samples that are likely to require banking, the decision by an ART unit to offer gonadal tissue cryopreservation to patients must be taken judiciously, after assessing the need. A multidisciplinary team should carefully consider all the factors necessary to provide a safe and secure service.

A European Union directive is currently being drafted, in order to 'Set standards of quality and safety for the donation, procurement, testing, processing, storage and distribution of human tissues and cells' (http://europa.eu.int). This Directive will cover all banked tissues used in therapy, including gametes, embryos and stem cells. If this is adopted as legislation, the standards for storage of embryos and gametes will be brought into line with those for other tissues. It is therefore essential that all clinics practising assisted conception treatment should strive to apply and maintain stringent high standards of total quality management in all aspects of their procedures, in order to offer all fertility patients a safe and effective service.

REFERENCES

Barrat, C. L., Englert, Y., Gottlieb, B. & Jouannet, P. (1998). Gamete donation guidelines. The Corsendonk consensus document for the European Union. *Human Reproduction*, **13**: 500–1.

Clarke, G. N. (1999). Sperm cryopreservation: is there a significant risk of cross-contamination? *Human Reproduction*, **14**: 2941–3.

Englert, Y. (ed.) (1998). Gamete donation: current ethics in the European Union. *Human Reproduction*, **13** (Suppl.2). Oxford: Oxford University Press.

Food and Drug Administration (FDA), USA: www.fda.gov/cber/tiss.htm

Fountain, D., Ralston, M., Higgins, N. *et al.* (1997). Liquid nitrogen freezers: potential source of haematopoietic stem cell contaminants. *Transfusion*, **37**: 585–91.

Gonzales, D. S., Jones, J. M., Pinyopummintr, T. *et al.* (1996). Trophectoderm projections: a potential means for locomotion, attachment and implementation of bovine, equine and human blastocysts. *Human Reproduction*, **11** (12): 2739–45.

Letur-Könirsch, H., Collin, G., Sifer, C. *et al.* (2003). Safety of cryopreservation straws for human gametes of embryos: a study with human immunodeficiency virus-1 under cryopreservation conditions. *Human Reproduction*, **18**(1): 140–4.

Royal College of Obstetricians and Gynaecologists, UK (2000). *Storage of Ovarian and Prepubertal Testicular Tissue: Report of a working party* www.rcog.or.uk.

Schnauffer, K., Measock, S., Neal, T. J., Lewis-Jones, D. I., Kingsland, C. R. & Troup, S. A. (2003). An investigation to determine the efficacy of CBS™ Cryobiostraws in preventing bacterial contamination. *Abstracts of the Association of Clinical Embryologists Annual Conference, 2003*, **05**: 9.

Stringfellow, D. A., Riddell, K. P., Galik, P. K., Damiani, P., Bishop, M. D. & Wright, J. C. (2000). Quality controls for bovine viral diarrhea virus-free IVF embryos. *Theriogenology*, **53**(3): 827–39.

Tedder, R. S., Zuckerman, A. H. & Goldstone, A. H. (1995). Hepatitis B transmission from contaminated cryopreservation tank. *Lancet*, **346**: 137–40.

FURTHER READING

A Code of Practice for Tissue Banks: providing tissues of human origin for therapeutic purposes. (2001). UK Department of Health, ISBN 1 84182 329 5. www.doh.gov.uk/humantissuebanking

Araneta, M. R. G., Mascola, L., Eller, A. *et al.* (1995). HIV transmission through donor artificial insemination. *Journal of the American Medical Association*, **273**: 854–8.

Berry, W. R., Gottesfeld, R. L., Alter, H. J. & Vierling, J. M. (1987). Transmission of hepatitis B virus by artificial insemination. *Journal of the American Medical Association*, **257**: 1079–81.

Bielanski, A., Nadin-Davis, S., Sapp, T. & Lutze-Wallace, C. (2000). Viral contamination of embryos cryopreserved in liquid nitrogen. *Cryobiology*, **40**(2): 110–16.

Bielanski, A., Sapp, T. & Lutze-Wallace, C. (1998). Association of bovine embryos produced by in vitro fertilization with a noncytopathic strain of bovine viral diarrhea virus type II. *Theriogenology*, **49**(6): 1231–8.

Booth, P. J., Stevens, D. A., Collins, M.E. & Brownlie, J. (1995). Detection of bovine viral diarrhoea virus antigen and RNA in oviduct and granulosa cells of persistently infected cattle. *Journal of Reproduction and Fertility*, **105**(1): 17–24.

Booth, P. J., Collins, M. E., Jenner, L. *et al.* (1998). Non-cytopathogenic bovine viral diarrhea virus (BVDV) reduces cleavage but increases blastocyst yield of *in vitro* produced embryos. *Theriogenology*, **50**(5): 769–77.

CDC (1990). HIV-1 infection and artificial insemination with processed semen. *Morbidity and Mortality Weekly Report*, **39**: 249–56.

Centifanto, Y. M., Drylie, D. M., Deardourff, S. L. & Kaufman, H. E. (1972). Herpesvirus type 2 in the male genitourinary tract. *Science*, **178**: 318–19.

Chauhan, M., Barratt, C. L. R., Cooke S. & Cooke, D. (1989). Screening for cytomegalovirus antibody in a donor insemination program: difficulties in implementing the American Fertility Society guidelines. *Fertility and Sterility*, **51**: 901–2.

Chiasson, M. A., Stoneburner, R. L. & Joseph, S. C. (1990). Human immunodeficiency virus transmission through artificial insemination. *Journal of Acquired Immune Deficiency Syndromes*, **3**: 69–72.

Clarke, G. N., Bourne, H., Hill, P. *et al.* (1997). Artificial insemination and in-vitro fertilization using donor spermatozoa: a report on 15 years of experience. *Human Reproduction*, **12**: 722–6.

Davis, L. E., Stewart, J. A. & Garvin, S. (1975). Cytomegalovirus infection: a seroepidemiologic comparison of nuns and women from a venereal disease clinic. *American Journal of Epidemiology*, **102**: 327–30.

Deture, F. A., Drylie D. M., Kaufman H. E. & Centifano, Y. M. (1978). Herpesvirus type 2: study of semen in male subjects with recurrent infections. *Journal of Urology*, **120**: 449–51.

Givens, M. D., Galik, P. K., Riddell, K. P., Brock, K. V. & Stringfellow, D. A. (1999). Quantity and infectivity of embryo-associated bovine viral diarrhea virus and antiviral influence of a blastocyst impede in vitro infection of uterine tubal cells. *Theriogenology*, **52**(5): 887–900.

Hamer, F. C., Horne, G., Pease, E. H., Matson, P. L. & Lieberman, B. A. (1995). The quarantine of fertilized donated oocytes. *Human Reproduction*, **10**(5): 1194–6.

Hartshorne, G. (2003). Future regulation of fertility banking in the UK. *Human Fertility*, **6**: 71–3.

Ho, D. D., Schooley, R. T., Rota, T. R., Kaplan, J. C. & Flynn, T. (1984). HTLV-II in the semen and blood of a healthy homosexual man. *Science*, **226**: 451–3.

Inami, T., Konomi, N., Arakawa, Y. & Abe, K. (2000). High prevalence of TT virus DNA in human saliva and semen. *Journal of Clinical Microbiology*, **38**: 2407–8.

Kelsen, J, Tarp, B. & Obel, N. (1999). Absence of human herpes virus 8 in semen from healthy Danish donors. *Human Reproduction*, **14**: 2274–6.

Lang, D. J., Kummer, J. F. & Hartley, D. P. (1974). Cytomegalovirus in semen: persistence and demonstration in extracellular fluids. *New England Journal of Medicine*, **291**: 121–3.

Leiva, J. L., Peterson, E. M., Wetkowski, M., De La Maza, L. M. & Stone, S. C. (1985). Microorganisms in semen used for artificial insemination. *Obstetrics and Gynecology*, **65**: 669–72.

Liesnard, C. A. (1998). Screening of semen donors for infectious disease. *Human Reproduction*, **13** (suppl.2): 12–24.

Mansat, A., Mengelle, C., Chalet, M. *et al.* (1997). Cytomegalovirus detection in cryopreserved semen samples collected for therapeutic donor insemination. *Human Reproduction*, **12**: 1663–6.

Marguant-Le Guienne, B., Remond, M., Cosquer, R. *et al.* (1998). Exposure of in vitro-produced bovine embryos to foot-and-mouth disease virus. *Theriogenology*, **50**(1): 109–16.

Marks, J. L., Marks, D. & Lipshultz, L. I. (1990). Artificial insemination with donor semen: the necessity of frequent donor screening. *Journal of Urology*, **143**: 308–10.

Mascola, L. (1987). Semen donors as the source of sexually transmitted diseases in artificially inseminated women: the saga unfolds. *Journal of the American Medical Association*, **257**: 1093–4.

Mascola, L. & Guinan, M. E. (1986). Screening to reduce transmission of sexually transmitted diseases in semen used for artificial insemination. *New England Journal of Medicine*, **314**: 1354–9.

Moore, D. E., Ashley, R. L., Zarutskie, P. W., Coombs, R. W., Soules, M. R. & Corey, L. (1989). Transmission of genital herpes by donor insemination. *Journal of the American Medical Association*, **261**: 3441–3.

Morris, J. (2003). Cryopreservation and contamination. *Assisted Reproductive Technology and Science*, **2**(4): 1–3.

Nagel, T. C., Tagatz, G. E. & Campbell, B. F. (1986) Transmission of *Chlamydia trachomatis* by artificial insemination. *Fertility and Sterility*, **46**: 959–60.

Olatunbosun, O., Deneer, H. & Pierson, R. (1995). Human papillomavirus DNA detection in sperm using polymerase chain reaction. *Obstetrics and Gynecology*, **97**: 357–360.

Olatunbosun, O. A., Chizen, D. R. & Pierson, R. A. (1998). Screening of potential semen donors for sexual transmitted diseases. *West African Journal of Medicine*, **17**: 19–24.

Pannekoek, Y., Westenberg, S. M., De Vries, J. *et al.* (2000). PCR assessment of *Chlamydia trachomatis* infection of semen specimens processed for artificial insemination. *Journal of Clinical Microbiology*, **38**: 3763–7.

Prior, J. R., Morroll, D. R., Birks, A. G., Matson, P. L. & Lieberman, B. A. (1994). The screening for cytomegalovirus antibody in semen donors and recipients within a donor insemination programme. *Human Reproduction*, **9**: 2076–8.

Russell, P. H., Lyaruu, V. H., Millar, J. D., Curry, M. R. & Watson, P. F. (1997). The potential transmission of infectious agents by semen packaging during storage for artificial insemination. *Animal Reproduction Science*, **47**: 337–42.

Schacker, T., Ryncarz A. J., Goddard J., Diem, K., Shaughnessy, M. & Corey, L. (1998). Frequent recovery of HIV-1 from genital herpes simplex virus lesions in HIV-1 infected men. *Journal of the American Medical Association*, **280**: 61–6.

Stewart, G. J., Tyler, J. P. P., Cunningham, A. L. *et al.* (1985). Transmission of human T-cell lymphotrophic virus type II (HTLV-II) by artificial insemination by donor. *Lancet*, **14**: 581–4.

Tjiam, K. H., Van Heijst, B. Y. M., Polak-Vogelzang, A. A., Rothbarth, H., Van Joost, T. & Michel, M. F. (1987). Sexually communicable microorganisms in human semen samples to be used for artificial insemination by donor. *Genitourinary Medicine*, **63**: 116–18.

Van Engelenburg, F. A., Van Schie, F. W., Rijsewijk, F. A. M. & Van Oirschot, J. T. (1995). Excretion of bovine herpesvirus 1 in semen is detected much longer by PCR than by virus isolation. *Journal of Clinical Microbiology*, **33**: 308–12.

Vanroose, G., Nauwynck, H., Van Soom, A., Vanopdenbosch, E. & de Kruif, A. (1998). Replication of cytopathic and non-cytopathic bovine viral diarrhea virus in zona-free and zona-intact in vitro-produced bovine embryos and the effect on embryo quality. *Biology of Reproduction*, **58**(3): 857–66.

Wald, A, Matson, P., Ryncarz A. & Corey L. (1999). Detection of herpes simplex virus DNA in semen of men with genital HSV-2 infection. *Sexually Transmitted Diseases*, **26**: 1–3.

Wallace, W. H. B. & Walker, D. A. (2001). Conference consensus statement: ethical and research dilemmas for fertility preservation in children treated for cancer. *Human Fertility*, **4**: 69–76.

Wortley, P. M., Hammett, T. A. & Fleming, P. L. (1998). Donor insemination and human immunodeficiency virus transmission. *Obstetrics and Gynecology*, **91**: 515–18.

Index